Carcinomas of the Head and Neck

Cancer Treatment and Research

WILLIAM L. MCGUIRE, *series editor*

Bennett J.M. (ed): Controversies in the Management of Lymphomas. 1983. ISBN 0–89838–586–5
Humphrey G.B., Grindey G.B. (eds): Adrenal and Endocrine Tumors in Children. 1983. ISBN 0–89838–590–3
DeCosse J.J., Sherlock P. (eds): Clinical Management of Gastrointestinal Cancer. 1984. ISBN 0–89838–601–2
Catalona W.J., Ratliff, T.L. (eds): Urologic Oncology. 1984. ISBN 0–89838–628–4
Santen R.J., Manni A. (eds): Diagnosis and Management of Endocrine-related Tumors. 1984. ISBN 0–89838–636–5
Costanzi J.J. (ed): Clinical Management of Malignant Melanoma. 1984. ISBN 0–89838–656–X
Wolf G.T. (ed): Head and Neck Oncology. 1984. ISBN 0–89838–657–8
Alberts D.S., Surwit E.A. (eds): Ovarian Cancer. 1985. ISBN 0–89838–676–4
Muggia F.M. (ed): Experimental and Clinical Progress in Cancer Chemotherapy. 1985. ISBN 0–89838–679–9
Higby D.J. (ed): Issues in Supportive Care of Cancer Patients. 1986. ISBN 0–89838–816–3
Surwit E.A., Alberts D.S. (eds): Cervix Cancer. 1987. ISBN 0–89838–822–8
Jacobs C. (ed): Cancers of the Head and Neck. 1987. ISBN 0–89838–825–2
MacDonald J.S. (ed): Gastrointestinal Oncology. 1987. ISBN 0–89838–829–5
Ratliff T.L., Catalona W.J. (eds): Genitourinary Cancer. 1987. ISBN 0–89838–830–9
Nathanson L. (ed): Basic and Clinical Aspects of Malignant Melanoma. 1987. ISBN 0–89838–856–2
Muggia F.M. (ed): Concepts, Clinical Developments, and Therapeutic Advances in Cancer Chemotherapy. 1987. ISBN 0–89838–879–5
Frankel A.E. (ed): Immunotoxins. 1988. ISBN 0–89838–984–4
Bennett J.M., Foon K.A. (eds): Immunologic Approaches to the Classification and Management of Lymphomas and Leukemias. 1988. ISBN 0–89838–355–2
Osborne C.K. (ed): Endocrine Therapies in Breast and Prostate Cancer. 1988. ISBN 0–89838–365–X
Lippman M.E., Dickson R. (eds): Breast Cancer: Cellular and Molecular Biology. 1988. ISBN 0–89838–368–4
Kamps W.A., Humphrey G.B., Poppema S. (eds): Hodgkin's Disease in Children: Controversies and Current Practice. 1988. ISBN 0–89838–372–2
Muggia F.M. (ed): Cancer Chemotherapy; Concepts, Clinical Investigations and Therapeutic Advances. 1988. ISBN 0–89838–381–1
Nathanson L. (ed): Malignant Melanoma: Biology, Diagnosis, and Therapy. 1988. ISBN 0–89838–384–6
Pinedo H.M., Verweij J. (eds): Treatment of Soft Tissue Sarcomas. 1989. ISBN 0–89838–391–9
Hansen H.H. (ed): Basic and Clinical Concepts of Lung Cancer. 1989. ISBN 0–7923–0153–6
Lepor H., Ratliff T.L. (eds): Urologic Oncology. 1989. ISBN 0–7923–0161–7
Benz C., Liu E. (eds): Oncogenes. 1989. ISBN 0–7923–0237–0
Ozols R.F. (ed): Drug Resistance in Cancer Therapy. 1989. ISBN 0–7923–0244–3
Surwit E.A., Alberts D.S. (eds): Endometrial Cancer. 1989. ISBN 0–7923–0286–9
Champlin R. (ed): Bone Marrow Transplantation. 1990. ISBN 0–7923–0612–0
Goldenberg D. (ed): Cancer Imaging with Radiolabeled Antibodies. 1990. ISBN 0–7923–0631–7

Carcinomas of the Head and Neck
Evaluation and Management

edited by

CHARLOTTE JACOBS, M.D.
Stanford University School of Medicine
Stanford, California, U.S.A.

1990 **KLUWER ACADEMIC PUBLISHERS**
BOSTON / DORDRECHT / LONDON

Distributors for North America:
Kluwer Academic Publishers
101 Philip Drive
Assinippi Park
Norwell, Massachusetts 02061 USA

Distributors for all other countries:
Kluwer Academic Publishers Group
Distribution Centre
Post Office Box 322
3300 AH Dordrecht, THE NETHERLANDS

Library of Congress Cataloging–in–Publication Data

Carcinomas of the head and neck : evaluation and management / edited by Charlotte Jacobs.
p. cm.—(Cancer treatment and research)
Includes bibliographical references.
ISBN 0–7923–0668–6
1. Head—Cancer. 2. Neck—Cancer. I. Jacobs, Charlotte. II. Series.
[DNLM: 1. Head and Neck Neoplasms—therapy. W1 CA693 / WE 707 C265]
RC280.H4C37 1990
616.99′491—dc20
DNLM/DLC
for Library of Congress

90-4035
CIP

Printed in the United States of America.

Contents

Head and Neck Oncology

Preface

It was not too many years ago that the role of chemotherapy for head and neck cancer consisted of single–agent methotrexate for selected patients with recurrent disease. In the past decade, multiple new agents, high–dose chemotherapy, combinations, and intra–arterial approaches have been used for the patient with recurrent disease. Wheeler critically assesses the current status of these approaches. When oncologists began testing chemotherapy in the combined modality approach, trials consisted of induction chemotherapy and use of single agents as radiosensitizers. Although a great deal has been learned from these trials, benefit in terms of survival has been marginal. Even more promising may be the concomitant use of combination chemotherapy and radiation. Taylor describes the encouraging results as well as the potential. Induction chemotherapy may have a second important goal in addition to improving curability—it could be used for organ preservation. Dimery et al., present the background for this approach in the patient with laryngeal cancer as well as a description of their randomized trial for voice preservation.

Head and neck squamous cancers are a heterogeneous group of diseases, and surgeons have long sought parameters that will help predict outcome. DNA content, determined by flow cytometry, can be correlated with outcome, as described by Ensely et al. Not only does it permit identification of subsets of patients with differing prognoses, but ploidy differences my help us understand the basic biology of this disease. Schantz et al. address three important aspects of humoral immunity—the role of the antibody in mediating cell kill, the role of circulating immune complexes and their use in predicting outcome, and the potential for monoclonal antibodies in diagnosis and therapy.

Finally, this is a disease for which there are known causative factors. as well as preliminary results and toxicity. Another technique to enhance local control is photodynamic therapy, and Gluckman and Zitsch critically evaluate the available photosensitizers, light sources, techniques, and applications.

The challenge of head and neck cancer stems from its significant morbidity because of location. Those patients who are cured often face a life unable to speak or swallow or with cosmetic defects. Head and neck teams are now focusing more on reconstruction and rehabilitation. Trudeau and Schuller review the multidisciplinary approach to improving vocal communication following total laryngectomy and compare tracheoesophageal speech, artificial devices, and esophageal speech. Hillel and Patten describe the evaluation of the eleventh nerve syndrome following neck dissection, its mobidity, and the importance of rehabilitation.

Thyroid cancers are the most common endocrine tumors, and are frequently managed by the head and neck team. Peterson and McDougall review and clarify controversial issues regarding the diagnosis and treatment of this disease.

Carcinomas of the head and neck have traditionally been of primary interest to otolaryngologists and radiation therapists. It is only in recent years that chemotherapists, radiologists, epidemiologists, and biologists have enthusiastically undertaken the study of this disease. This is reflected in the formation of combined modality teams for patient management and for the conduct of clinical trials, and in the increasing number of publications concerning head and neck cancer. In this volume we present some of the recent advances in staging, primary treatment, rehabilitation, chemotherapeutic approaches, and the clinical applications of basic biology.

Magnetic resonance imaging (MRI) has enhanced the ability to accurately evaluate extent of disease. Lufkin and Hanafee review the technique of MRI, its clinical usefulness, and the circumstances in which it is preferred to computed tomography (CT) and other imaging techniques. A significant problem in deciding if patients with advanced cancer are candidates for surgical resection is often determining whether or not the carotid artery is invaded. Gooding evaluates the merits of ultrasound, angiography, CT, and MRI in assessing invasion.

The management of head and neck cancers with surgical resection is constantly evolving. In this volume, Levine describes craniofacial resection and reconstruction for cancers of the ethmoids and superior nasal vault, in particular esthesioneuroblastoma, and Fee presents the techniques and results of nasopharyngectomy for recurrent nasopharyngeal cancer. Although most skin cancers can be easily managed with surgical resection, advanced squamous and basal cell cancers present a challenge to the head and neck team. Weber et al., present the multidisciplinary approach to this disease including optimal surgical techniques, radiation therapy, chemotherapy, and retinoids.

Local control is a major problem for patients with stage III and IV head and neck cancer despite optimal surgery and radiation. New techniques, such as interstitial irradiation and hyperthermia, have shown promise, and more recently the two have been combined with encouraging results. Welton et al., present the biologic basis for this combination and methodology, Jacobs reviews etiologic considerations for head and neck cancer and stresses the importance of prevention. Thus, progress continues in the field of head and neck oncology. The significant morbidity of this disease continues to challenge clinicians and researchers.

C. Jacobs

Contributing Authors

BYERS, Robert M., Department of Head and Neck Surgery, The University of Texas MD Anderson Cancer Center, 1515 Holcombe Avenue, Houston, TX 77030

de BRAUD, Filippo, Division of Hematology/Oncology, Wayne State University School of Medicine, P.O. Box 02188, Detroit MI 48201–1998

DIMERY, Isaiah W., Department of Medical Oncology, The University of Texas MD Anderson Cancer Center, 1515 Holcombe Blvd, Houston TX 77030

ENSLEY, John F., Division of Hematology/Oncology, Wayne State University School of Medicine, P.O. Box 02188, Detroit MI 48201–1998

FEE, Willard E., Jr., Division of Otolaryngology/Head and Neck Surgery, Stanford University School of Medicine, Stanford CA 94305

GLUCKMAN, Jack L., Dept of Otolaryngology and Maxillofacial Surgery, Univ of Cincinnati Medical Center, 231 Bethesda Avenue, Cincinnati OH 45267

GOFFINET, Donald R., Department of Radiation Oncology, Stanford University School of Medicine, Stanford CA 94305

GOODING, Gretchen A.W., Department of Radiology, University of California, Veterans Administration Medical Center, 1450 Clement Street, San Francisco CA 94121

HANAFEE, William, Department of Radiological Sciences, UCLA Medical Center, Los Angeles CA 90024–1721

HILLEL, Allen, Department of Otolaryngology/Head and Neck Surgery, University of Washington Seattle Veterans Hospital, 1660 S Columbian Way, Seattle WA 98108

HONG, Waun Ki, Department of Medical Oncology, The University of Texas MD Anderson Cancer Center, 1515 Holcombe Blvd, Houston TX 77030

JACOBS, Charlotte D., Division of Medical Oncology—M211, Department of Medicine, Stanford University School of Medicine, Stanford CA 94305

KAPP, Daniel S., Department of Radiation Oncology, Stanford University School of Medicine, Stanford, CA 94305

KRAMER, Alan M., Department of Medical Oncology, The University of Texas MD Anderson Cancer Center, 1515 Holcombe Blvd, Houston TX 77030

LEE, Norris K., Department of Head and Neck Surgery, The University of Texas MD Anderson Cancer Center, 1515 Holcombe Blvd, Houston TX 77030

LEVINE, Paul A., Department of Oncology/Head and Neck Surgery, University of Virginia Medical Center, Charlottesville VA 22908

LIPPMAN, Scott M., Department of Medical Oncology, The University of Texas MD Anderson Cancer Center, 1515 Holcombe Blvd, Houston TX 77030

LUFKIN, Robert B., Department of Radiological Sciences, UCLA Medical Center, Los Angeles CA 90024–1721

McDOUGALL, I. Ross, Division of Nuclear Medicine, Stanford University Medical Center, Stanford CA 94305

McNEESE, Marsha D., Department of Radiotherapy, The University of Texas MD Anderson Cancer Center, 1515 Holcombe Blvd, Houston TX 77030

MACIOROWSKI, Zosia, Division of Hematology/Oncology, Wayne State University School of Medicine, P.O. Box 02188, Detroit MI 48201–1988

PATTEN, Carolynn, Department of Otolaryngology/Head and Neck Surgery, University of Washington Seattle Veterans Hospital, 1660 S. Columbian Way, Seattle WA 98108

PETERSEN, Margaret M., Division of Nuclear Medicine, Stanford University Medical Center, Stanford CA 94305

PIETRASZKIEWICZ, Haline, Division of Hematology/Oncology, Wayne State University School of Medicine, P.O. Box 02188, Detroit MI 48201–1998

SAKR, Wael, Department of Pathology, Wayne State University School of Medicine, Detroit MI 48201

SAVAGE, Howard E., Department of Head and Neck Surgery, The University of Texas MD Anderson Cancer Center, 1515 Holcombe Blvd, Houston TX 77030

SCHANTZ, Stimson, Department of Head and Neck Surgery, The University of Texas MD Anderson Cancer Center, 1515 Holcombe Blvd, Houston TX 77030

SCHULLER, David E., Department of Otolaryngology, The Ohio State University, 456 West 10th Ave, Columbus OH 43210–1240

TAYLOR, Samuel G., IV, Section of Medical Oncology, Rush Presbyterian St. Luke's Medical Center, 1725 W Harrison St., Suite 830, Chicago IL 60612

TRUDEAU, Michael D., Department of Otolaryngology and Division of Speech and Hearing Science, The Ohio State University, 4100 University Hospitals Clinic, 456 West Tenth Ave, Columbus OH 43210–1240

WEBER, Randal S., Department of Head and Neck Surgery, The University of Texas MD Anderson Cancer Center, 1515 Holcombe Ave, Houston TX 77030

WELTON, Patrick L., Department of Radiation Oncology, Stanford University School of Medicine, Stanford, CA 94305

WENDT, Charles D., Department of Clinical Radiotherapy, The University of Texas MD Anderson Cancer Center, 1515 Holcombe Blvd, Houston TX 77030

WHEELER, Richard H., Univ of Alabama 211 Tumor Institute, University Station, Birmingham AL 35291

ZITSCH, Robert P., Department of Otolaryngology and Maxillofacial Surgery, University of Cincinnati Medical Center, 231 Bethesda Ave, Cincinnati OH 45267

I

Advances in Staging and Primary Treatment

1. Magnetic Resonance Imaging of Head and Neck Cancer

Robert Lufkin and William Hanafee

Magnetic resonance (MR) has revolutionized head and neck imaging and has largely replaced computed tomography (CT) as the study of choice for malignancies of the extracranial head and neck. Magnetic resonance imaging (MRI) easily surpasses CT in its ability to differentiate subtle differences in soft tissue boundaries and extensions of tumors of the head and neck. The beam hardening artifacts on CT images from dental amalgam and dense cortical bone of the mandible, skull base, shoulders and other areas are also not a problem with MRI. Multiplanar imaging capabilities and lack of ionizing radiation make MR the preferred imaging study for many head and neck processes that would have in the past required a CT scan.

The role of any imaging modality in most head and neck cancers is to identify deep infiltration of tumors. Mucosal changes are, for the most part, best evaluated by direct inspection during physical examination. Physiologic studies of motion and fixation are beyond the capability of present day MRI techniques, but blood flow and vascularity determinations can be performed with MRI, eliminating the need of many invasive angiographic procedures.

Probably nowhere else in the body do anatomical boundaries provide such important clues to the natural history of a disease process. Even when the exact nature of the offending process cannot be determined, disruptions of facial planes and muscle interfaces help to define surgery or radiation therapy management of the patient.

Technique

Perhaps the most significant factor in the superiority of MR over CT scanning in the head and neck is the superior soft tissue contrast resolution of MR. By changing the pulse sequence parameters (TR, TE, Theta), MR image contrast can be manipulated in many ways not possible with CT scanning. This results in images which emphasize MR relaxation properties of the tissues known as T1 and T2. The resulting images are referred to as 'T1 or T2 weighted'. Unlike the CNS, where virtually no MR signal from fat is present, the abundance of fat–water interfaces in the extracranial head

Jacobs, C. (ed): Carcinomas of the Head and Neck: Evaluation and Management.

and neck, which literally defines the anatomy of this region, greatly influences the selection of pulse sequences for optimum image contrast.

The high signal levels available on T1 weighted images permit anatomical details to be detected that are often not seen on CT. This improved contrast resolution plus the availability of easy coronal, sagittal and oblique viewing greatly enhances the information obtained by axial scanning. The vast majority of head and neck imaging is performed with T1 weighted pulsing sequences. T2 weighted pulsing sequences are used when more information is required regarding tumor infiltration into muscle, fluid collections, and obstructed sinuses.

The use of CT–guided aspiration cytology of deep or clinically occult lesions has improved the workup of many patients with head and neck tumors. Aspiration cytology is now possible with MR guidance using specially developed MR compatible needles (E–Z–EM Corporation, Westbury, New York) [1,2,3].

The role of the new contrast agent gadolinium–DTPA (Magnevist, Berlex, New York) in MR examinations of the head and neck is currently under investigation [4]. Preliminary studies show that although tumor enhancement occurs, little clinically relevant information is added in many cases. When intracranial extension is present, however, the gadolinium can improve the detection of blood brain barrier and leptomeningeal pathology.

Nasopharynx

The lack of motion and abundant facial planes of the nasopharynx result in high–quality magnetic resonance imaging [5,6]. Retropharyngeal adenopathy, tumor infiltration beyond the pharyngobasilar fascia, and hypertropic lymphoid tissue are all identified with greater ease on magnetic resonance than on CT (figure 1) [7]. T1 weighted images are usually adequate for examining the nasopharynx because of the abundance of loose areolar tissue between various muscle groups and bundles. Tumors with inflammatory changes can be identified as low signal regions in these loose areolar planes.

Usually seven axial sections will adequately cover from the soft palate up to the skull base and the floor of the middle cranial fossa. An additional seven coronal views may be helpful to give better coverage of the posteriorly located nodal changes following the jugular vein in the anterior extremities of the nasopharynx at the junction of the nasal conchae.

If sagittal projections are obtained, at least seven sections should be performed so that the lateral extremities of the cavernous sinuses and the foramen lacerum regions can be completely examined. If a patient has symptoms of cranial nerve IX, X, XI, or XII involvement, more than seven sections will be needed to adequately evaluate these more peripheral regions.

In particular, the direct coronal and sagittal MR scans are valuable to assess craniocaudal extension of tumor in skull base involvement. While CT

Figure 1. Nasopharyngeal squamous carcinoma.

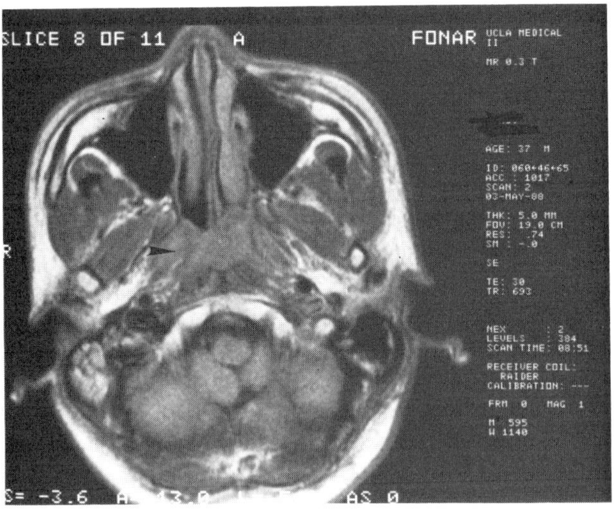

Figure 1a. Axial views (SE/700/30) through the nasopharynx reveal a mass with obliteration of the surrounding fascial planes, and crossing of the pharyngobasilar fascia (arrowhead).

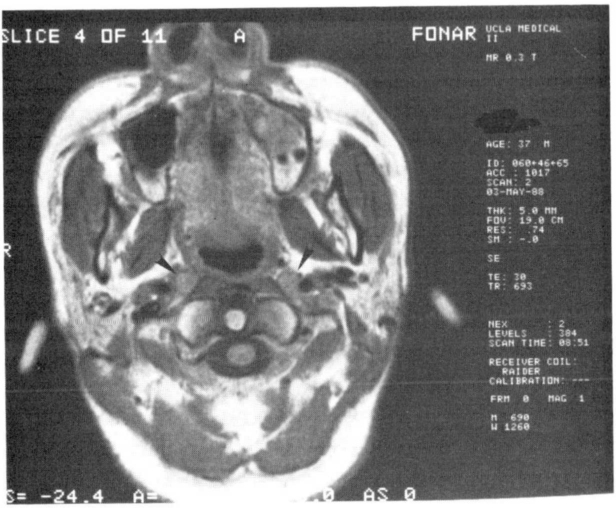

Figure 1b. Axial section with the same parameters obtained through the level of Passavant's muscle shows no evidence of primary tumor, however, large bilateral retropharyngeal lymph nodes (arrowhead) are present.

scanning is unquestionably more accurate in detecting small amounts of calcification *per se*, the magnetic resonance examination is adequate to evaluate skull base invasion. Abnormalities of the skull base are detected by replacement of the normal low signal cortical bone with higher signal neoplasm. The capability of multiplanar imaging and the far superior soft tissue resolution of magnetic resonance make MR the clear imaging study of choice to evaluate the nasopharynx.

The configuration of the nasopharynx is dominated by a very tough fascial membrane called the pharyngobasilar fascia. This tough fascia represents a continuation of the pharyngeal constrictor muscles and extends from the level of the soft palate to the base of the skull. Its function is to maintain the airway as an open channel for breathing during normal activities and during chewing. During the act of swallowing the soft palate obliterates the lumen produced by the pharyngobasilar fascia.

The pharyngobasilar fascia is pierced anteriorly by the eustachian tube. The eustachian tube passing from the middle ear cavity communicates with the nasopharynx through an opening just behind the anterior attachment of the pharyngobasilar fascia to the medial pterygoid plate. Only malignant tumors and very aggressive inflammatory processes such as mucor will pass from the mucosa of the nasopharynx through the pharyngobasilar fascia to involve the structures within the paranasopharyngeal space. The first anatomical structure to become involved is usually the tensor veli palatini muscle which lies immediately lateral to the medial pterygoid plate and takes its origin from the skull base.

The tensor veli palatini muscle is enveloped in a fascial plane of its own which divides the paranasopharyngeal space into two compartments [8]. The tensor veli palatini muscle fascia passes posterior to the styloid process and divides the space into a lateral compartment which is spoken of as the prestyloid space and a medial compartment which is spoken of as a post–styloid space. This terminology comes from surgical approaches because the surgeons encounter the more lateral space as they come in from the side, and hence they see this space before the styloid process. The more medially placed space is visualized after the styloid process has been seen, and hence it is the post–styloid space. This post–styloid space communicates anteriorly between the pharyngobasilar fascia and the tensor veli palatini fascia, and posteriorly it goes back to the carotid artery. In the more lateral compartment (prestyloid compartment) lies the deep lobe of the parotid gland. The amount of parotid tissue in this region, between the tensor veli palatini muscle fascia and the fascia covering the medial pterygoid muscle, is quite variable. These two fascial planes generally fuse just before their attachment to the base of the skull. Their skull base attachment is immediately medial to the foramen ovale.

The nasopharynx remains an area that is obscure to casual clinical examination. Its proximity to the skull base makes cancers in this region particularly devastating. Most malignancies of the nasopharynx are squamous cell carcinomas with varying degrees of differentiation. The tumors may affect all age groups, including children and teenagers. Plasmocytomas, lymphomas, and occasionally rhabdomyosarcomas are also encountered. These tumors tend to be bulkier and infiltrate more widely than squamous carcinoma.

The presenting symptoms of nasopharyngeal carcinoma vary widely. The most common complaints of patients presenting with nasopharyngeal tumors are nasal obstruction, local invasion of cranial nerves, serous otitis media, and cervical lymph node metastases (figure 2) [9]. In general, patients fall into two main categories for nasopharyngeal MR examination:

1. to delineate the extent of a known malignancy, and
2. the search for the presence of the tumor to explain symptoms or clinical findings.

Clinical examination may be extremely difficult due to gag reflex or poor patient cooperation. Visualization of the vault of the nasopharynx and regions surrounding the eustachian tube can be difficult under the best of circumstances. Prominent, chronically inflamed adenoidal tissue may obscure much of the nasopharynx even if the structure is reasonably accessible to inspection. Nasopharyngeal tumors have a tendency to infiltrate beneath the mucosa and extend over wide areas with little superficial evidence of their presence. This is especially true in recurrent disease following therapy where the mucosa can return to relatively normal status but where deep infiltrations persist. MR is particularly well suited to compliment the clinical examination in this situation.

Unknown Primary

The patient presenting with the solitary, enlarged cervical lymph node presents one of the most interesting challenges in head and neck diagnosis. This is the so–called unknown primary, when only the metastasis to the node is clinically evident. Sound surgical principles dictate that the primary tumor should be managed at the same setting as the metastasis. Statistics suggest that failure to follow this principle leads to a logarithmic jump in postoperative complications and treatment failures.

Unfortunately there are no clear–cut MR signal changes to indicate malignant adenopathy. The morphological size criteria used in CT may also be applied to MR (figure 3) [10,11,12,13]. Under no circumstances should an open biopsy of the lymph node be performed until all areas of the head and neck have been ruled out as a source of the primary tumor [14]. Since the nasopharynx presents such a difficult area to examine clinically, MR performs a vital task in showing the presence or absence of a deeply infiltrating tumor.

Figure 2. Diagnosis by MR guided aspiration cytology of recurrent squamous carcinoma of the parapharyngeal space extending to the skull base.

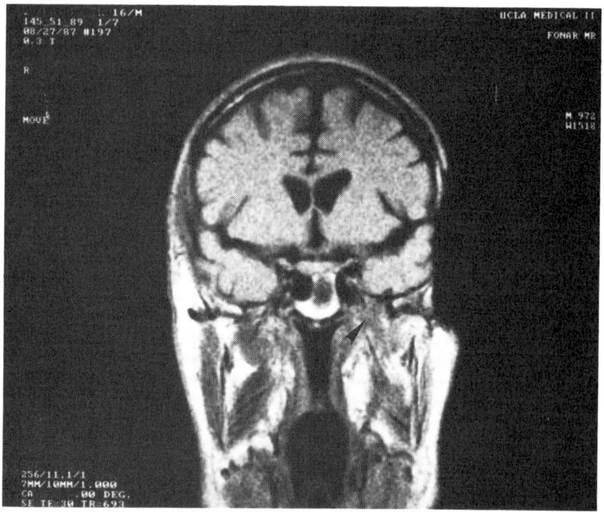

Figure 2a. Coronal image (SE/700/300) shows mass in the high infratemporal fossa (>).

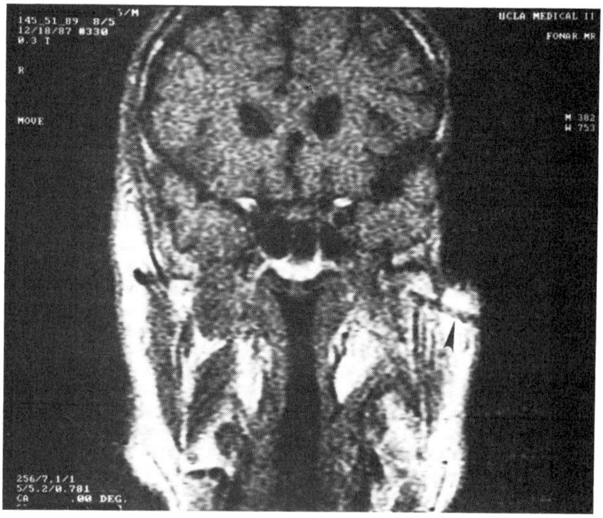

Figure 2b. Follow–up fast gradient echo image after needle placement. Although image quality is less with rapid scanning techniques (SE/173/10/60° flip angle), the needle is well visualized (arrowhead) and scan time is reduced to 48 seconds.

Figure 3. Recurrent squamous cell carcinoma of the neck. Adenopathy with central necrosis and extracapsular extension following partial glossectomy and radical neck dissection.

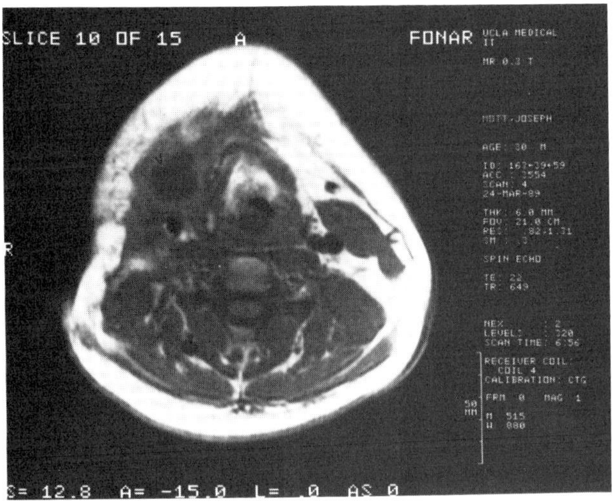

Figure 3a. Axial T1 weighted image (SE/649/22) reveals a soft tissue mass lateral to the thyroid cartilage with obliteration of fascial planes and low intensity center (arrowhead). The sterno-cleidomastoid muscle and jugular vein are absent following radical neck dissection.

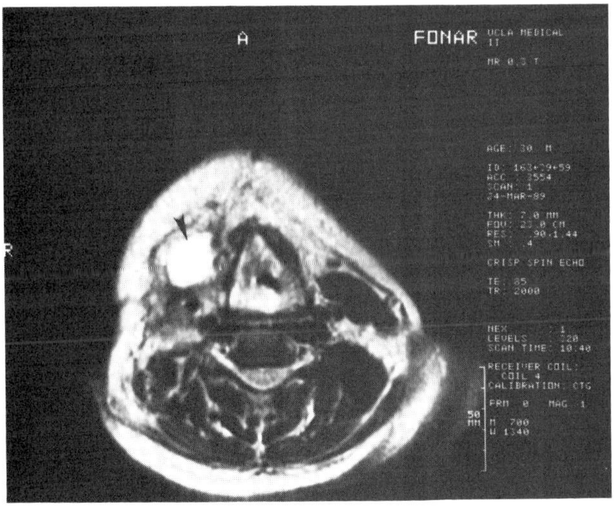

Figure 3b. Axial T2 weighted images at the same level (SE/2000/85) reveal high–signal intensity within the mass again confirming central necrosis (arrowhead).

Tongue and Oropharynx

The imaging information that MR now provides is superior to that possible with CT and is considered the imaging study of choice to evaluate masses in the tongue and oropharynx [15,16]. The tongue is one area in the head and neck where T2 weighted pulse sequences are extremely valuable. The musculature of the tongue is of low signal on both T1 and T2 weighted images. Tumors produce a very similar signal on T1 weighted images. By prolonging the study to obtain late echoes, the tumors with longer T2 give an increased signal relative to the tongue musculature. For this reason we use axial scanning with T2 weighting to obtain sections from the tongue and soft palate region to a level below the inferior pole of the tonsil to include the pre–epiglottic space of the larynx.

Anatomic details of the midline are best obtained by coronal T1 weighted images. The T1 weighting allows us to survey lymph nodes in the loose areolar tissue surrounding the jugular vein and digastric tendons. This fibrofatty tissue gives a very bright signal on both T1 and T2 weighted images. On T1 weighted images the tumor will stand out as a low signal structure. On T2 weighted images the tumor increases in signal and becomes difficult to distinguish from the areolar tissue, carotid artery, and jugular vein.

Squamous cell carcinomas account for well over 90% of the malignancies of the tongue [17]. The remaining lesions are lymphomas, leukemic infiltrations, rhabdomyosarcomas, and an assortment of benign tumors and inflammatory processes. Their behavior is largely governed by their location and the lymphatic drainage of the region.

Squamous cell carcinomas of the tongue, tonsillar bed and posterior pharyngeal wall are the lesions most likely to require radiologic imaging. Occasionally an infiltrating tumor of the hard palate may have spread to the nasopharynx so that additional imaging is needed prior to surgical management. Adenoid cystic carcinomas almost invariably extend along perineural lymphatics so that some type of imaging can at times be helpful. Unfortunately, since the most central spread of these tumors is microscopic in nature, it cannot be reliably detected by present imaging methods. The remaining anterior lesions of the cheek, retromolar trigone, alveolar ridge, and lips are readily visible by inspection or available to the palpating finger, and imaging studies are seldom necessary.

Tongue and tonsillar fossa tumors can be considered together since the anatomic structures to be visualized are all seen on the same projections. Frequently, the exact site of origin of a lesion cannot be determined and will involve both regions. Posterior pharyngeal wall tumors are quite rare. They infiltrate locally and extend to the retropharyngeal lymphatics and jugular nodes. The primary tumors are easily seen by clinical examination, but at times their extensions may be obscure. Nodal spread constitutes the principal indication for radiologic investigation. When the nodes show extracapsular spread to adjacent structures, prognosis worsens markedly. Tumor *totally* surrounding the carotid artery is generally considered a contraindication to surgery. A case is not called inoperable if only one side of a carotid artery is involved because the surgeon may be able to find a plane of dissection.

Two anatomic regions need defining in order to plan surgical management. One is the neurovascular bundles which are intimately involved with the muscles comprising the lateral border of the tongue. The second anatomical region is the midline fibrous septum that separates the two lateral halves of the tongue. Integrity of these structures is necessary for the surgeon to perform a hemiglossectomy. At least one hypoglossal nerve and one lingual artery must be retained. A total glossectomy is a much more involved procedure for selected patients and ideally requires specialized preoperative planning.

Axial sections with T2 weighting will show whether the tumor has spread from the anterior and middle thirds of the tongue into the base (figures 4–5). The relationship of the tumor to the lingual artery and nerve is easily visible since these lie in intimate relationship to the interdigitation of the styloglossus and hyoglossus muscle. Here the base of the fibrous septum becomes deficient, and tumors have easy access to spreading across to the opposite side. Disruption of fascial planes of the diaphragm of the floor of the mouth (the mylohyoid muscle) in a bilateral fashion clearly indicates a far advanced tumor.

Anterior third of the tongue and floor of mouth tumors are readily available to inspection and palpation and seldom require imaging studies. Middle third of the tongue tumors, like anterior third of the tongue tumors, tend to have unilateral nodal drainage. Their incidence of metastases at the time of admission is slightly higher than anterior tongue because they are usually discovered late. The intimate association of the lateral portion of the tongue with the glossopalatinus muscle and glossopharyngeal sulcus means that these tumors have ready access to the tonsillar beds by direct extension. Frequently it is impossible to state whether the tumor originated in the tongue, the glosspharyngeal sulcus, or the tonsillar bed.

Carcinomas of the posterior third of the tongue are particularly troublesome. Because of their inaccessibility, they are usually not discovered until relatively late. Seventy–six percent of the tumors are reported to have metastases at the time of initial examination. Nodal disease is frequently bilateral because of the bilateral drainage of the posterior third of the tongue.

Approximately 25% of patients with tongue cancers that present for MR imaging studies due to nodal disease have tumors in the posterior third of the tongue not visible or palpable by clincial examination. Tumors of the base of the tongue have a propensity to spread laterally into the glossopharyngeal sulcus and tonsillar bed regions and anteriorly into the vallecula and pre–epiglottic space. Therefore MR investigations of the tongue and oropharynx fall into three categories:

Figure 4. Squamous carcinoma of the tongue base. MR imaging with and without gadolinium.

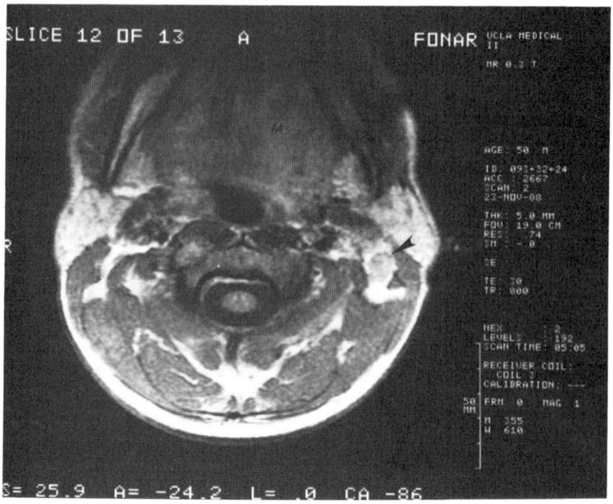

Figure 4a. Axial T1 weighted image (SE/800/30) through the high tongue base reveals mass effect on the left (M) and associated adenopathy (arrowhead).

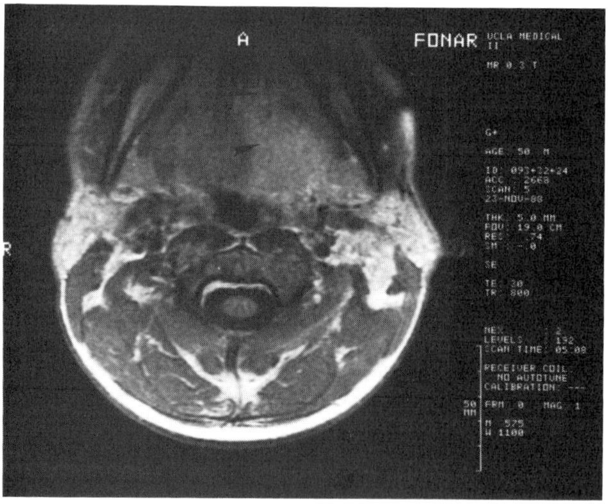

Figure 4b. Similar level and pulse sequence following administration of gadolinium DPTA reveals mild enhancement of the tongue base mass (arrowhead) with slightly decreased visualization of the lymph node.

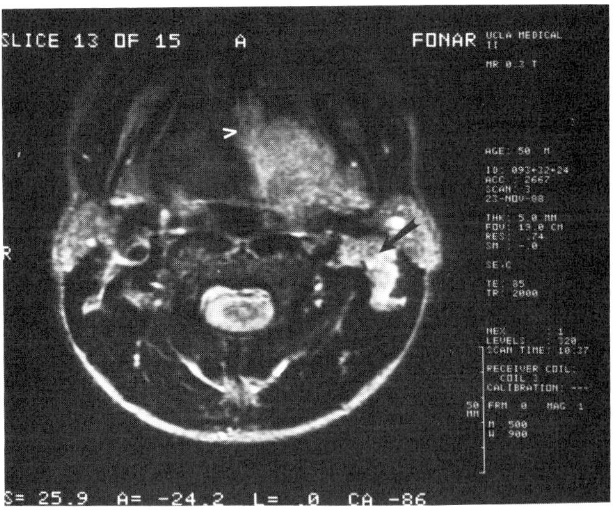

Figure 4c. T2 weighted image (SE/2000/85) without gadolinium reveals high signal in the tongue base mass (arrowhead) and also increased signal in the region of the adenopathy (arrow) similar to that seen with gadolinium on the T1 weighted images.

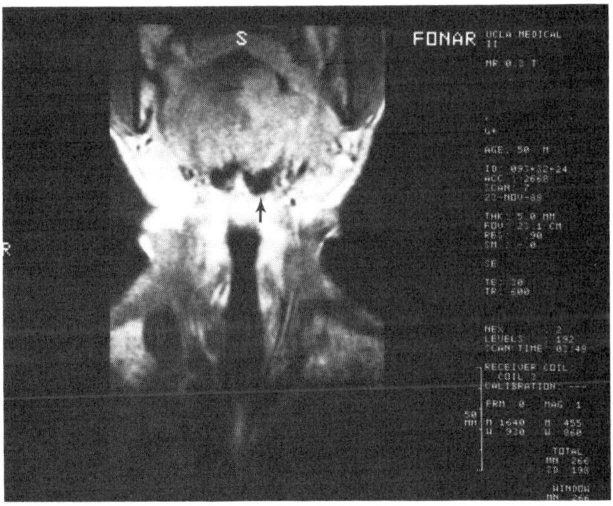

Figure 4d. The coronal T1 weighted image is useful for defining the extent of the mass (arrowhead) and showing that there is no extension to the supraglottic larynx. The vallecula is free of tumor (arrow).

Figure 5. Recurrent squamous carcinoma of the right tonsil.

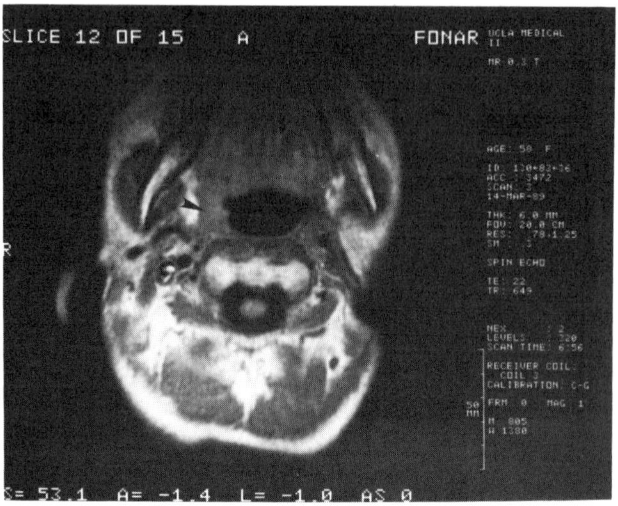

Figure 5a. Axial T1 weighted image (SE/649/22) reveals postsurgical changes in the left neck as well as right sided tonsillar fullness (>).

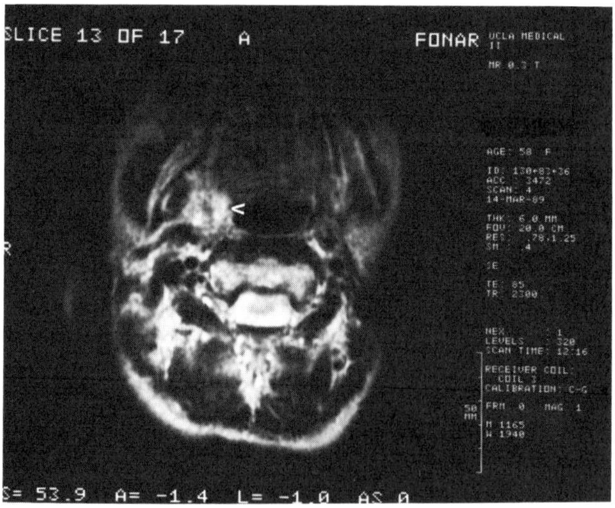

Figure 5b. T2 weighted image (SE/2300/85) at the same level reveals an increased signal in the region of the tonsil (arrowhead) consistent with recurrent tumor, although edema or post biopsy changes could appear the same.

1. patients with known cancers in whom we wish to delineate the extent of the tumor and nodal metastases,
2. patients presenting with atypical pain syndromes or nodal disease in whom we are searching for the primary tumor, and
3. patients with evidence of recurrent disease following treatment.

Many surgeons feel that total glossectomy is an option in only select patients because following surgery, the patient is left unable to swallow or manage secretions. Laryngectomy is usually also required as part of this procedure, leaving the individual without a natural voice.

Therefore, limited conservational surgical resections of the tongue are performed when possible, and these require the preservation of one lingual artery and one hypoglossal nerve. These hemiglossectomies are only possible when the tumor has not crossed the midline or only minimally extends to the opposite side. Since most tongue and floor of mouth cancers tend to extend along vascular pathways, this limitation proves crucial in many instances. MR studies are thus directed to the tumor mass, its extent, and to the integrity of the midline.

In general, MR produces better soft tissue detail in evaluating the tongue and oropharynx than CT. MR is therefore considered the study of choice in this area. Lack of artifact from dental amalgam and beam hardening artifact from the mandible on MR also eliminates two major shortcomings of CT in the examination of this area. Finally, the ability of MR to obtain direct coronal and sagittal scan planes is a distinct advantage in recognizing intrinsic tongue musculature and assessing tumor volume and spread for treatment planning.

Larynx and Hypopharynx

Rarely does any radiologic imaging modality play a significant role in reaching a diagnosis of malignancy in the larynx and hypopharynx. These regions are so readily accessible to clinical examination that visual inspection usually strongly indicates the diagnosis of cancer as confirmed by biopsy. Therefore, the primary role of MR is the same as that of CT in imaging the larynx and hypopharynx: to define the extent of the disease. While laryngoscopy can show mucosal surfaces and masses involving the lumen, deep extensions are difficult to detect from clinical examination alone, yet, in several areas, these extensions have profound implications for the management of disease. CT and now MR to an even greater extent, can define this important deep anatomy [18,19,20,21,22,23,24,25,26].

Relatively T1 weighted images are ideal for the study of the larynx. T1 weighted sequences maximize contrast between loose areolar tissue of the parapharyngeal and preepiglottic spaces, the neck, and most tumors. The higher signal intensity of squamous carcinoma on T2 weighted images is a disadvantage in the larynx because the high signal areolar tissue within the larynx becomes isointense with the tumor on these pulse sequences. The lower signal to noise of the T2 weighted images also limits the use of thin sections and high in plane spatial resolution which are so valuable in the study of this region.

Axial and coronal scanning of the larynx will demonstrate the intrinsic musculature of the larynx as low signal regions lying sandwiched between the bright signal of mucosa and submucosa glands with bright signal of the loose areolar tissue separating the intrinsic muscle from the overlying thyroid cartilage. Infiltration of the intrinsic muscles or the adjacent bright signal areolar tissue planes indicate deep infiltration and spreading tumor.

The space lying anterior to the epiglottis must consist of very loose areolar tissue in order for the epiglottis to invert during the act of swallowing. This loose areolar tissue creates an extremely bright signal which is displaced by a low signal when tumors infiltrate the region. In the midline lie the low signal ligaments that attach the epiglottis to the hyoid bone and thyrohyoid membrane, forming a barrier between the right and left sides of the larynx [27]. Tumor masses rarely extend from one side to the other unless they have crossed the midline along the mucosal surface.

The vertical spread of tumors is even more exacting, and surgeons feel quite comfortable with a 2–3 millimeter margin of tumor free region adjacent to excisional planes because of the abrupt transition between supraglottic and glottic lymphatics. Only in advanced lesions do the tumors spread down the inferior margin of the epiglottis to the anterior commissure and subglottic region or else from superior to inferior in the paralaryngeal space. Coronal and sagittal MRI scans with T1 weighted pulsing sequences readily demonstrate these spreads (figure 6).

The primary function of the larynx is a sphincter rather than an organ for making noise. This sphincter action requires a complicated system of coordinated muscular movements over cartilaginous plates and fascial planes. The embryology of the larynx itself is quite unique and bears careful attention when evaluating patients for voice conservation surgery or precision radiation therapy. A horizontal cleavage plane of origin occurs at the level of the laryngeal ventricle, creating a supraglottic larynx and a glottic (true vocal cords) and subglottic region. The supraglottic larynx is embryologically part of the buccopharyngeal anlage, and its lymphatic drainage is shared with the tongue. The spread of tumors follows the lymphatic drainage and extends superiorly, laterally and posteriorly to nodes in intimate association with the jugular vein at the level of the hyoid bone.

The true vocal cords and subglottic region act more like the trachea with some of the lymphatic drainage being directly anterior from the anterior portion of the true vocal cords while the majority of the lymphatic drainage is posteriorly, inferiorly and laterally. The lymphatic drainage of the lower subglottic space is circumferential in its pathways and communicates freely with the tracheal lymphatics. The supraglottic larynx is further divided in the

Figure 6. Transglottic carcinoma in a 77 year old woman.

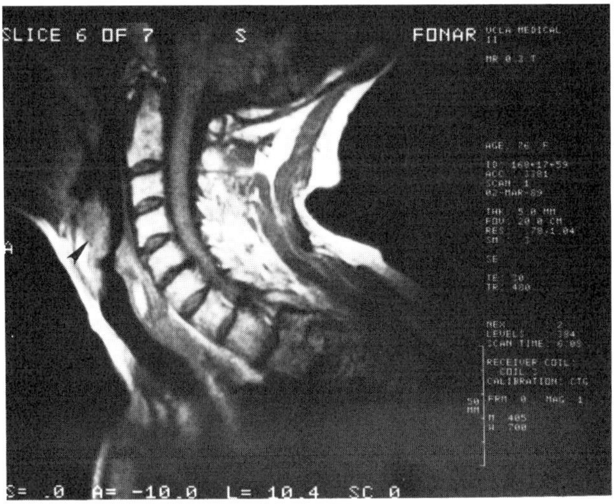

Figure 6a. Sagittal T1 weighted image (SE/480/30) reveals anterior lobulated soft tissue mass (arrowhead) narrowing the airway.

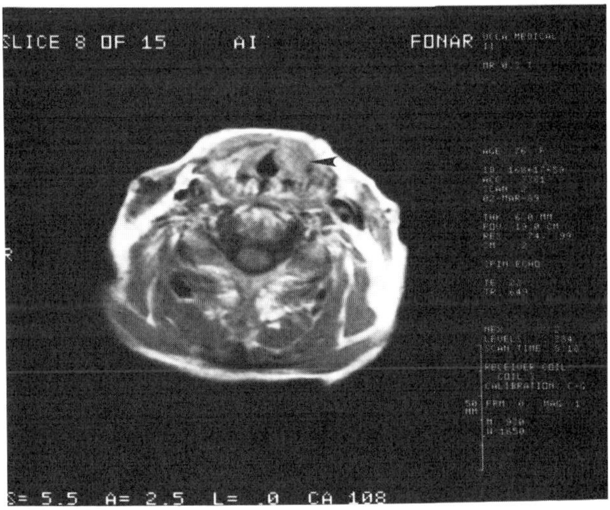

Figure 6b. Axial T1 weighted image at the undersurface of the true vocal cords shows subglottic extension with additional involvement of the anterior soft tissue of the neck (arrowhead).

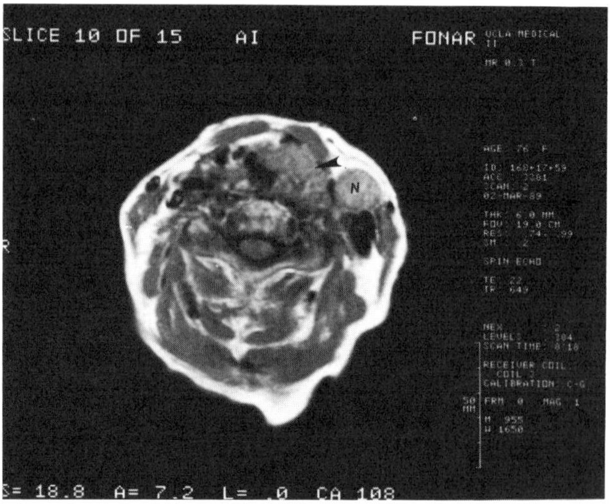

Figure 6c. Axial T1 weighted image of the high false vocal cords shows involvement of the left paralaryngeal space and adjacent soft tissues (−>). A large lymph note is also present (N).

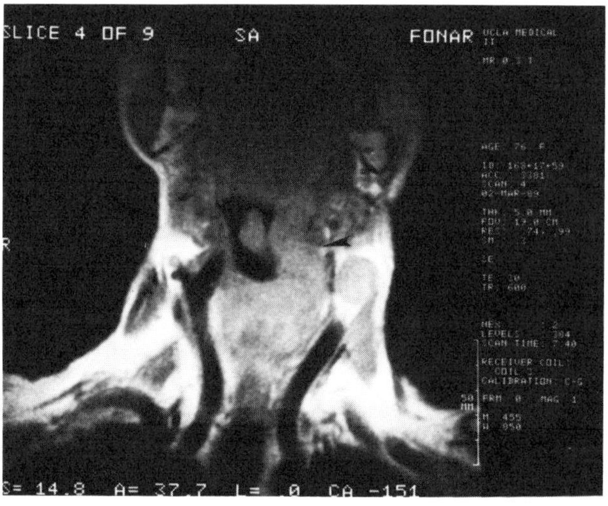

Figure 6d. Coronal T1 weighted image (SE/600/30) of the posterior larynx reveals left sided mass and associated node.

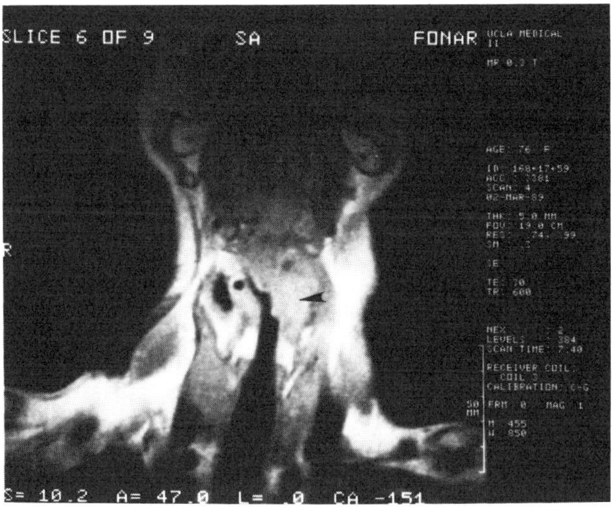

Figure 6e. Coronal T1 weighted images (SE/600/30) through the airway again shows left sided soft tissue component with airway compromise (arrowhead).

midline by ligaments which pass from the epiglottis to the thyrohyoid membrane and the hyoid bone.

The very early true cord tumor can be readily evaluated on indirect clinical examination and does not generally require an imaging study. The more advanced lesions that show extension to the anterior commissure regions above or below the vocal cord are quite a different matter. They require imaging techniques to show deep infiltration and full extent of the tumor.

The patient is ideally biopsied after the imaging examination. However, if a biopsy has already taken place, the imaging study should be delayed four to five days or until edema subsides. The disruption of facial planes and edema due to the biopsy can closely mimic tumor extension on MR studies of this and other regions of the head and neck.

Important anatomic considerations to be delineated by MR are cartilage invasion, vocal cord infiltration, preepiglottic space disease, and superior extension to the base of tongue or inferiorly to the subglottic space. The final decision whether to offer voice conservation surgery, radical surgery or radiation therapy will depend on these factors [28].

The loss of natural voice function resulting from a total laryngectomy can be devastating to many individuals. Less radical laryngeal resections that allow the preservation of natural speech and the protective sphincter mechanism of the larynx have been developed for certain smaller laryngeal tumors. Planning for any of these conservation laryngeal surgeries depends on an accurate preoperative knowledge of the precise extent of the disease within the larynx. Specifically, all techniques require an intact cricoid cartilage and at least one mobile arytenoid on which to construct the functional voice box. CT and now MR can provide this essential information. To plan this type of operation, the direct coronal and direct sagittal imaging capabilities of magnetic resonance far surpass axial CT images in the ability to define critical information regarding the cranial–caudal extent of the tumors.

The recognition of tumor spread of other areas also markedly affects patient management. In the case of spread of the supraglottic tumor to involve the tongue base, a partial glossectomy may have to be performed in addition to the primary surgery. In other areas, extraorgan spread may render the tumor unresectable. Supraglottic cancers tend to spread superolaterally while true cord tumors and pyriform sinus cancers tend to spread posteriolaterally and inferiorly (figure 7) [29,30]. A shift of centering or extra sections are necessary to show these nodal spreads. Finally, when cartilage invasion is present, cure with radiation therapy is often not possible. Therefore, the overall management of the patient must be reconsidered.

Compared to CT, MR consistently shows superior soft tissue definition. The use of direct coronal and sagittal scan planes allows the visualization of intrinsic laryngeal musculature in addition to better defining cranial caudal tumor extension. Thus, MR is now the imaging study of choice for the evaluation of cancer of the larynx. The role of magnetic resonance can also be extended to replace CT scanning for the evaluation of the laryngeal airway and for the evaluation of benign lesions of the larynx.

Figure 7. Squamous carcinoma of the piriform sinus.

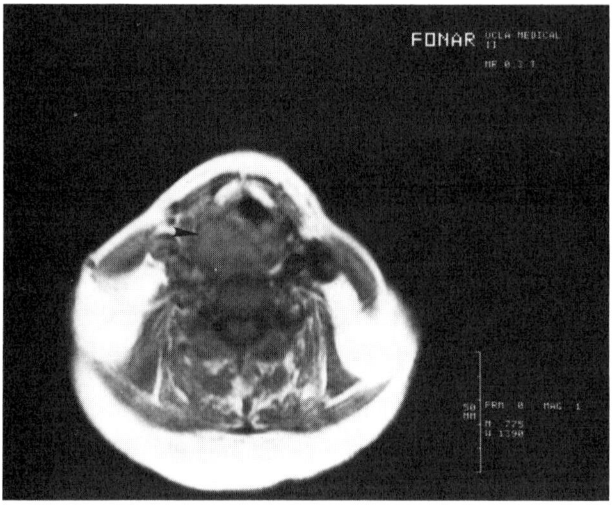

Figure 7a. Axial sequence (SE/500/30) shows soft tissue mass (arrowhead) arising in the piriform sinuses extending anteriorly.

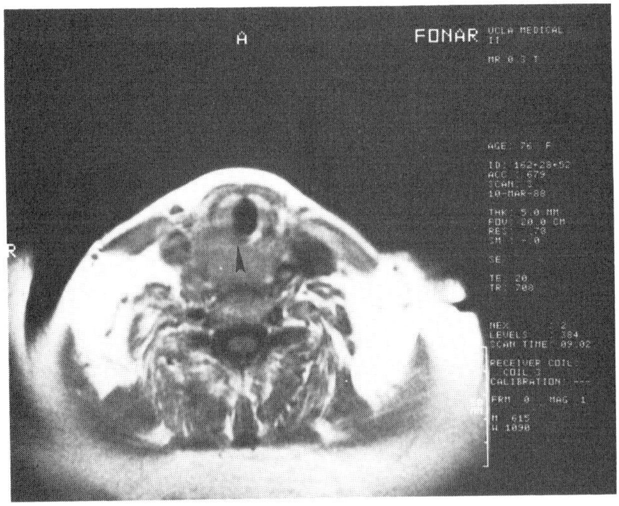

Figure 7b. Axial section through the level of cricoid cartilage shows replacement of high–signal marrow suggesting cartilage invasion by the tumor (arrowhead).

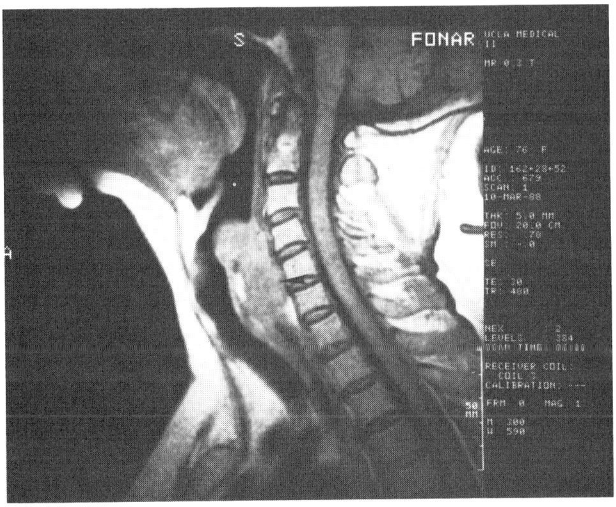

Figure 7c. Sagittal view shows full cranial caudal extent of the mass extending to the postcricoid region (arrowhead).

Salivary Glands

The preferred method of imaging the salivary glands has evolved with new developments in imaging technology as well as clinical needs. While intraductal contrast plain film sialography is still used to evaluate inflammatory lesions of the salivary glands, early CT scanners quickly replaced plain films for evaluation of masses. As CT technology improved spatial resolution, intravenous contrast replaced intraductal contrast for the CT sialogram evaluation of salivary gland masses. Now magnetic resonance has replaced CT scanning for the imaging evaluation of the majority of masses in the major salivary glands [31,32,33,34,35,36].

The approach to the study of masses in this area has been to use surface coils whenever possible and to obtain T1 weighted images in the axial plane. These views are supplemented with coronal or sagittal views when there is suggestion of temporal bone involvement. Complex, cystic, or unusual lesions are also evaluated with additional T2 weighted sequences when necessary.

Since 80% of major salivary gland tumors occur in the parotid gland, we will focus our attention on this particular region. The three main clinical goals for examining parotid masses are:

1. differentiation between benign and malignant tumors;
2. differentiation between extrinsic parapharyngeal space masses presenting as a parotid mass and actual intrinsic parotid masses; and
3. definition of the relationship of the facial nerve to the parotid tumor. Is the tumor superficial, deep or combined?

The policy at UCLA is to perform fine needle aspiration cytology on most tumors. This means that the first two goals are often achieved for superficially located tumors with a combination of clinical palpation and cytology in the clinic before any imaging studies are requested.

Magnetic resonance can only rarely suggest the histology of tumors, such as lipomas by their characteristic fat appearance or the possibility of a Warthin tumor in multilobulated cystic masses of the parotid. In the majority of cases magnetic resonance is not any more accurate than CT in predicting the histology of parotid lesions. This is in part due to the unusual histology of salivary gland tumors.

Therefore, the value of magnetic resonance in most cases, like CT, is to define the gross morphologic characteristics of the tumor outline. Although poor tumor margination may be a clue to malignancy, it is certainly not a reliable finding in MR (or CT) studies. Deep parapharyngeal space involvement may be demonstrated with CT; however, MR provides much better soft tissue contrast resolution. The real advantage of magnetic resonance in evaluating parotid masses is its ability to more accurately define the extent of the masses, to localize the tumor as extraparotid or intraparotid and to determine whether the intraparotid tumor is superficial or deep (figure 8).

With CT, only a rough estimate of the relationship of the parotid tumor

Figure 8. Recurrent adenocarcinoma of the parapharyngeal space. Both sequences are T1 weighted (SE/800/30).

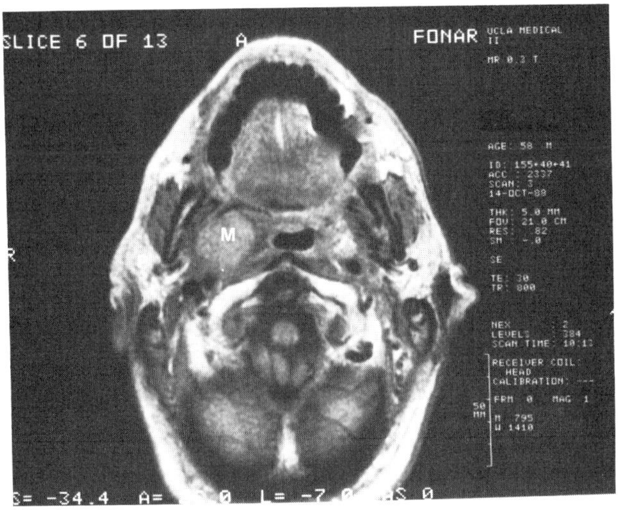

Figure 8a. The axial view through the level of the plate reveals a soft tissue mass arising in the right parapharyngeal space (M) which distorts the pharyngeal airway, but does not invade it. The parotid gland (P) is unremarkable.

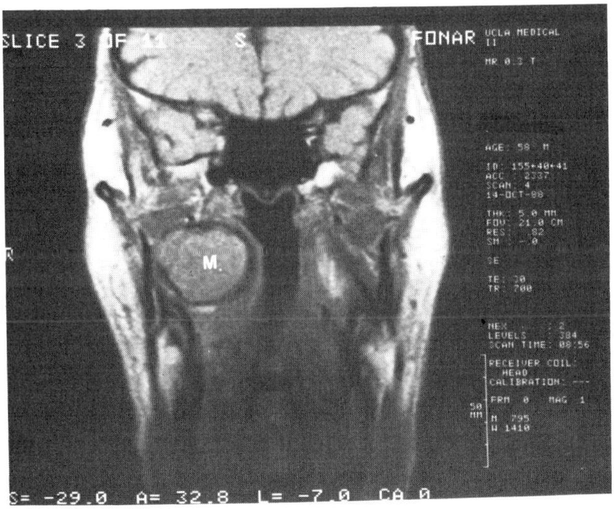

Figure 8b. The coronal view also shows the relationships of the mass (M) to the adjacent displaced pharyngeal wall and surrounding parapharyngeal space structures.

to the facial nerve can be made. CT as well as other imaging techniques prior to MRI have failed to accomplish imaging of the intraparotid facial nerve. T1 weighted MR images using surface coils can be used to demonstrate the major trunk of the facial nerve within the parotid gland, which on axial images, can be seen as a structure of slightly lower signal intensity lying within the high signal of the fatty parotid parenchyma. Its course from the stylomastoid foramen passing laterally to the retromandibular vein is characteristic. Coronal images are sometimes useful to determine the distance of the parotid mass from the stylomastoid foramen.

The relationship of parotid tumors to the facial nerve, which courses through and divides within the parotid gland, is of obvious value in planning the surgical approach and in order to more thoroughly appreciate the potential morbidity of operation preoperatively. Malignant tumors in close relation to the facial nerve may require excision of part of that structure and subsequent microsurgical repair or transposition of the VII nerve. Access to larger, deeper lesions may require division and reflection of the ramus of the mandible.

Paranasal Sinuses

At first glance it would appear that magnetic resonance would not be suitable to examine the paranasal sinuses. Since cortical bone and air do not return a signal on MR, one might assume that CT or other x–ray procedures would be needed to adequately visualize the sinus walls. Actually, most diseases affecting the paranasal sinuses are primarily soft tissue abnormalities of the lining of these cavities rather than the bones themselves.

Changes in the bony walls of the sinuses are generally secondary manifestations of the mucosal disease. In fact, the sclerotic, thickened margins of the sinuses interfere with visualization of mucosa. If bone destruction is present, it is usually a late manifestation of malignant disease of the mucosa. Deformed and displaced bony septa may contribute to or be the result of disease. MRI is actually an excellent imaging modality in this situation because bony septa are lined by mucosa which gives a high signal. The bony septum can be visualized as a negative shadow, a lower signal between the layers of high signal soft tissue.

It is, therefore, not surprising that MR is extremely valuable in evaluating masses of the paranasal sinuses. MR allows excellent delineation of solid tissue masses surrounded by secretions within the paranasal sinuses. Erosions of the bony walls are also well demonstrated on MR as the absence of signal void normally present in cortical bone (figure 9). For extension outside the bony sinuses, MR is the clear study of choice because it differentiates skeletal muscle from tumor extension, which can be difficult on CT studies (figure 10). In cases where there is a question of extension to the anterior or middle cranial fossa, MR with gadolinium enhancement remains the study of choice.

Figure 9. Squamous carcinoma of the maxillary sinus in a 41 year old male.

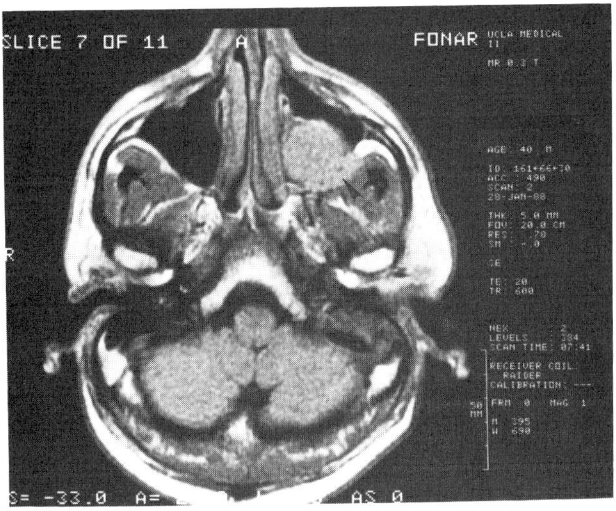

Figure 9a. Pre–gadolinium T1 weighted image (SE/600/20) shows the mass in the maxillary sinus with erosion of the posterior sinus wall (>).

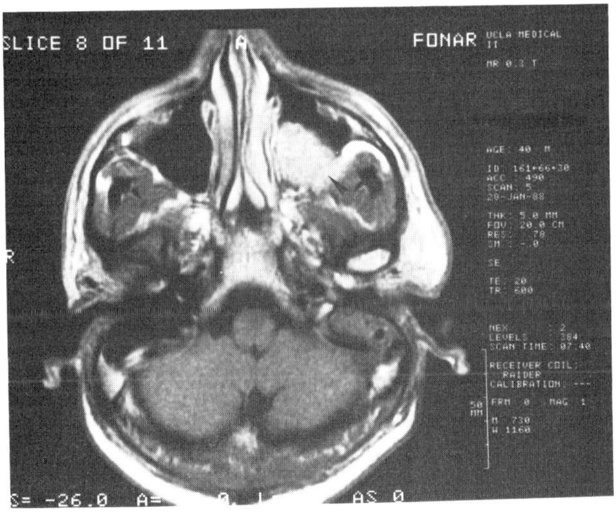

Figure 9b. Post–gadolinium image shows mild increased signal intensity of the tumor.

Figure 10. Squamous carcinoma of the maxillary sinus. All images are T1 weighted. (SE/800–500/30).

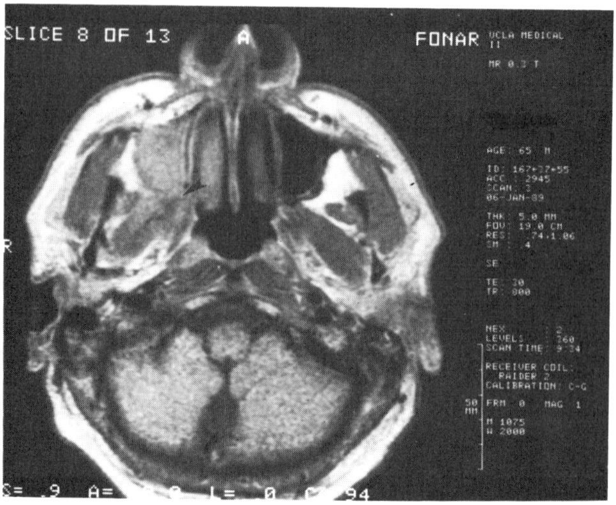

Figure 10a. Axial view through the midantrum shows opacification with bony destruction posteriorly through the ptyerigoid plates, invading the adjacent muscle (arrowhead).

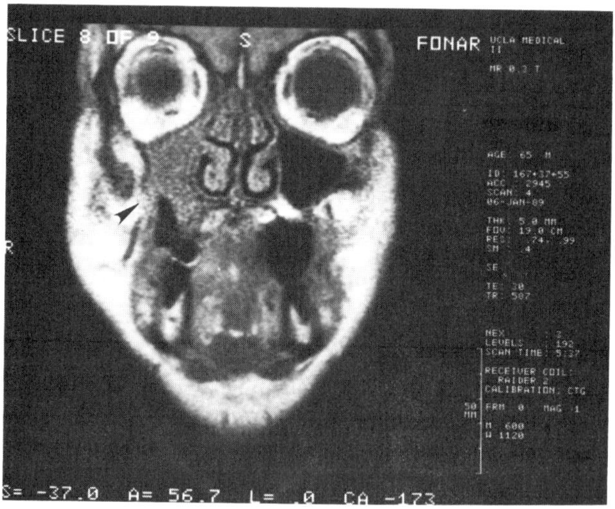

Figure 10b. Coronal view confirms this information and additionally shows involvement of the orbital floor and destruction of lateral maxillary sinus wall (arrowhead).

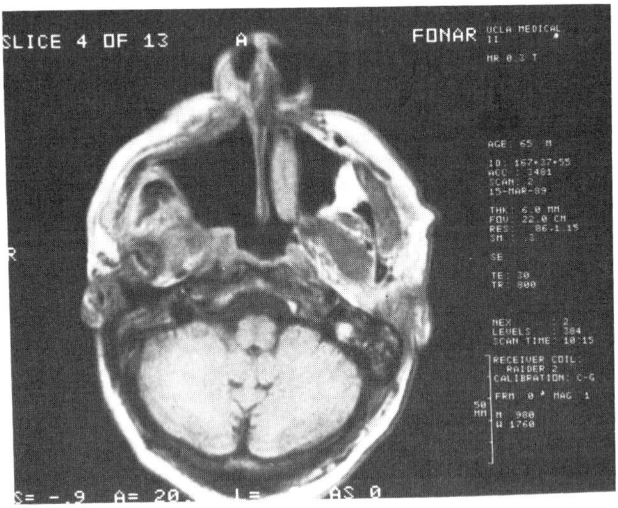

Figure 10c. Axial view following total resection shows satisfactory removal of the mass.

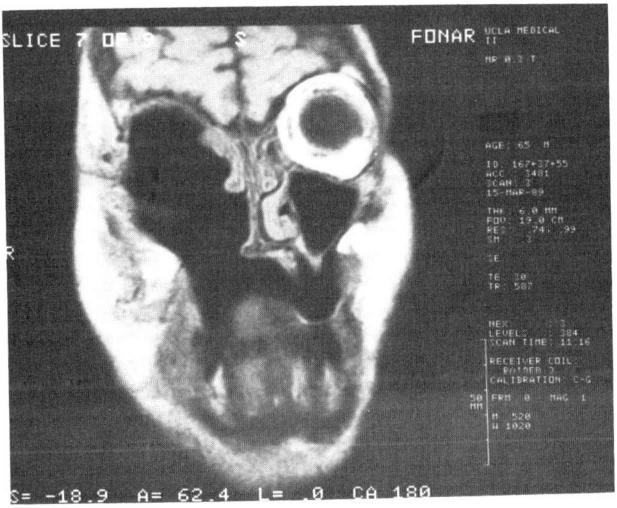

Figure 10d. Coronal view also confirms successful gross total removal.

The high soft tissue contrast capabilities of MR in distinguishing low protein fluids, high protein fluids, soft tissues, and normal musculature make MR ideal for display of malignant paranasal sinus disease. Frequently the very ill patient is just the individual who requires coronal or sagittal projections that are difficult or impossible to obtain with most CT equipment.

While the mainstay for imaging inflammatory paranasal sinus disease will continue to be plain x–rays because of their relative low cost, MR can now be substituted for CT scanning to evaluate advanced lesions in this area in most cases. With continued development of faster, lower cost MR scanners, it is not impossible that magnetic resonance will eventually even replace plain x–rays in the evaluation of this area.

Conclusions

Experience over the last six years indicates that magnetic resonance is now the imaging modality of choice to investigate the nasopharynx, tongue, oropharynx, larynx, hypopharynx, and the majority of miscellaneous lesions of the neck [37]. CT can be used in the same regions; however, information obtained from CT is not as clearly demonstrated and in some situations, such as malignancies of the tongue, the lesions may be missed entirely. Difficult clinical cases in which the two studies are complimentary will still be present but will definitely be in the minority.

MR guided aspiration cytology is now a reality through the use of specially developed MR compatible needles. Gadolinium DTPA shows only limited promise for use in head and neck cancer although its final role remains to be defined.

References

1. Lufkin R, Teresi L, Hanafee W: New needle for MRI guided aspiration cytology. American Journal of Roentgenology 149:380–382, 1987.
2. Lufkin R, Teresi L, Chui, Hanafee W, Teresi L, Chiu L, Hanafee W: A technique for MR guided needle placement in the head and neck. American Journal of Roentgenology 151:193–196, 1988.
3. Duckwiler G, Lufkin R, Teresi L, Spickler E, Dion J, Vinuela F, Bentson J, Hanafee W: Head and neck lesions: MR–guided aspiration biopsy. Radiology 170:519–522, 1989.
4. Robinson JD, Crawford S, Teresi L, Schiller VL, Lufkin RB, Harnsberger HR, Dietrich RB, Crim JR, Duckwiler GR, Spickler E, Hanafee W: Gadolinium MR imaging in the head and neck. Radiology (in press).
5. Dillon WP, Mills CM, Kjos B, et al.: Magnetic resonance imaging of the nasopharynx. Radiology 152:731–738, 1984.
6. Teresi LM, Lufkin RB, Vinuela F, et al.: MR imaging of the nasopharynx and floor of the middle cranial fossa. Part I. Normal anatomy. Radiology 164:811–816, 1987.
7. Teresi LM, Lufkin RB, Vinuela F, et al.: MR imaging of the nasopharynx and floor of the middle cranial fossa. Part II. Malignant tumors. Radiology 164:817–821, 1987.

8. Curtin HD: Separation of the masticator space from the parapharyngeal space. Radiology 163:195–204, 1987.
9. Cachin YU, Sancho–Garnier H, Micheau C, Marandas P: Nodal metastases from carcinomas of the nasopharynx. Otolaryngol Clin North Am 12:145–154, 1979.
10. Mancuso AA, Maceri D, Rice D, Hanafee W: CT of cervical lymph node cancer. AJR 136:381–385, 1981.
11. Mancuso AA, Harnsberger HR, Muraki AS, et al.: Computed tomography of cervial and retropharyngeal lymph nodes: normal anatomy. Radiology 148:709–714, 1983.
12. Dooms GC, Hricak H, Crooks LE, Higgins CB: Magnetic resonance imaging of the lymph nodes: comparison with CT. Radiology 153:719–728, 1984.
13. Dooms GC, Hricak H, Moseley MD, Bottles K, Fisher M, Higgins CB: Characterization of lymphadenopathy by magnetic resonance relaxation times: preliminary results. Radiology 155:691–697, 1985.
14. Mancuso AA, Hanafee W: Elusive head and neck carcinomas beneath intract mucosa. Laryngoscope 93:133–139, 1983.
15. Unger JM: The oral cavity and tongue: magnetic resonance imaging. Radiology 155:151–153, 1985.
16. Lufkin R, Hanafee W, Wortham D, Hoover L: MRI of the tongue and oropharynx using surface coils. Radiology 161:69–75, 1986.
17. Batsakis JG: Tumors of the Head and Neck: Clinical Pathological Consideration, ed 2. Baltimore: Williams & Wilkins, 1979.
18. Stark DD, Moss AA, Gamsu G, Clark OH, Gooding GW, Webb WR: Magnetic resonance imaging of the neck. Part 1. Normal anatomy. Radiology 150:447–454, 1983.
19. Lufkin R, Hanafee W, Wortham D, Hoover L: MRI of the larynx and hypopharynx using surface coils. Radiology 158:747–754, 1986.
20. Lufkin RB, Hanafee W: Application of surface coils to NMR anatomy of the larynx. American Journal of Neuroradiology: AJR 491–497, 1985.
21. Lufkin R, Larsson S, Hanafee W: NMR anatomy of the larynx and tongue. Radiology 148:173–175, 1983.
22. Glazer HS, Niemeyer JH, Balfe D, et al.: Neck neoplasms: MR imaging. Part II Posttreatment evaluation. Radiology 160:349–354, 1986.
23. Glazer HS, Niemeyer JH, Balfe D, et al.: Neck neoplasms: MR imaging. Part I. Initial evaluation. Radiology 160:343–348, 1986.
24. Stark DD, Moss AA, Gamsu G, Clark OH, Gooding GW, Webb WR: Magnetic resonance imaging of the neck. Part 2. Pathologic anatomy. Radiology 150:455–462, 1983.
25. McArdle CB, Bailey BJ, Amparo EG: Surface coil magnetic resonance imaging of the normal larynx. Arch Otolaryngol Head Neck Surg 112:616–622, 1986.
26. Castelijns JA, Gerritsen GJ, Kaiser MC, et al.: MRI of normal or cancerous laryngeal cartilages: Histopathologic correlation. Laryngoscope 97:1085–1093, 1987.
27. Last RJ: Anatomy: regional and applied. 6th ed. New York: Churchill Livingstone, 1978.
28. Burstein FD, Calcaterra TC: Supraglottic Laryngectomy: Series Report and Analysis of Results. Laryngoscope 95, 7:833–836, 1985.
29. Kirchner JA: Two hundred laryngeal cancers: patterns of growth and spread as seen in serial section. Laryngoscope 87:474–482, 1977.
30. Larsson SV, Mancuso A, Hoover L, Hanafee W: Differentiation of pyriform sinus cancer from supraglottic laryngeal cancer by computed tomography. Radiology 141:427–432, 1981.
31. Teresi L, Lufkin R, Kolin E, Hanafee W, et al.: MRI of the intraparotid facial nerve. American Journal of Neuroradiology 8(2):253–259, 1987.
32. Teresi L, Lufkin R, Wortham D, Abemayor E, Hanafee W: Parotid masses: magnetic resonance imaging. Radiology 163(2):405–409, 1987.
33. Casselman JW, Mancuso AA: Major salivary gland masses: comparison of MR imaging and CT. Radiology 165:183–189, 1987.
34. Mandelblatt SM, Braun IF, Davis PC, et al.: Parotid masses: MR imaging. Radiology 163:411–414, 1987.

35. Rice DH, Becker T: Magnetic resonance imaging of the salivary glands. Arch Otolaryngol Head Neck Surg 113:78–80, 1987.
36. Mirich DR, McArdle CB, Kulkarni MV: Benign pleomorphic adenomas of the salivary glands: surface coil MR imaging verus CT. J Comput Assist Tomogr 11:620–623, 1987.
37. Lufkin R, Hanafee W: MR Atlas of Head and Neck Anatomy, New York, Raven Press, 1989.

2. Diagnostic Imaging in the Diagnosis of Malignant Invasion of the Carotid Artery: Ultrasound, Computed Tomography, Magnetic Resonance Imaging

Gretchen A.W. Gooding

Anatomy of Carotid Artery

The carotid artery arises at the bifurcation of the brachiocephalic artery on the right and from the aortic arch on the left and courses superficially in the neck posterior to the sternocleidomastoid muscle, dividing into internal and external branches near the angle of the jaw. The walls of the carotid artery are composed of the internal intima, the media, and the outer adventitia. All are contained in the carotid sheath. The carotid sheath is continuous with the deep cervical fascia and contains not only the carotid artery where it is thick and dense, but also the adjacent lateral jugular vein and the vagus nerve which lies between the two in a posterior position. The carotid artery is relatively impervious to invasion by malignancy. The adjacent and usually lateral jugular vein is not as resistant to malignant invasion and may become flattened or distorted and eventually invaded by adjacent cancer [1].

Physical Signs

Physical examination of the neck is not a reliable indicator of malignant carotid invasion [1]. While many neck masses are readily palpated, a palpable mass in the neck with transmitted pulsation is not a reliable indicator of frank invasion of the carotid artery and can be confused with other abnormalities, such as a carotid artery aneurysm. In fact, from palpation alone, bulky calcific plaque in the carotid bulb may be confused with metastatic neck disease clinically because of the hard and fixed nature of the carotid bulb in this situation.

Etiology

Carotid invasion by malignancy is usually secondary to squamous cell carcinoma, since that is the cause of 90% of head and neck cancers. This catastrophic event, which is associated with a very poor prognosis, is most likely to occur from recurrence of squamous cell carcinoma which may originate from a number of sources above the clavicle, including the tongue,

Jacobs, C. (ed): Carcinomas of the Head and Neck: Evaluation and Management.

nasopharyynx, oropharynx, and tonsils. The cancer may spread by local invasion of the primary lesion, and while there is potential for direct invasion of the carotid artery, it is a rare occurrence, probably because of the protective nature of the thick, deep cervical fascia that surrounds it.

Besides local extension, squamous cell carcinoma metastasizes to the local lymph nodes of the neck and may aggressively extend regionally. Local lymph node metastasis may impinge upon the carotid artery and at times locally invade, again rarely. A review of the records of 508 patients who had had radical neck surgery for squamous cell carcinoma showed 5.5% to have had tumor attached to the carotid arterial system [2]. Neoplastic extension may track along the cranial nerves into the skull foramina or in the opposite direction peripherally. Distal hematogenous spread is not likely to be associated with carotid invasion of the neck.

Diagnostic Imaging

Computed tomography (CT), magnetic resonance imaging (MRI), and ultrasound (US) can be used to define neck nodes. Plain films of the neck may show bulges in soft tissues from adenopathy or displacement of the trachea but are otherwise not useful for the detection of adenopathy in the neck.

Benign neck nodes by sonography are usually oval, hypoechoic, of greater dimension in transverse diameter than in anterior-posterior plane and may have a central linear echogenic line caused from normal fat in the hilus. Malignant nodes tend to be larger and more bulky. A sonographic study of postoperative patients with thyroid cancer [3] suggests that there is considerable overlap in the determination of benign versus malignant disease based on size alone. Small nodes in the neck may be malignant, and large ones can be caused by inflammatory disease rather than malignancy [3].

Malignant nodes tend to have a greater anterior-posterior diameter [4]. An echogenic line from fat in the hilus found in the length of the mid portion of a node suggests a benign node. Calcific punctate densities in nodes have been associated with medullary thyroid cancer in three patients [3].

Nodes on CT and MRI are of soft tissue density. Neck nodes on MRI tend to enhance on T–2 weighted images to become brighter. Size is used as an indicator of malignancy, but not an absolute one, since inflammatory processes may result in large nodes. Malignant nodes have no absolute pathognomonic pattern by CT, US, or MRI, but large bulky nodes in the neck are suspect, particularly when poorly defined and poorly marginated. These findings suggest infiltration and penetration of adjacent tissues [5].

CT requires intravenous contrast injection to define the vascular structures, determine tumor margination, and differentiate the normal from abnormal soft tissues. CT, US and MRI define the relationship of the tumor to the carotid artery, but CT is not particularly sensitive for defining invasion.

Classically the carotid artery has been visualized noninvasively by angiography which can depict the vessel and its branches in full length in two planes at 90 degrees in longitudinal axis. With the advent of CT and MRI, axial images became possible, with coronal planes and other obliquities from reconstructed images also feasible, although time—consuming to achieve.

Ultrasound

Ultrasound of the carotid artery is limited to visualization in the neck above the clavicles and below the angle of the jaw. It may be further limited when the patient cannot extend his neck as in ankylosing spondylitis which further reduces the window of scanning. When the patient has a high bifurcation of the carotid artery, only a few millimeters of the internal and external branches may be seen. With the advent of the Doppler duplex technique, and more recently, the addition of color coded Doppler imaging, ultrasound has become a well accepted, proven technique to evaluate the vessel, particularly in atherosclerosis, providing both an image as well as a spectral analysis of velocity profiles [6,7]. For most effective evaluation, ultrasound requires a transducer of high frequency, 7.5–10 MHz, to register the image from the reflected echoes generated by the instrumentation. The carotid artery is well defined, classically in longitudinal and transverse images, as an anechoic tube with bright walls of high echo intensity which represent the intima, media, and adventitia. Duplex Doppler combines the capability of an image of the vessel with the capability to interrogate the flow by spectral analysis to determine velocity, spectral broadening, and, in some instances, from a measure of the diameter or the area, make a calculation of flow. The introduction of color coded Doppler has furthered the understanding of the shear forces at play in the carotid artery. At the bulb, in late systole and early diastole, flow reversal is normally present in the slower turbulent flow along the periphery. Forward flow of high shear force is red; reversed flow is blue. The diagnosis of carotid invasion, however, is based on the gray scale image of wall integrity.

The normal carotid artery has, by sonography, a bright wall interface (figure 1). The carotid artery lumen is anechoic on standard black and white images and red on color coded Doppler.

In the evaluation of carotid artery invasion by ultrasound, the examiner relies primarily upon the visual grey scale image of the vessel and subtle abnormalities of the wall (figure 2). Mass effect may be obvious from adjacent metastatic nodes that may encircle the carotid artery or its branches. The jugular vein tends to be compressed by adjacent masses. The carotid arteries

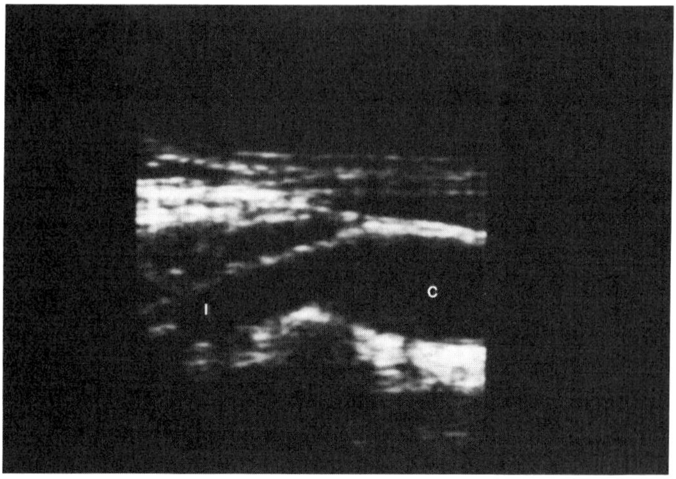

Figure 1. A longitudinal 10 MHz sonogram of a normal carotid bulb and internal carotid artery demonstrates the bright vascular walls and the anechoic black lumen. I = internal carotid, c = common carotid.

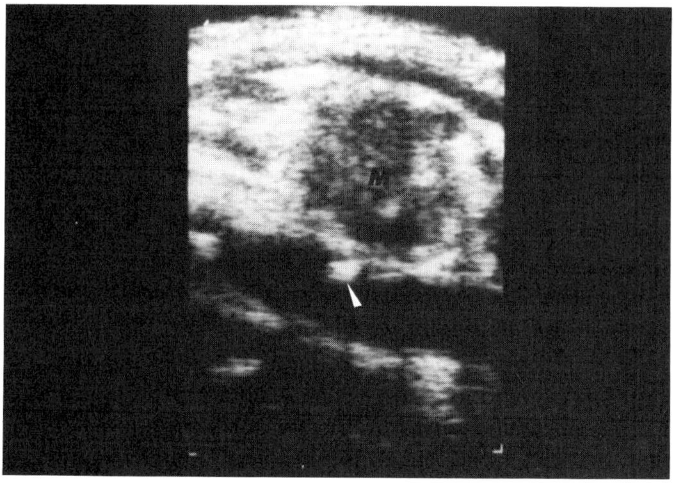

Figure 2. A longitudinal sonogram of 10 MHz demonstrates irregular bright plaque along the vessel wall acess and a clear interface between the carotid artery and the adjacent hypoechoic mass of squamous cell carcinoma. m = mass.

are resistant to compression effects. The artery may be entirely surrounded by mass, but have the bright interface of its walls intact, uninvaded by malignancy. A loss in continuity of the wall of a few millimeters, on only one plane, may be artifactual, not real. Wall abnormalities must be documented in two planes.

A break in the hyperechoic carotid wall with an actual step off in continuity is a reliable sonographic sign of invasion of adjacent tumor. A gross incursion of tumor into the lumen with a break through the normal hyperechoic intact walls is also evidence of malignant invasion (figure 3). A mass adjacent to the carotid artery may attenuate the acoustic beam and artefactually produce a loss of carotid wall echogenicity which has the potential to give a false positive (figure 4). Also, on transverse scan a normal loss of wall interface on both lateral margins of the carotid wall may be falsely ascribed to carotid invasion. This lack of bright definition of the lateral carotid walls on transverse scan is caused by the acoustic beam striking the wall in tangent rather than at the perpendicular as it does in the anterior–posterior plane.

When the examiner is uncertain as to whether carotid invasion has occurred or not, MRI is the study of choice. Ultrasound tends to lead the examiner to a diagnosis of malignant invasion accurately when obvious signs are present. When subtle changes of the carotid wall are the only evidence sonographically, false positive evaluations become more common.

From the clinician's standpoint, if the ultrasound examination shows no evidence of malignant invasion of the carotid artery, that is a reliable indicator of no carotid invasion and can be relied upon to make clinical decisions. There were no false negative ultrasound examinations in our original studies [8]. If there is some question of carotid invasion by sonography, MRI is the next step, since ultrasound is more likely to be falsely positive than MRI. The specificity of ultrasound in this situation is 75% and of MRI, 87%. Both have sensitivities of 100% [9].

In the thyroid, ultrasound is more effective than CT in defining small lesions within the parenchyma of the thyroid gland. Enhancement of thyroid tissue by CT is so dramatic that small lesions may be obscured by partial volume effects. However, ultrasound is not effective in defining abnormalities surrounding the oral cavity, the pharynx, trachea, or esophagus, because these are air–filled structures, and air causes the acoustic beam to scatter instead of providing an orderly image from echoes reflected from the tissues. Preliminary work has used the modality to study the tongue [10]. Potential exists for the intraoral use of ultrasound to study the deep parotid, medial to the mandible. Initial early work has demonstrated its usefulness in detecting thyroid cartilage invasion in aggressive laryngeal cancer [10].

Sonography is not appropriate to examine the bones of the neck. Sound travels very well in bone, but the acoustic energy is lost at the bone–soft tissue interface because of intense absorption and refraction, and no image is therefore produced.

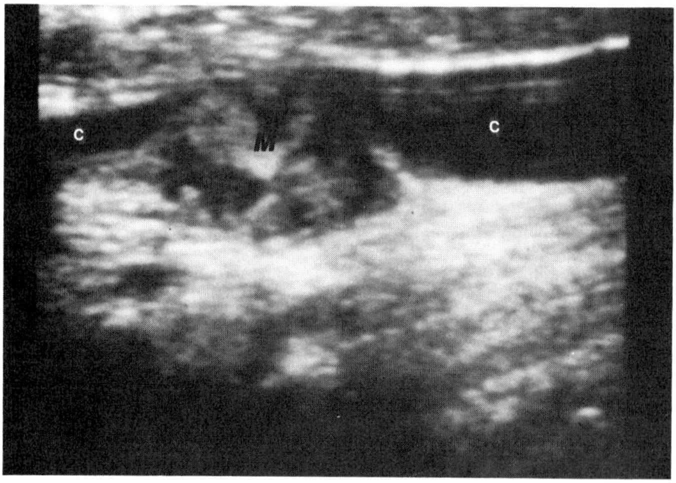

Figure 3. A longitudinal sonogram of 10 MHz demonstrates a tumor mass directly invading the wall of the carotid artery. c = common carotid, m = mass.

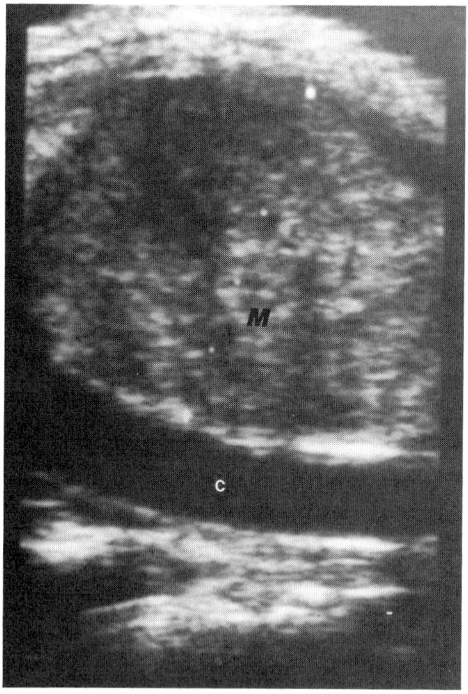

Figure 4. A longitudinal sonogram of 10 MHz demonstrates a large mass that is anterior to the carotid artery. On the right side of the image, the carotid artery is directly perpendicular to the acoustic beam and the carotid walls are bright. On the left, as the vessel turns upward and the acoustic beam is more tangential than perpendicular, the walls of the carotid artery become less distinct. This is not carotid artery invasion.

Angiography

By angiography, head and neck tumors tend to cause displacement, narrowing and slower flow in the carotid artery noted from mass effect. With prior radiation, the vessel may have a ratty appearance which is also the effect of early invasion of the carotid by malignancy. Tumor vascularity is variable, from the typical homogeneous highly vascular benign chemodectoma to the poorly vascular malignant necrotic mass. Most tumors do not have a particular angiographic thumbprint that is unique, and biopsy is required for pathologic diagnosis.

Angiography, usually by the digital subtraction technique, is indicated when carotid resection, reconstruction, or bypass is a consideration. Also, angiography is appropriate when carotid aneurysm is a possibility [11] or chemodectoma which has a highly characteristic hypervascular appearance. Bilateral studies are the norm and indicate the state of collateral vasculature both in the neck and in the brain.

Angiography is not effective in defining carotid artery invasion by malignancy. Angiography basically defines the internal lumen of the carotid artery, not the wall thickness or integrity. Vessels may be distorted from mass effect and irregularity of the wall may be present, but angiography is primarily used to define the vascularity of the neck mass itself rather than its invasive characteristics on local anatomy.

Computed Tomography

Readily available, computed tomography is the current gold standard by which other modalities are evaluated in the diagnosis of head and neck tumors. With the patient supine and the neck hyperextended, 5 mm thick axial slices every 5 mm are obtained from the clavicle to the skull base during a rapid drip intravenous infusion of centrast media.

With CT, the anatomy from the skull base to the mediastinum is well defined, including the glandular structures of the thyroid, the enlarged parathyroid, the salivary glands, the larynx, the aerodigestive tract, (esophagus, pharynx, parapharyngeal spaces), the neurovascular bundle, the retropharyngeal space and the vertebrae. Laryngography has been all but replaced by CT. Cortical bone disease can be recognized by CT which is not possible with US and MRI.

The carotid sheath, which is not seen *per se* by CT, is within the neurovascular compartment of the neck, distinct from the visceral compartments and the prevertebral area, in the superficial layer of the deep cervical fascia along with the parotid gland, the submandibular gland, the sternocleidomastoid muscle and the trapezius muscle. By CT, the carotid artery is well defined, as is the more lateral jugular vein and the vagus nerve, posterior in position to the jugular vein and the carotid artery (figure 5). Sympathetic

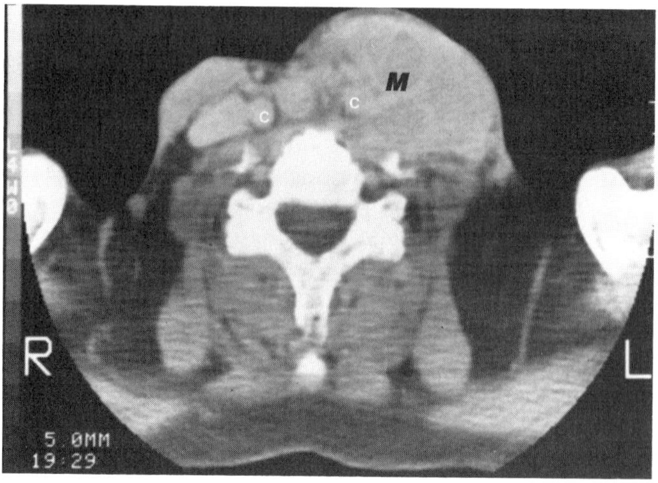

Figure 5. A CT scan demonstrates a large left neck mass that encompasses the left carotid artery. This suggests invasion. The right carotid artery has a fine low–density circumferential band of fat about it which is of normal appearance.

fibers are also present in the carotid sheath and little lymph nodes which may be seen as punctate white areas on the scans in the region.

Normally, there are several chains of lymph nodes in the head and neck regions, all of which are susceptible to metastatic invasion by malignant tumor. Those most likely to involve the carotid sheath are the deep cervical, but nodal involvement with tumor may be extensive and involve widespread areas of the anterior, superficial, and deep nodal areas. Adenopathy may extend from the cervical salivary glands to involve the carotid artery. These nodes are evaluated on CT primarily by size. Nodes under 1 cm are considered benign, but may not always be. Large nodes over 2 cm are considered malignant when infectious etiologies can be excluded. Contrast infusion is essential in the head and neck CT examination to differentiate vessels from lymph nodes. This is not the case for ultrasound or MRI.

Nodes by CT may not enhance after contrast injection or may have only peripheral rim enhancement which may be thick or thin. A thickened enhanced rim suggests nodal capsular or extracapsular extension [12]. Malignant nodes often have a low attenuation center with an enhanced periphery, but this pattern can also occur with infectious processes such as tuberculosis. Deep infiltration of neoplasia of the head and neck, whether direct or metastatic, may obliterate the carotid sheath [12].

Supraclavicular nodes may be an indication of metastatic disease below the clavicle, from lung, breast, stomach, ovary, prostate, colon, pancreas, uterus, liver, or kidney. There is nothing from the CT appearance, other than location, that distinguishes these from the nodes metastatic from a head and neck primary cancer. Both have potential to invade the carotid artery, but that is a rare occurrence in either case.

Both CT and US are appropriate localizers of neck masses for image directed percutaneous biopsies [13]. The biopsy can thereby be directed away from areas of necrosis where positive pathologic data is less likely to be obtained.

CT excels in the definition of malignancy of the nasopharynx, pharynx, parapharyngeal space, and infratemporal fossa [14]. It provides the surgeon and the radiation oncologist with a map of the site of origin, the localization for appropriate biopsy, and the extent of spread. While ultrasound is excellent for soft tissue and local vascular assessment in the neck above the clavicle and below the angle of the jaw, CT has the advantage in determining bony metastasis, muscle atrophy from cranial nerve denervation from tumor, and visualization of the carotid artery and its branches from its origin at the aortic arch to the vasculature of the brain. When a fine low–density plane of fat surrounds the carotid artery, the vessel is considered not invaded by adjacent tumor [15]. Intravenous contrast is essential, even though invasive and with potential for contrast reaction, because it allows differentiation of various tissues on the basis of density changes, and as such defines the carotid artery and its branches as bright contrast enhanced structures.

However, when adjacent tumor is also bright and contrast enhanced, the two structures may visually seem to merge, and the distinction of whether or not there is carotid invasion becomes a moot point, that is not possible to define with assurance [16] (figures 6, 7). With CT, both axial and coronal scans are possible, just as with MRI, but special programming, which is time consuming, is necessary when coronal views are needed.

CT of the head and neck is used to detect an abnormality on the basis of mass effect, replacement, distortion and displacement of anatomic structures, or focal muscle atrophy. Muscular atrophy suggests denervation from neoplastic cranial nerve involvement [14].

Magnetic Resonance Imaging

Vessels are identified by MRI and distinguished from soft tissue structures without contrast agents. Early preliminary work in MRI suggests that carotid imaging to detect flow abnormalities is feasible but at the present time, is elusive [17]. However, its applicability in the head and neck is rapidly developing, primarily because of excellent soft tissue contrast, and in the future it may supplant CT in the evaluation of the oncologic patient [18,19]. Image acquisition in multiple planes has a distinct advantage for a three dimensional approach to the extent of disease. Further improvements are predicted with the advent of new imaging strategies with and without contrast agents such as gadolinium – DTPA, faster scan times, improved spatial resolution, and developments in surface coil technology [20]. MRI has

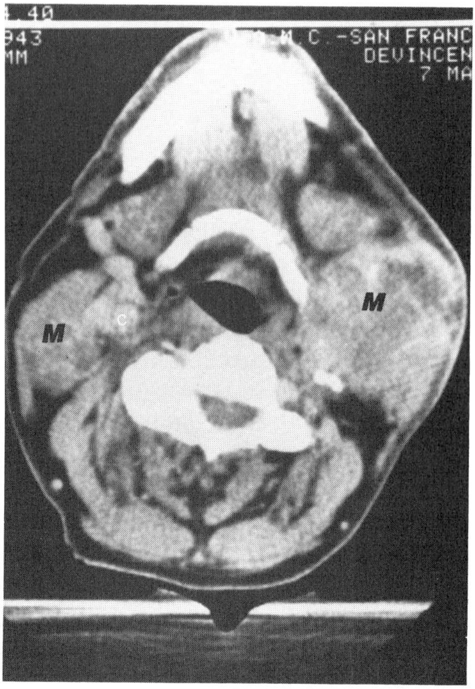

Figure 6. A CT scan demonstrates marked bilateral adenopathy of the neck, left greater than right. The left carotid artery is not seen and the question of carotid invasion is raised because of the inability to define the vessel. The right carotid artery appears at least partially intact. This patient is the same as in figure 3, which shows sonographic unequivocal invasion of the carotid artery on the left.

superior soft tissue definition when compared with CT. Teresi, et al., consider it the imaging study of choice for evaluation of cancer of the larynx, placing it in perspective with the realization that the clinical examination in conjunction with cytology are the primary measures in diagnosis in the area [21]. MRI has replaced CT as the primary study for parapharyngeal space masses [22]. This is based on superior soft tissue resolution.

In paranasal sinus and nasal cavity disease, increased accuracy with MRI has resulted from the finding that disparate T2–relaxation values can help to distinguish inflammation from malignancy with better precision [23]. Precise absolute tissue specificity from the imaging data by CT, MRI, or ultrasound is not possible.

Although MRI is sensitive to changes in bone marrow, the chief disadvantage of MRI in the head and neck is the poor demonstration of cortical bone and the inability to show calcifications [24]. Just as with CT, MRI is dependent upon the absence of motion during the image acquisition and in some situations both technologies in concert have a complementary role in the depiction of the disease.

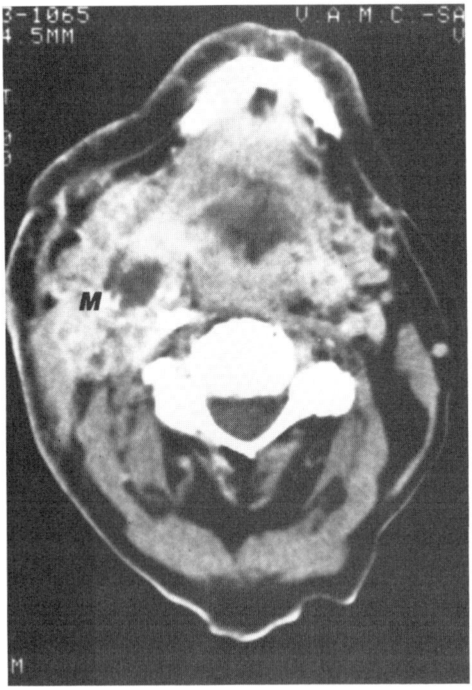

Figure 7. A CT scan demonstrates a large inhomogeneous neck mass extending from the base of the tongue on the right along the sternocleidomastoid muscle and the vascular space. The mass surrounds the vascular structures on the right which are difficult to distinguish from the adjacent soft tissues. This is recurrent squamous cell carcinoma invading the carotid artery.

Patients having MRI must be free of any ferromagnetic material such as a pacemaker, shrapnel, or metal prosthetic device. They must be able to tolerate prolonged immobility in cramped quarters while in the scanner. Motion artifact degrades the image, just as with CT.

In the investigation of the question of carotid artery invasion, axial and coronal scans are obtained with the patient supine using an anterior saddle shaped surface coil. Five mm slices are obtained with a 2.5 mm gap between slices from the clavicles to the mid nasopharynx, using a 1.5 Tesla imaging system [9].

In the detection of carotid artery invasion, early experience [9] with MRI suggests that any effacement of any part of the carotid wall by tumor is consistent with carotid invasion. Of 18 cases studied with MRI who were suspected of carotid invasion, (of whom three patients actually had carotid invasion at surgery), MRI had a sensitivity of 100% and a specificity of 87% [9] (figures 8, 9, 10). MRI was equivalent to US in detecting carotid invasion, but had an advantage in demonstrating that the carotid artery was free of malignant infiltration. One advantage may be that MRI has potential

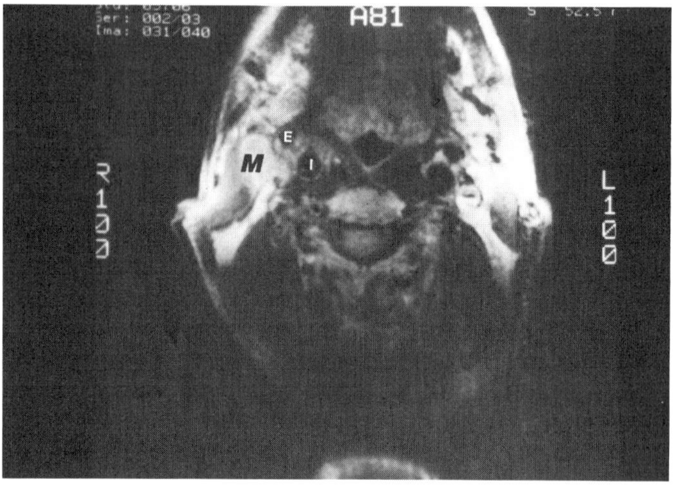

Figure 8. An MRI (axial plane) demonstrates a right sided mass that invades the external carotid and partially invades the internal carotid artery. m = mass, I = internal carotid artery, E = external artery (contributed by Dr. William P. Dillon, Department of Radiology, University of California, San Francisco, California).

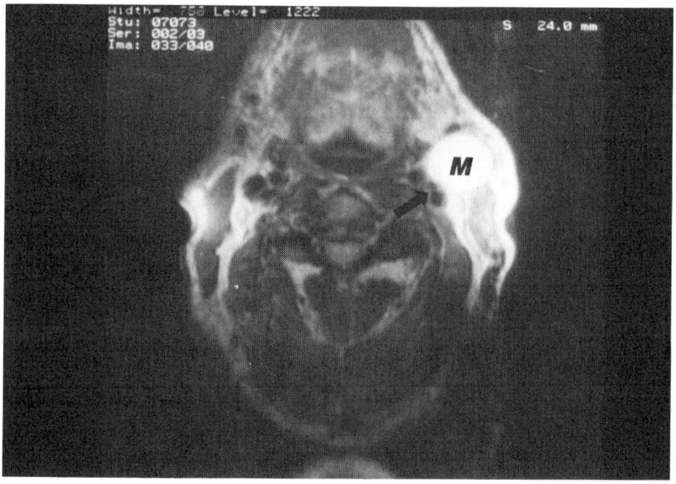

Figure 9. An MRI (axial plane) of a T–2 weighted image shows a left sided neck mass invading the carotid artery (arrow), the margins of which are poorly defined.

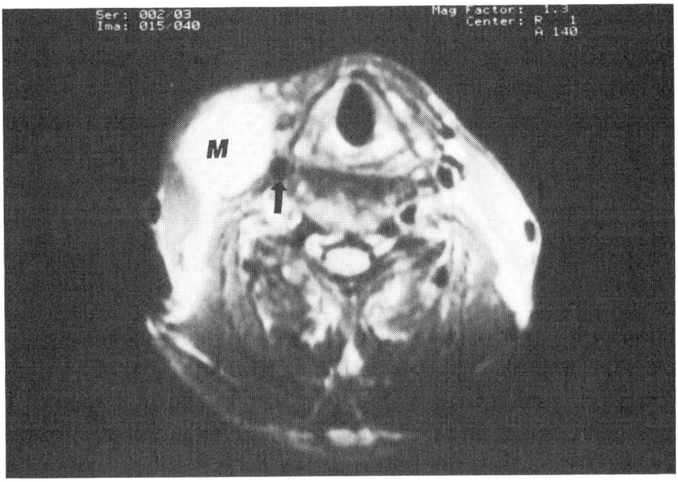

Figure 10. An MRI (axial plane) of a T–2 weight image demonstrates a new mass adjacent to, but separate from, the right carotid artery (arrow). (Figures 9 and 10 are contributed by Dr. Alan Langman, Department of Otolaryngology, University of Michigan, Ann Arbor, Michigan).

to distinguish the lower intensity signal of fibrosis from the usually higher signal intensity of tumor on T–2 weighted images [25].

The Silent Malignancy of the Head and Neck

Imaging modalities of CT, US, and MRI may not always detect the silent head and neck neoplasm which is apt to be a small lesion not visible to inspection in the nasopharynx, the base of the tongue, in the walls of the vallecula, the pyriform sinus, the laryngeal surface of the glottis, the laryngeal ventricle, the thyroid, or the hypopharynx. If a microscopic focus of malignancy is present, imaging modalities will not detect an abnormality. In the aerodigestive areas of the oropharynx, pharynx, larynx or esophagus, surface abnormalities of flat mucosal lesions may not be detected.

Surgical Considerations

Head and neck cancer, when associated with carotid artery invasion, has an extremely poor prognosis, and patients have historically not been considered surgical candidates. Resection of the carotid artery in these situations is hazardous, since hemiplegia from acute ligation may occur. In fact, stroke is highly likely in this situation. However, preoperative prediction of tolerance to the resection using carotid arteriography, temporary balloon occlusion of the internal carotid artery, and xenon computed tomography cerebral blood flow mapping has been used to identify those who may be candidates for the procedure [26]. Carotid artery bypass holds promise [27]. Removal of the tumor and the adjacent affected carotid artery followed by reconstruction of the carotid artery with bypass allows unimpeded perfusion to the brain. Stump pressures at the time of surgery aid in the prediction of the adequacy of cross blood flow at the time of the procedure. These procedures are preferentially performed with autonomous vein, such as the saphenous vein and may extend from the axillary artery to the internal carotid artery [28]. The bypass may thereby be outside the field of radiation and may even be at a distance from the wound closure and therefore less likely to be susceptible to carotid blowout from prior radiation, infection, or fistula. A high incidence of graft failure occurs in carotid artery graft procedures when the patient has had prior radiation.

Conclusions

In summary, CT, US, and MRI have specific indications in the examination of the head and neck. For assessment of carotid artery invasion by malignancy, US and MRI offer distinct advantages over CT. Ultrasound, which is relatively inexpensive, well tolerated and non–invasive, requires no contrast agents, offers multiple planes of visualization, and can be obtained and repeated, if necessary, expeditiously. A negative sonogram is a reliable indicator of absence of carotid artery invasion. MRI is expensive and time consuming, and, as such, is not as appropriate as a screen for carotid invasion as US. However, MRI can visualize the carotid artery superiorly beyond the limitation of US at the angle of the jaw and is likely to yield fewer false positive examinations in instances of prior surgery, radiation, and fibrosis. When the issue of carotid artery invasion is not clear–cut with one study or another, US and MRI used in concert are the complimentary combination that is likely to provide the clinician with the most helpful information in making the final decision as to appropriate therapy.

References

1. Bruneton JN, Roux P, Caramella E, Demard F, Vallicioni J, Chauvel P: Ear, nose, and throat cancer: ultrasound diagnosis of metastasis to cervical lymph nodes. Radiology 152:771–773, 1984.
2. Kennedy JT, Krause CJ, Loevy S: The importance of tumor attachment to the carotid artery. Arch Otolaryngology 103:70–73, 1977.
3. Sutton RT, Reading CC, Charboneau JW, James EM, Grant CS, Hay AD: US–guided biopsy of neck masses in postoperative management of patients with thyroid cancer. Radiology 168: 769–772, 1988.
4. Sakai F, Kiyono K, Sone S, Kondo Y, Oguchi M, Watanabe T, Kakai Y, Imai Y, Takeda

S, Yamamoto K, Ohta H: Ultrasonic evaluation of clinical metastatic lymphadenopathy. J Ultrasound Med 7:305–310, 1988.
5. Hajek PC, Salomonwitz E, Turk R, Tscholakoff D, Kumpan W, Czembirek H: Lymph nodes of the neck: Evaluation by US. Radiology 1588:739–742, 1986.
6. Erickson SJ, Mewissen MW, Foley WD, Lawson TL, Middleton WD, Quiroz FA, Macrander SKJ, Lipchik LO: Stenosis of the internal carotid artery: assessment using color doppler imaging compared with angiography. American Journal of Roentgenology 152:1299–1305, 1989.
7. Hallam MJ, Reid JM, Cooperberg PL: Color–flow doppler and conventional duplex scanning of the carotid bifurcation: prospective, double–blind, correlative study. American Journal of Roentgenology 152:1101–1105, 1989.
8. Gooding GAW, Langman AW, Dillon WP, Kaplan MJ: Malignant carotid artery invasion: sonographic detection. Radiology 171:435–438, 1989.
9. Langman AW, Kaplan MJ, Dillon WP, Gooding GAW: Radiologic assessment of tumor and the carotid artery: correlation of MRI, US, and CT with surgical findings. Head and Neck 11:443–449, 1989.
10. Gritzmann N, Fruwald F: Sonographic anatomy of the tongue and the floor of the mouth. Dysphagia 2:196–202, 1988.
11. Grevers G: Bilateral carotid artery aneurysms in extensive cancer of the base of the tongue. A rare differential diagnosis in cervical swellings. Larygologie, Rhinologie, Otologie 66:534–535, 1987.
12. Mancuso AA, Som PM: The upper aerodigestive tract (nasopharynx, oropharynx, and floor of the mouth). In: Head and Neck Imaging, Excluding the Brain. Chapter 10. Bergeron RT, Osborn AG, Som PM, CV Mosbey (eds). St. Louis: pp 374–401, 1974.
13. Parker SH, Hopper KD, Yakes WF, Gibson MD, Ownbey JL, Carter TE: Image–directed percutaneous biopsies with a biopsy gun. Radiology 171:663–669, 1989.
14. Carter B: Upper aerodigestive tract and neck. In: Computed Tomography of Whole Body. Haaga JR, Alfidi RJ, CV Mosbey (eds). St. Louis: 445–488, 1988.
15. Adams GL: Treatment of head and neck cancer with combined modalities. Investigative Radiology 24:562–567, 1989.
16. Rothstein S, Persky MS, Horii S: Evaluation of malignant invasion of the carotid artery by CT scan and ultrasound. Laryngoscope 98:321–324, 1988.
17. Masaryk TJ, Modic MT, Ruggieri PM, Ross JS, Laub G, Lenz GW, Tkach JA, Haacke EM, Selman WR, Harik SI: Three–dimensional (volume) gradient–echo imaging of the carotid bifurcation: preliminary clinical experience. Radiology 171, 801–806, 1989.
18. Dillon WP. Applications of magnetic resonance imaging in the head and neck. Seminars in US, CT, MRI 7:202–215, 1986.
19. Lufkin RB, Hanafee W: Magnetic resonance imaging of head and neck tumors. Cancer and Metastasis Reviews 7:19–38, 1988.
20. Kassel EE, Keller MA, Kucharczyk J: MRI of the floor of the mouth, tongue, and orohypopharynx. Radiologic Clinics of North America 27:331–51, 1989.
21. Teresi LM, Lufkin RB, Hanafee WN: Magnetic resonance of the larynx. Radiologic Clinics of North America 27:393–406, 1989.
22. Cross RR, Shapiro MD, Som PM: MRI of the parapharyngeal space. Radiologic Clinics of North America 27:353–378, 1989.
23. Shapiro MD, Som PM: MRI of paranasal sinuses and nasal cavity. Radiologic Clinics of North America 27:447–475, 1989.
24. Lore' JM Jr: The neck: cervical lymph nodes. In: an atlas of head and neck surgery. Philadelphia: W.B. Saunders 645–702, 1988.
25. Glazer HS, Lee JKT, Levitt RG, et al.: Radiation Fibrosis: differentiation from recurrent tumor by MR imaging. Radiology 156:721–726, 1985.
26. Sekhar LN, Janecka IP, Schramm VL Jr, Horton JA, Eibling DE: Elective resection of the internal carotid artery without reconstruction. Laryngoscope 98:960–966, 1988.

27. Okamura H, Naakamura HK, Yanagihara N: Reconstruction of the carotid artery in radical neck dissection. Auris, Nasus, Larynx 12 (Suppl 2):103–106, 1985.
28. Carabasi RA, DeLaurentis DA: Axillo–internal carotid artery bypass in the treatment of neck metastatic. Journal of Vascular Surgery 2:578–580, 1985.

3. Craniofacial Resection for Tumors of the Ethmoid and Superior Nasal Vault

Paul A. Levine

The development and acceptance of the feasibility of surgical resection of the anterior skull base in conjunction with the superior nasal vault has revolutionized the treatment for malignancies in this anatomic locus [1,2]. Prior to this era, complete tumor removal was performed using the limited facial approach, and the addition of the frontal craniotomy not only permitted a safe, controlled resection of the cribriform plate/fovea ethmoidalis region, but also allowed for an accurate evaluation of resectability of the neoplasm in conjunction with a direct route for an oncologic resection of bone, dura, and potentially, brain. This chapter deals with the evaluation and treatment of these rare, difficult malignancies as we treat them at the University of Virginia Health Sciences Center, Department of Otolaryngology–Head and Neck Surgery.

The malignancy that we have had the most experience in treating in this region has been the esthesioneuroblastoma, but the differential also includes any of the other sinonasal malignancies, such as adenoid cystic carcinoma, sinonasal undifferentiated carcinoma, squamous cell carcinoma, and malignant melanoma [3]. Since the differential for these neoplasms should also include lymphoma, plasmocytoma, and sarcoma, an accurate diagnosis may require multiple biopsies and electron microscopy [4].

Two of the more difficult differentiations to make may be that of an esthesioneuroblastoma and the recently described sinonasal undifferentiated carcinoma (SNUC) [5]. The light microscopic findings of an esthesioneuroblastoma include:

1. plexiform intracellular neurofibrils,
2. poorly defined to nonexistent cytoplasm,
3. round to oval nuclei, and
4. palisading sheets of neoplastic cells, separated by slender vascular septae into a lobular pattern [6].

Though neurofibrils must be present to make the proper diagnosis, the presence of the Homer–Wright rosette or pseudorosette does not have to be present in the biopsy specimen to make the diagnosis [7]. Electron microscopy may be necessary to confirm the diagnosis [8]. In spite of our experience in diagnosing these tumors, one patient in our review of craniofacial

Jacobs, C. (ed): Carcinomas of the Head and Neck: Evaluation and Management.

resections, who was initially thought to have esthesioneuroblastoma, was later found to have malignant melanoma postoperatively, and another, also thought to be esthesioneuroblastoma, was found to be malignant lymphoma at necropsy. This supports the concept that the pathologic diagnosis may be difficult, even by an experienced pathologist [3].

The other tissue diagnosis that may be difficult to make is that of sinonasal undifferentiated carcinoma, the so–called SNUC tumor. This pathologic diagnosis is based upon the findings of extensive necrosis with invasion of blood vessels. Under light microscopy, the sheet–like cellular configuration of the tumors shows wide trabeculae with nests [5]. Antibodies to cytokeratin and SNUC show immunoreactivity, and often there is binding to epithelial membrane antigen and neuron–specific enolase [9].

Once the pathology has been confirmed, the treatment plan should not be formulated until the full extent of the disease has been determined. Our approach to tumors in this region mandates a multidisciplinary approach, including an otolaryngologist–head and neck surgeon, hematologist–oncologist, radiation therapist, neurosurgeon, and neuro–opthalmologist. Initial examination requires a complete head and neck evaluation, including an examination for cervical metastases and for ocular disturbances. Radiologic evaluation of the tumors is imperative, since often they are significantly more extensive than clinically appreciated. Until the more recent advances in MRI scanning techniques, high resolution CT scanning was the procedure of choice. Since CT scanning and MRI appear to provide equivalent information for those tumors not eroding through the cribriform plate or roof of the ethmoids, we obtain a CT scan first. For those with more extensive disease, we also obtain an MRI scan, since it provides better soft tissue contrast, especially with Gadolinium–EDTA enhancement [10]. This is important when evaluating the involvement of vascular structures, such as the cavernous sinus and carotid siphon [11]. It appears that bone destruction, initially thought to be better employing CT scanning [11], is equally accurate on MRI, but bone detail remains superior on the CT scan, in spite of the MRI's ability to provide direct coronal images [12].

Adjuvant Therapy

The basic philosophy at the University of Virginia Health Sciences Center for treatment of head and neck neoplasms is to treat with chemotherapy and/or radiation therapy in a preoperative manner. While the controversy with pre–versus postoperative adjuvant therapy still continues, we have found what we believe to be distinct advantages in treating all of these patients in a preoperative mode. One has been a shrinkage, and, in many cases, a pathologic sterilization of tumor prior to surgical resection [13,14], the survival significance of which we are unable to comment upon at this writing. The other advantage has been the ability to spare an orbital resection in 36 of 41 patients who had pre–therapy erosion of the medial wall of the orbit. We have found, with accurate frozen section control at the time of surgery, that the eye can be spared, with or without periorbital resection and grafting, in almost 90% of our patients, significantly lessening the functional and cosmetic morbidity of the surgical resection, without jeopardizing the survival [15].

While no staging system has been used by us for nonesthesioneuroblastoma patients, we follow the system established by Kadish et al. for esthesioneuroblastomas and practice similar principals for treating the other neoplasms in this region. Utilizing this system, stage A is involvement of the nasal cavity only; stage B is involvement of the nasal cavity and one or more paranasal sinuses; and stage C is involvement outside the nasal cavity including orbit, base of skull, or intracranial cavity, cervical nodes, or distant metastases [16].

Since esthesioneuroblastomas have been found to be radiosensitive [17], radiotherapy has been used preoperatively for all cases, with the addition of preoperative chemotherapy for stage C disease. 50 Gy of radiation therapy is delivered in 25 fractions as described by Million et al. [18]. The critical issue with radiotherapy is whether the eye can be shielded from the radiation. With significant orbital invasion, the entire orbit is irradiated and subject to all of the attendant risks of therapy, such as cataracts and a dry eye. If there is no orbital invasion, the medial 25% of the globe is within the high–dose volume to insure adequate treatment of the ethmoid complex. If there is minimal invasion of the medial wall, most of the lacrimal gland can be shielded, obviating the dry eye [19].

Our present chemotherapy regimen includes a 28 day cycle of cyclophosphamide 650 mg/M^2 intravenously(IV) and vincristine 1.5 mg/M^2 IV on days 1 and 8 for patients with stage C disease. If, after two courses, there is a significant response, both clinically and on repeat CT scan, one or two additional courses are administered. If there is no significant tumor regression, the patient proceeds to radiotherapy [13]. The basis for this treatment plan was the work of Wade et al. in which five cases of Stage B and C disease were treated with chemotherapy, and eight additional cases were analyzed, with an overall response rate of 62% [20]. We are now trying a more aggressive regimen given every 21 days with cyclophosphamide 1,000 mg/M^2 IV, vincristine 1.5 mg/M^2 IV, and doxorubicin 40 mg/M^2 IV on day one. Postoperatively, chemotherapy, instituted three to four weeks after the completion of surgery, is given to those patients who responded to the initial treatment and can be given for six months [19].

Surgical Approach

The combined craniofacial approach to the anterior skull base is the safest method to evaluate and resect tumors involving the roof of the nasal vault and the ethmoid complex. Prior to the acceptance of this concept, local resection via lateral rhinotomy without the anterior craniotomy was associated with a high local recurrence rate due to inadequate tumor resection [21].

During our twelve–year experience with the craniofacial resection at the University of Virginia Health Sciences Center, improvements in the surgical technique continue to evolve. The neurosurgical team has altered the craniotomy approach. Most of the patients have had a frontal or bifrontal craniotomy with either a large laterally–based frontal bone flap or, more recently, an osteoplastic flap of the frontal sinus with extension through the posterior wall. The supraorbital rim approach, developed at our institution [22], has been replaced by the transfrontal sinus approach. This was done because of the incidence of mid–forehead depressions secondary to burr holes for the supraorbital rim approach which became evident twelve or more months following the surgery. The facial portion of the resection has been performed utilizing the lateral rhinotomy. The facial degloving technique has been recently supported [23], and this may prove to have applicability in future cases. Internally, the structures resected include the cribriform plate, ethmoid complex, nasal septum, and the involved portions of the maxillary and/or sphenoid sinuses, as dictated by each specific tumor's location.

The greatest surgical challenge is not the resection, but the reconstruction. The adequacy of the separation of the sinonasal cavity from the cranial contents dictates the degree of postoperative complications. Unlike Schuller [24], we have not found it necessary to provide rigid support in the surgical defect to prevent the potential of brain herniation. The mainstay of our reconstruction involves the use of a laterally–based pericranial flap placed between the repaired dura and a split thickness skin graft placed from below. In addition, we have employed abdominal fat–fascia free grafts as an extra layer between the pericranium and skin, and we have used fibrin glue as an additional method of repairing dural leaks. The number of cases is presently too small to support their usage by statistical analysis [3]. Additional techniques that require homograft transplantation, such as the utilization of lyophilized dura to replace resected dura, have been abandoned.

Conclusions

It is difficult to compare survival rates due to the rarity of these lesions and the variation in treatment regimens from institution to institution. If one examines the survival rate of esthesioneuroblastomas, for example, we find a two–year determinate survival rate of 88%, as compared to 50% in the era prior to the craniofacial resection, suggesting an improvement in local control with more aggressive initial therapy. Most recurrences presented within the first two years, as with most head and neck cancers, with the longest disease–free interval before recurrence being almost eight years after definitive treatment. Aggressive salvage therapy has been important, including surgery, radiation therapy, and chemotherapy. We have taken a novel approach to inoperable or recurrent lesions, using high–dosage chemotherapy followed by autologous bone marrow transplantation. Although this approach has provided palliation from seven months to five years, the ultimate place that this type of therapy will fill in our treatment armamentarium is still unclear [19].

Since the potential complications of this type of surgery are significant, one cannot determine the value of this procedure without scrutinizing the complication rate. In our recent published series of 25 craniofacial resections, the mortality rate was 4%. Five patients developed postoperative cerebrospinal fluid leaks, but only one required surgical intervention. Three patients developed symptomatic pneumocephalus, with the most aggressive therapy for this condition being re–intubation and intraoperative evacuation in one patient. One patient required an operative evacuation of an epidural hematoma [3].

As mentioned earlier, in no esthesioneuroblastoma patient was the globe resected. With adjuvant preoperative therapy and frozen section control of the periorbita, at most, a portion of the periorbita was resected in 88% of the 41 craniofacial patients studied. The complication of restricted extraocular motility or enophthalmos developed in those patients who required periorbital resection [3], but in none of these patients was the sparing of the eye found to be reason for treatment failure [15].

Infectious complications were significant, in spite of the usage of perioperative antibiotic coverage for gram positive, gram negative, and anaerobic bacteria which was continued until the nasal packing was removed, usually on the tenth postoperative day. One patient had a subgaleal and epidural abscess with an infected bone flap, and another, an epidural abscess with bone flap infection. Four patients had fevers of unknown etiology that resolved after removal of the packing and combination antibiotic coverage [3].

Our patients' complication rate compares favorably with others [25], in spite of the fact that only one of our 25 resectioned patients did not receive preoperative therapy. As important is the fact that analysis of our patients undergoing craniofacial resection for all types of malignant neoplasms, including esthesioneuroblastoma, adenoid cystic carcinoma, and adenocarcinoma, showed that 72% of the patients were alive without disease at 34 months. Whether these data mean that we are ultimately curing more of these patients is unclear at this time, since extended follow–up is necessary, especially for patients with esthesioneuroblastoma and adenoid cystic carcinoma. We are providing significantly improved palliation and quality of life for these patients, who were once thought to have incurable lesions. Continued surgical experience and controlled clinical trials will permit us to better cope with the challenges posed by malignancies of the superior nasal vault and ethmoid region.

References

1. Smith RR, Klopp CT, Williams JM: Surgical treatment of cancer of the frontal sinus and adjacent areas. Cancer 7:991–994, 1954.
2. Ketcham AS, Wilkins RH, Van Buren JM, Smith RR: A combined intracranial approach to the paranasal sinuses. Am J Surg 106:698–703, 1963.
3. Levine PA, Scher RL, Jane JA, Persing JA, Newman SA, Miller J, Cantrell RW: The craniofacial resection—eleven year experience at the University of Virginia: problems and solutions. Otolaryngology–Head and Neck Surg, (in press).
4. Newbill ET, Johns ME, Cantrell RW: Esthesioneuroblastoma: Diagnosis and management. South Med J 78:275–282, 1985.
5. Levine PA, Frierson HF, Mills SE, Stewart FM, Fechner RE, Cantrell RW: Sinonasal undifferentiated carcinoma. A distinctive and highly aggressive neoplasm. Laryngoscope 97:905–908, 1987.
6. Obert GJ, Devine KD, McDonald JR: Olfactory neuroblastoma. Cancer 13:205–215, 1960.
7. Schenck ML, Ogura JM. Esthesioneuroblastoma. Arch Otolaryngol 96:322–324, 1972.
8. Taxy JB, Hidvegi DF: Olfactory neuroblastoma. Cancer 39:131–138, 1977.
9. Frierson HF, Mills SE, Fechner RE, Taxy JB, Levine PA: Sinonasal undifferentiated carcinoma: an aggressive neoplasm derived from schneiderian epithelium and distinct from olfactory neuroblastoma. Am J Surg Pathol 10:771–779, 1986.
10. Phillips CD, Gay SB, Newton RL, Levine PA: Gadolinium (DPTA)—enhanced magnetic resonance imaging of tumors of the head and neck. Head and Neck (in press).
11. Levine PA, Paling MR, Black WC, Cantrell RW: MRI versus high-resolution CT scanning: Evaluation of the anterior skull base. Otolaryngol Head Neck Surg 96:260–267, 1987.
12. Virapongse C, Mancuso A, Fitzsimmons J: Value of magnetic resonance imaging in assessing bone destruction in head and neck lesions. Laryngoscope 96:284–291, 1986.
13. Levine PA, McLean WC, Cantrell RW: Esthesioneuroblastoma. The University of Virginia experience 1960-1985. Laryngoscope 96:742–746, 1986.
14. Kaplan MJ, Hahn SS, Johns ME, Stewart FM, Constable WC, Cantrell RW: Mitomycin and fluorouracil with concomitant radiotherapy in head and neck cancer. Arch Otolaryngol 111:220–222, 1985.
15. Perry C, Levine PA, Williamson BR, Cantrell RW: Preservation of the eye in paranasal sinus cancer surgery. Arch Otolaryngol Head Neck Surg 114:632–634, 1988.
16. Kadish S, Goodman M, Wang CC: Olfactory neuroblastoma: A clinical analysis of 17 cases. Cancer 37:1571–1576, 1976.
17. Elkon D, Hightower SI, Lim ML, Cantrell RW, Constable WC: Esthesioneuroblastoma. Cancer 44:1087–1094, 1979.
18. Million RR, Cassisi NJ, Hamlin DJ: Nasal vestibule, nasal cavity, and paranasal sinuses. In: Million RR, Cassisi NJ (eds). Management of head & neck cancer—A multidisciplinary approach. Philadelphia: JB Lippincott, 173–208, 1984.
19. Stewart FM, Frierson HF, Levine PA, Spaulding CA: 1988. Esthesioneuroblastoma. In: Williams CJ, Krikorian JG, Green MR, Raghaven D (eds). Textbook of uncommon cancer. New York: John Wiley & Sons 631–652, 1988.
20. Wade PM, Smith RE, Johns ME: Response of esthesioneuroblastomas to chemotherapy. Report of five cases and review of literature. Cancer 53:1036–1041, 1984.
21. Elner A, Koch A: Combined radiological and surgical therapy of cancer of the ethmoid. Acta Otolaryngol 78:270–276, 1974.

22. Johns ME, Kaplan MJ, Park TS, Jane JA, Cantrell RW: The supraorbital rim approach to the anterior skull base. Laryngoscope 94:1137–1139, 1984.
23. Maniglia AJ: Indications and techniques fo midfacial degloving. A 15 year experience. Arch Otolaryngol Head Neck Surg 112:750–752, 1986.
24. Schuller DE, Goodman JH, Miller CA: Reconstruction of the skull base. Laryngoscope 94:1359–1364, 1984.
25. Sundaresan N, Shah JP: Craniofacial resection for anterior skull base tumors. Head Neck Surg 10:219–224, 1988.

4. Surgical Resection for Recurrent Nasopharynx Cancer

Willard E. Fee, Jr.

The primary treatment for nasopharynx cancer has been irradiation therapy; by convention, it has long been considered inaccessible to surgeons for reasons that are not clear. What is clear is that radiation therapy produces very good results for primary treatment, perhaps better than surgical excision although randomized trials have not been performed. For those patients who recur in the neck, a neck dissection has long produced the best results. An optional approach for nasopharynx recurrence is less clear, although re–irradiation has been the standard treatment.

Results of Re–irradiation

Re–irradiation of patients with recurrent nasopharynx cancer results in permanent control in 10–25% [1–3]. Although higher survival rates have been recorded, it is probable that many of these patients were living with disease. Fu, et al. [4] showed that 16 of 33 patients treated for recurrence were alive at three years, but the local control rate was only 5 patients of 33 (15%). Wang [5] reported the results of 51 patients retreated with radiation therapy. Those who received less than 60 Gy had a three–year survival of 15% with 0% survival at five years. Thirty–eight patients who were treated with 60 Gy or more had a five–year survival of 45% and a ten–year survival of 39%. He reported a 38% five–year survival for patients with T_1 and T_2 lesions vs. 15% for T_3 and T_4; it is difficult to reconcile these numbers. In any case, it is probable that many of these patients reported alive are actually living with disease.

The most detailed paper and the largest in the world comes from Yan, et al. [6] from the Chinese Academy of Medical Sciences in Beijing, China, where 219 patients with recurrences were reported. One hundred and sixty–two patients had disease localized in the head and neck. The five–year survival was 23%, and the five–year cure rate without evidence of disease was 14%. Those who presented with distant metastasis had a five–year survival of 3%, and none of these patients were without evidence of disease at five years. They had 20 patients who had disease isolated to the

Jacobs, C. (ed): Carcinomas of the Head and Neck: Evaluation and Management.

Table 1. Retreatment Complications.

Radiation Myelitis	12%
Radiation	8%
Cranial nerve palsy	7%
Osteoradionecrosis	2%
Soft tissue necrosis	5%
Subcutaneous fibrosis	16%
Otitis media	19%
Trismus	29%

nasopharynx; 16 of the 20 re–recurred; thus, only 20% survived free of disease in the most favorable of cases. Interestingly, Yan, et al. [6] studied 276 patients with a recurrence of nasopharynx cancer who did not receive any specific treatment, and one of these patients was alive at the end of the fifth year.

Table 1 shows the complications of those patients who were retreated and who survived for more than five years according to Yan, et al. [6]. McNeese and Fletcher [7] retreated 30 patients with irradiation therapy and noted hearing loss in eight, severe trismus in four, necrosis of the nasopharynx in two, and mandibular necrosis in one patient. One patient died of skull base necrosis, and one patient had documented hypopituitarism.

Results of Chemotherapy

Lynn, et al. [8] treated 44 patients prospectively with bleomycin, vincristine methotrexate and cyclophosphamide and compared their survival with 81 patients with recurrence who refused chemotherapy and, presumably, received no therapy. The overall mean survival for the treated patients was 14.8 months compared to 8.3 months for controls, and the three–year survival was less than 5% for those treated vs 0% for controls. Decker, et al. [9] presented their ten–year experience with various combinations of chemotherapy in 17 patients with recurrent nasopharynx cancer. Their medial survival was 293 days (range 149–942 days). Only three patients achieved complete remission with cisplatin–based combination; one patient was living 653+ days apparently free of disease, while the other two remissions were of short duration.

The association of nasopharynx cancer with Epstein–Barr virus has led several investigators to treat with interferon but, unfortunately, with disappointing results [10]. Treuner, et al. [11], however, have reported six pediatric patients treated with beta interferon with one complete response lasting two–and–a–half years.

Thus, it would appear that chemotherapy and immunotherapy have some, but limited, activity against this disease. Experimentation should continue, particularly in patients who have metastatic disease.

Results of Surgical Therapy

The surgical approach to the nasopharynx has been a time–honored technique for benign tumors of the nasopharynx such as angiofibroma or cordoma. Wilson [12] has a classic article on the numerous approaches.

Sooy [13] reported a 50% disease–free survival following electrical desiccation and 40–60 Gy of intracavitary cobalt. Fisch [14] reported seven patients with T_4 recurrent disease who had extensive neurological deficits with cranial nerve involvement. Using the lateral approach, complete tumor removal was not possible in these patients due to infiltration of the dura and cranial nerves, and all patients were dead of disease within two to three years; he did achieve 'excellent palliation', particularly with regard to pain. The morbidity of surgery with this approach is not discussed, although his technique involves preservation of the mandible and the facial nerve. He presented an additional six patients with 'persistent' (regretfully, not defined) T_1 or T_2 lymphoepithelial carcinoma following irradiation therapy who underwent surgical resection and were all alive and free of disease two to five years following therapy.

Panje and Gross [15] reported eight patients who underwent a lateral resection for recurrent T_3 or T_4 disease; one patient was surviving 38 months following surgery, which included a total temporal bone resection, upper ramus of the mandible, and the posterior maxilla. Five died of their primary disease, two with distant metastases and three with local recurrence; no time intervals were reported, nor are the details of the remaining two patients given. This approach was associated with considerable morbidity. All patients required facial nerve rehabilitation and had sensory nerve deafness; five patients had unilateral laryngeal paralysis; six required oral prosthetic restitution; three developed CSF leaks which resolved spontaneously without meningitis, and three required a gastrostomy for nutrition. The mean hospitalization was 22 days.

Tu, et al. [16] reported nine patients who underwent salvage surgery for centrally located lesions on the posterior superior wall. In two patients, a lateral rhinotomy approach was utilized as tumor intruded into the nasal cavity; neither of these patients survived five years. Seven patients were explored through a palatal fenestration, and tumor removal included the periosteum and eustachian tube, if necessary; electrocautery was applied to the bony surface. Four of seven patients survived five years.

In 1988, I reported nine patients who underwent an intraoral transpalatal and transmaxillary resection of their recurrent nasopharynx cancer of the posterior and lateral walls after irradiation failure [17]. All of the patients had recurrent, poorly differentiated carcinoma (World Health Organization Classification III). Two of the patients were resected for palliation only as they had disease which could not be removed completely: one of these patients died within a year, and although had some pain relief, the overall result was unsatisfactory. The other patient achieved significant palliation (elimination of pain, epistaxis, and airway obstruction). She is living with disease over four years since her surgical resection. The other seven patients were all treated for cure with one patient five–and–one–half years post–resection free of disease, and two others over three years free of disease. The remaining four patients have all recurred either locally or intracranially and are living with disease. The morbidity of the procedure is minor with all patients swallowing between one to three days postoperatively, and the mean hospital stay was 8.7 days (range 2–30 days). Only two patients did not require resection of their soft palate and were able to swallow without difficulty and without velopharyngeal insufficiency. The remaining patients all required a soft palate obturator to enable them to speak and eat without velopharyngeal insufficiency.

The transoral technique produces results which are at least as good, if not better, than irradiation or the lateral surgical approaches. The length of hospital stay and morbidity from the transoral approach appear to be less than that described for the lateral approach. However, in some selected cases, the transoral approach may need to be combined with the lateral approach with limited temporal or infratemporal fossa involvement to achieve cure. It is also possible that patients will achieve better local control rates if surgery is followed by intracavitary radiation therapy. We have treated one patient with a re–recurrence with surgical resection followed by intracavitary radiation four weeks postoperatively which he tolerated well.

Conclusion

Recurrent nasopharyngeal carcinoma after irradiation failure poses a challenge to therapists. The results of re–irradiation produce no better than 10–20% cure rates while that of chemotherapy is disappointing. Surgical resection can be performed safely with high cure rates, although local re–recurrences continue to develop. It is our plan to continue the transoral approach for surgical resection and follow it with intracavitary re–irradiation.

References

1. Dickson RI, Flores AD: Nasopharyngeal carcinoma: an evaluation of 134 patients treated between 1971–1980. Laryngoscope 95:276–283, 1985.
2. Hoppe RT, Goffinet DR, Bagshaw MA: Carcinoma of the nasopharynx: Eighteen years' experience with megavoltage radiation therapy. Cancer 37:2605–2612, 1976.
3. Vaeth JM: Radiation therapy of locally recurrent nasopharyngeal cancer. Radio Clin North Am 33:72–76, 1964.
4. Fu KK, Newman H, Phillips TL: Treatment of locally recurrent carcinoma of the nasopharynx. Therapeutic Radiology 117:425–431, 1975.

5. Wang CC: Re–irradiation of recurrent nasopharyngeal carcinoma–treatment techniques and results. Int J Radiat Oncol Biol Phys 13:953–956, 1987.
6. Yan JH, Hu YH, Gu XZ: Radiation therapy of recurrent nasopharyngeal carcinoma. Acta Radiol (Oncol) 22 (Fasc.1):23–28, 1983.
7. McNeese MD, Fletcher GH: Retreatment of recurrent nasopharyngeal carcinoma. Radiology 138:191–193, 1981.
8. Lynn TC, Huang SC, Tu SM: Treatment of nasopharyngeal carcinoma. Excerpta Med Int Congr Ser 571:408–417, 1982.
9. Decker DA, Drelichman A, Al–Sarraf M, et al.: Chemotherapy for nasopharyngeal carcinoma—a ten year experience. Cancer 52:602–605, 1983.
10. Connors JM, Jacobs C: Nasopharyngeal carcinoma: Relationship to Epstein–Barr Virus and treatment with interferon. In: Cancers of the Head and Neck. Jacobs C (ed). Boston: Martinus Nijihoff Publishers, pp 167–175, 1987.
11. Treuner J, Niethammer D, Dannecker G, et al.: Successful treatment of nasopharyngeal carcinoma with interferon. Lancet 1:817–818, 1980.
12. Wilson CP: Observations on the surgery of the nasopharynx. Ann Otol Rhinol Laryngol 66:5–40, 1957.
13. Sooy FA: Experimental treatment of recurrent carcinoma of the nasopharynx with electrodesiccation, radioactive cobalt and x–ray radiation. Ann Otol Rhinol Laryngol 65:723–735, 1956.
14. Fisch U: The infratemporal fossa approach for nasopharyngeal tumors. Laryngoscope 93:36–44, 1983.
15. Panje WR, Gross CE: Treatment of tumors of the nasopharynx: surgical therapy. In: Comprehensive Management of Head and Neck Tumors, vol 1. Thawley SE and Panje WR (eds). Philadelphia: WB Saunders, pp 662–683, 1987.
16. Tu Gy, Hu YH, Xu GZ, Ye M: Salvage surgery for nasopharyngeal carcinoma. Arch Otolaryngol Head Neck Surg 114:328–329, 1988.
17. Fee WE, Gilmer PA, Goffinet DR: Surgical management of recurrent nasopharyngeal carcinoma after radiation failure at the primary site. Laryngoscope vol 98(11) 11:1220–1226, 1988.

5. Advanced Basal and Squamous Cell Carcinomas of the Skin of the Head and Neck

Randal S. Weber, Scott M. Lippman and Marsha D. McNeese

Although the skin of the head and neck accounts for less than 10 percent of the body surface area, a large proportion of cutaneous malignancies occur in this region. This factor is directly related to the greater amount of actinic radiation this region receives compared with the remainder of the skin surface. In the more than 500,000 patients with nonmelanoma skin cancer treated every year [1], basal and squamous cell carcinomas, in a ratio of 3 to 1, are the most frequently encountered histologic types; they usually occur on areas such as the nose, ear, and forehead that receive the greatest amount of sun exposure [2]. As a result of greater sun exposure in occupational and recreational activities, the incidence of skin cancer seems to be increasing and the initial age at presentation decreasing. About 50 percent of patients are older than 65, and 25% have multiple lesions [3]. The median delay between occurrence of initial symptoms to the patient's presentation for treatment is three years. Skin cancer incidence also varies with geography, climate, and skin color, fair–skinned persons of Scandinavian descent being especially susceptible.

About 7,800 deaths are attributable yearly to cutaneous malignancies; the morbidity is many–fold greater, however, in terms of medical costs, cosmetic deformity, and loss of function [4]. Treatment is protracted by the recurrent nature of the disease, the need for repeated reconstructive efforts, and the propensity of second primary skin cancers to occur. Most early basal and squamous cell cancers are successfully controlled with conservative local therapy on the first attempt. But advanced skin cancer of the head and neck, is a great challenge to the head and neck oncologist and has tremendous influence on the patient's psychological well–being.

Advanced skin cancer may be arbitrarily defined as a large tumor, usually greater than 2 cm, invading bone, muscle, or nerves. Other criteria for advanced disease include involvement of the regional lymphatic glands, and the existence of neoplasms for which surgical resection would involve removal of a cosmetic structure or functional unit such as the lip, eyelid, nose, or pinna. In this chapter we review the multidisciplinary management of advanced skin cancer of the head and neck.

Jacobs, C. (ed): Carcinomas of the Head and Neck: Evaluation and Management.

Basal Cell Carcinoma

Several different histological types of basal cell carcinoma (BCC) have been described, but the impact of tumor morphology on biologic behavior is unclear. Probably the single most important factor for predicting recurrence is the anatomic site of origin [5,6]. The growth pattern may be infiltrative or well delineated. Most basal cell carcinomas grow in a circumscribed pattern of interanastomosing lobules with pushing margins, nuclear palisading at the periphery, and surrounding dermal retraction. The key cell layer closely resembles the basal cell layer of skin that occasionally displays appendageal differentiation. Some basal cell carcinomas have an infiltrative growth pattern from the outset, which may extend some distance from the apparent margin. In infiltrative cancers the peripheral palisading is lost.

Clinically, basal cell carcinomas follow three types of growth: nodular or nodular ulcerative, morpheaform, and superficial multicentric. The nodular type, which has raised borders, comprises 80 percent of basal cell carcinomas. Its surface has a pearly translucency with superficial telangectatic capillaries. Long-standing nodular basal cell carcinomas may be ulcerated at the center, which accounts for the term *rodent ulcer*.

Morpheaform basal cell carcinoma, present in 10 percent of patients, appears flat or slightly depressed, firm, and fibrotic [7]. These tumors are more extensive, tend to be thicker, and often extend farther peripherally than is clinically apparent. Noncontiguous fingerlike projections of tumor extend outwardly and are surrounded by sclerotic bands of collagen. The ambiguity of the margins must be considered when treating a patient for this type of basal cell carcinoma.

The superficial multicentric basal cell carcinomas (BCC) arise from the epidermis in several areas as tiny buds and resemble chronic dermatitis; they generally do not invade deeply.

Regional lymph node metastases from basal cell carcinoma have been reported, as have systemic spread to bone, lung, and liver, and perineural and perivascular invasion [8].

Squamous Cell Carcinoma

Squamous cell carcinomas (SCC) of the skin occur less frequently than basal cell carcinomas, and when preceded by actinic skin changes, they tend to remain localized. By comparison, squamous cell carcinomas arising de novo or induced by ionizing radiation, thermal injury, or chemical burns behave more aggressively locally and have a higher incidence of lymph node metastasis [9]. The recurrence rate is higher when tumors invade the reticular dermis or deeper underlying tissues [10].

Squamous cell carcinomas may be well to poorly differentiated and display various growth patterns such as adenoid squamous, spindle cell and clear cell. In adenoid squamous carcinoma, cords or nests of cells are arranged in a glandular or ductal pattern, whereas spindle and clear cell squamous carcinomas demonstrate their respective descriptive cell types. The principal feature of squamous cell carcinoma is the presence of malignant keratinocytes in the dermis, which, depending on degree of differentiation, displays either a high or low degree of keratinization. In poorly differentiated tumors the histogenesis may be determined by the presence of intracellular bridges or immunohistochemical staining for keratins.

Large or recurrent squamous cell carcinomas extend locally into muscle, bone and cartilage. Lymph node metastasis is uncommon in the case of lesions smaller than 2 cm in diameter, but for larger tumors the incidence of metastasis increases to 15 percent and influences the patient's survival [11]. Because the parotid gland serves as a lymphatic watershed for the skin of the forehead, cheek, and midface structures, intraparotid lymph nodes are frequently the site of metastatic involvement [12]. Metastases to the upper cervical lymph nodes may also occur, and the submaxillary triangle lymph nodes are at risk for primary tumors of the cheek, lip, and nose. Lymph node metastasis may occur concomitantly with the skin primary tumor or develop later after apparently successful local therapy.

Neurotropism in squamous cell carcinoma of the skin occurs in about 2 to 15 percent of patients and is an ominous finding [13,14]. The mechanism of perineural extension is not well understood, but it is unrelated to the perineural lymphatics system [15]. In patients with nerve invasion, the control rate decreases to about 30 percent [12]. Some histologic morphologic characteristics of neurotropism correlate with an increased risk of perineural spread, adenoid squamous and spindle cell variants having a higher incidence of perineural spread than keratinizing squamous cell carcinomas. A correlation between nerve invasion and lymph node metastasis has been reported [14].

All patients with squamous cell carcinomas of the skin should be questioned carefully regarding the presence of numbness, tingling, or paralysis. Clinical examination should document the proximity of the tumor to any major nerve trunks, diminished areas of sensation, or the presence of paralysis; however, even patients with major nerve trunk invasion may have no symptoms. In patients suspected of having perineural invasion, magnetic resonance imaging may be helpful in identifying enlarged nerve trunks and intracranial extension of tumor along neural pathways.

Advanced Skin Cancer

Between 1977 and 1982, 134 patients with advanced basal and squamous cell carcinomas of the skin of the head and neck were seen at The University of Texas M.D. Anderson Cancer Center. The majority had been untreated, but 15 patients had undergone excisional biopsies before their referral to us.

Table 1. Patient Characteristics.

Patients	Basal cell carcinoma	Squamous cell carcinoma	Total
	89	45	134
Male: Female Ratio	2.1:1.0	4.6:1.0	2.6:1.0
Median age (years)	65	64	65
Previous skin cancer	24 (27%)	16 (36%)	40 (30%)

Table 2. Site distribution of basal cell carcinoma.

Site	No. of patients (%)
Nose	32 (36)
Periauricular Area	12 (13)
Ear	7 (8)
Canthus	7 (8)
Nasolabial Area	7 (8)
Eyelid	6 (7)
Miscellaneous	18 (20)
Total	89

Table 3. Site distribution of squamous cell carcinoma.

Site	No. of patients (%)
Nose	12 (27)
Periauricular Area	8 (18)
Ear	6 (13)
Temple	5 (11)
Lip	4 (9)
Miscellaneous	10 (22)
Total	45

All patients were considered to have advanced tumors as defined in the foregoing. The demographic data of this patient cohort are shown in Table 1. Patients with basal cell carcinomas outnumbered those with squamous carcinoma, and men predominated in the case of both neoplasms, but this was most striking among patients with squamous cell carcinomas. The median follow–up for patients with BCC and SCC was 25 and 38 months, respectively.

The most commonly involved sites in patients with BCC were the nose and periauricular regions (Table 2). In patients with SCC the most frequent sites of origin were the nose, periauricular region, and the ear (Table 3).

Wide surgical excision was the only treatment modality used for 88 patients with basal cell carcinoma. One additional patient with a deeply invasive BCC of the mental region involving the mandible required exten-

Table 4. Recurrence sites of squamous cell carcinoma according to size of primary tumor.[a]

Tumor size	No. of patients	Local	Sites of recurrence regional	Distant
<2 cm	11	1	0	0
≥2 cm	13	10	7	2

a) Size of primary tumor was unknown in one patient.

sive resection, partial mandibulectomy, and postoperative radiation. Of 89 patients, seven (8%) had positive margins following surgery, two patients showed perineural invasion, and one patient had histologically proved lymph node metastasis. Surgical defects were reconstructed with primary closure in five (6%) patients, split–thickness skin grafts in 54 (61%) patients, and local flaps in thirty (33%) patients. Four patients required prosthetic appliances for their rehabilitation.

Among the entire group of 89 patients there was one recurrence. This patient had an 8–cm periauricular tumor with lymph node metastasis and perineural invasion. When local recurrence developed, the patient was treated successfully with a radical parotidectomy and lateral temporal bone resection.

Surgical intervention alone was the initial treatment for 33 (73%) of our 45 patients with squamous cell carcinoma. Postoperative radiotherapy was used for 12 (27%) patients with lymph node metastasis, positive margins or perineural disease. The final surgical margins were positive in eight (18%) patients, while five (11%), two (4%), and six (13%) patients had perineural, bone, and muscle invasion, respectively. Regional lymph node dissections were performed in seven (15%) patients, but histologically positive metastasis was demonstrated in only two. In five patients primary closure was possible, the rest required skin grafts or local flap repair. Recurrences developed in 14 (31%) patients as follows: five locally, three regionally, four locally and regionally and two locally and distantly.

Certain factors such as the size of the primary tumor, lymph node metastasis, and perineural invasion correlated with the risk of recurrence for patients with squamous cell carcinoma (Table 4). Of 11 patients whose tumors were smaller than 2 cm, only one developed recurrent disease, as opposed to 13 (38%) of 34 patients with larger primaries who had recurrences ($p < 0.05$). In five patients with perineural disease, four developed recurrences, and in six patients with muscle invasion three developed recurrences. In patients with any one of the adverse factors (nerve, bone, muscle invasion or lymph node metastasis) the recurrence rate was 70% (seven of 10), but if none of these factors was present, the risk of recurrence was 20% (seven of 35) ($p < 0.008$). Combined therapy, given to three patients with perineural disease, was successful in two. Of two patients with perineural invasion treated by surgery alone, both recurred, which, compared with our results of combined therapy, suggests some potential benefit for postoperative radiotherapy in this situation.

Surgical salvage was successful in three of four patients with recurrent tumors. In five additional patients, salvage was attempted with surgery and radiotherapy, and the disease was controlled in three patients. At last contact, 25 (56%) of the 45 patients were alive and free of disease, whereas 10 (22%) patients were either dead of disease or living with disease, and 10 (22%) had died of other causes but were free of disease.

Surgical Therapy

Although early skin cancers are amenable to various forms of local management such as electrodesiccation and curettage, laser ablation, Mohs' chemosurgery, topical chemotherapy, and cryosurgery, all with a high–probability of cure, advanced lesions require aggressive and at times radical treatment to ensure control. Ill–planned and –executed treatment will result in a high failure rate and a cosmetically unacceptable result. Nothing is more distressing for the patient and physician than recurrent and uncontrollable skin cancer of the head and neck [16].

In many instances of advanced skin cancer, single–modality therapy is preferable to multiple modalities. When planning treatment one must take into account several factors in outcome including the feasibility of surgical resection, resultant cosmetic deformity, potential functional deficits, and the possibility of regional lymphatic or perineural spread. Obviously, the most important goal is cure with the least morbidity. Cosmetic factors are of secondary importance. The first attempt to control the disease is always the best, and when surgery is chosen for the initial modality, wide excision with clear margins is mandatory. Before resection, a biopsy is obtained to confirm the clinical diagnosis. The extent of the tumor is estimated and the planned area of excision outlined, allowing for a margin of normal tissue. The minimum resection margin for basal cell carcinoma is 2 to 5 mm [17]. The incidence of recurrence for positive margins is 30 percent, 12 percent for close margins (within two high–power fields), and less than 5 percent for free margins [18].

For squamous cell carcinoma the surgical margins must be more generous, with a minimum of 5 mm for tumors smaller than 1 cm and margins of 1 to 2 cm for larger tumors. As a rule of thumb, the larger the primary, the more generous the margin of normal tissue required. For lesions of the eyelid and medial canthal region, wide margins may not be feasible.

The deep margin is clinically estimated; however, deep invasion can be expected in certain areas such as the nasolabial fold, the base of the columella, and the medial canthal region [5]. Cartilage and bone invasion are difficult to ascertain clinically but may be elucidated preoperatively by computed tomography with bone settings. Because the skin overlying the nasal and ear cartilages is thin, invasion occurs frequently and should be anticipated when resecting cancers in these areas.

After the tumor is removed, the specimen is oriented for the pathologist, and the adequacy of the margins is determined by frozen–section examination of the fresh tissue. Any margin involved by tumor should be cleared by obtaining additional tissue, which is then examined to ensure complete resection. Resected bone, which must be decalcified before histologic examination, will delay the final assessment of margins. Because perineural invasion may not be seen on the tumor's examination by frozen section, it is important to examine sensory nerve branches by biopsy if they are located near the tumor. This is especially so for squamous cell carcinomas of the lower lip and infraorbital and supraorbital regions. If a nerve branch is involved, the main nerve trunk is identified and followed in a retrograde fashion to obtain a clear margin. At times this may necessitate partial mandibulectomy, maxillectomy, or orbital exploration. When cranial nerves are involved by tumor, intracranial extension along neural pathways is not rare.

Mohs' chemosurgery or controlled excision of skin cancers was first described by Frederick Mohs [19], and refers to in situ fixation of the tissue with zinc chloride, followed by serial excision and microscopic examination of the margins until complete removal is accomplished. The Mohs' technique has been modified and currently refers to examination of fresh tissue by serial histologic sectioning. Cure rates with this technique are high, especially for basal cell carcinoma in such problematic areas as the nasolabial fold, eyelid and medial canthus. Another advantage is the excision of a small amount of uninvolved tissue. Disadvantages include the time required for serial examination of large lesions and the cost of multiple histologic sections. The Mohs' technique is not useful for large squamous cell carcinomas for which wide margins are important. Although our method for excising advanced skin cancers is similar to the fresh–tissue Mohs' technique, a major difference is that during the initial resection, we attempt to remove all tumor with clear margins. Confirmation is obtained by frozen section control. This method seems more practical for advanced skin cancer; it is less time–consuming and less expensive, and it offers a high rate of cure.

The incidence of regional lymph node metastasis is low for squamous cell carcinoma of the skin. Metastasis may occur concomitantly with the primary tumor, or it may appear later after apparently successful treatment of the local disease. Although elective lymph node dissection is not indicated, at times it is necessary for adequate extirpation of the primary tumor. Skin cancer arising on the cheek or preauricular area, for example, may invade deeply into the parotid gland, and although there are no palpable lymph nodes, the gland and periparotid lymph nodes must be removed to obtain an adequate deep margin [20].

When clinically evident lymph node metastases are present, a parotidectomy with sparing of the facial nerve, if possible, should be performed.

Incontinuity neck dissection is also indicated [12]. A particular effort should be made to remove the superficial lymph node of the external jugular vein and the perivascular facial lymph nodes, both frequent sites of metastatic deposits from skin cancers.

The complex issues of reconstructing surgical defects resulting from the removal of advanced skin cancer are beyond the scope of this chapter, and we shall review only general principles. The head and neck surgeon is, at times, forced to compromise the cosmetic result to avoid camouflaging a tumor recurrence. If the completeness of tumor resection is uncertain or if the risk of local recurrence is great, these factors must be considered when selecting the type of reconstruction. Options include primary closure, skin grafts, healing by second intention, and the use of local or distant tissue flaps. In every situation, covering a surgical defect at high–risk for recurrence with a local bulky flap is to be avoided. Detecting tumor recurrence beneath tissue flaps is difficult and may not be established until effective treatment is no longer possible.

The type of defect, location, tumor factors (primary or recurrent), and functional considerations determine the appropriate type of reconstruction. The medial canthus, for instance, may be left to heal by second intention with an excellent cosmetic result. For total rhinectomy an interim nasal prosthesis will provide cosmetic rehabilitation during the high risk period of tumor recurrence, and later a total nasal reconstruction may be performed safely. Split–thickness skin grafts have widespread application to the head and neck and will provide immediate coverage [21]. Later the skin graft may be removed and a more sophisticated and cosmetically acceptable reconstruction performed, if indicated. Surgical defects that expose vital structures or create severe functional deficits will mandate immediate reconstruction. Total eyelid resection, for example, requires immediate repair to prevent exposure keratitis and vision loss. Full–thickness scalp defects with or without exposed dura must be resurfaced with scalp rotation flaps or distant myocutaneous flaps (figures 1–3). For large, complex defects, reconstruction is best managed by close cooperation between the head and neck surgeon and the reconstructive specialist.

Radiotherapy

Skin cancers may be treated by a number of modalities with comparable success rates, the most appropriate being dictated by the cosmetic and functional results of the treatment. Radiation in some instances has an advantage over the other methods because of the ability to treat subclinical disease at the periphery of the tumor without removing the surrounding normal tissue, therefore ensuring generous treatment margins without gross defect.

Various types of equipment are available for irradiation of skin lesions.

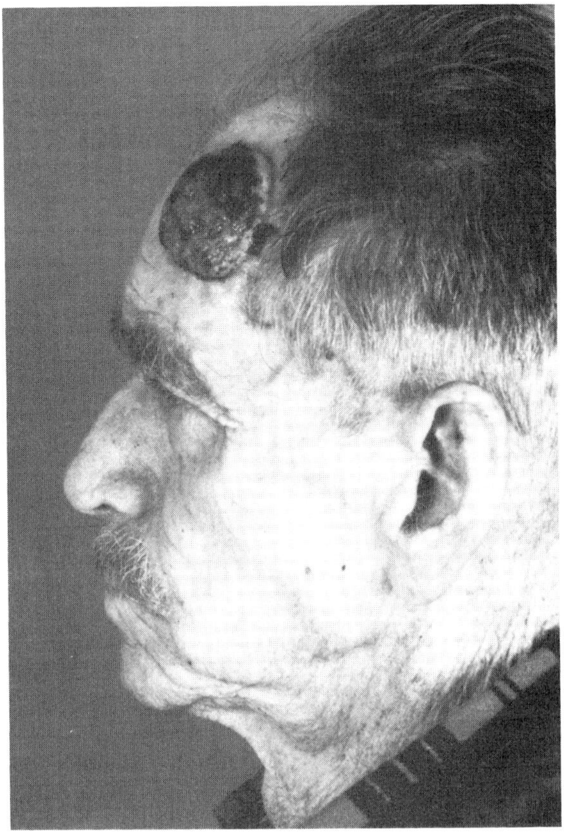

Figure 1. An 85–year–old patient with a fungating 4–cm squamous cell carcinoma of the forehead. The lesion was resected down to the skull with clear margins. The supraorbital nerve was examined by frozen section and found to be free of tumor.

Current treatment is most frequently given with the electron beam or with a combination of electrons and photons. Treatment planning and execution are complex and sophisticated [22]. Although skin cancers may be treated adequately with superficial X–rays, low–energy electrons are used at our institution because of their nearly ideal depth–dose characteristics. Treatment volume is defined by a custom–made lead mask with the treatment area cut out. The lesion is encompassed with a 5– to 10–mm margin of normal tissue around the lesion. In many instances, treatment with the electron beam is a superior modality because of its rapid dose build–up and sharp fall–off, which treats skin but spares the underlying tissues. The depth of treatment may be adjusted by varying the beam's energy. In some instances, as for massive lesions of the skin of the face or scalp, the use of

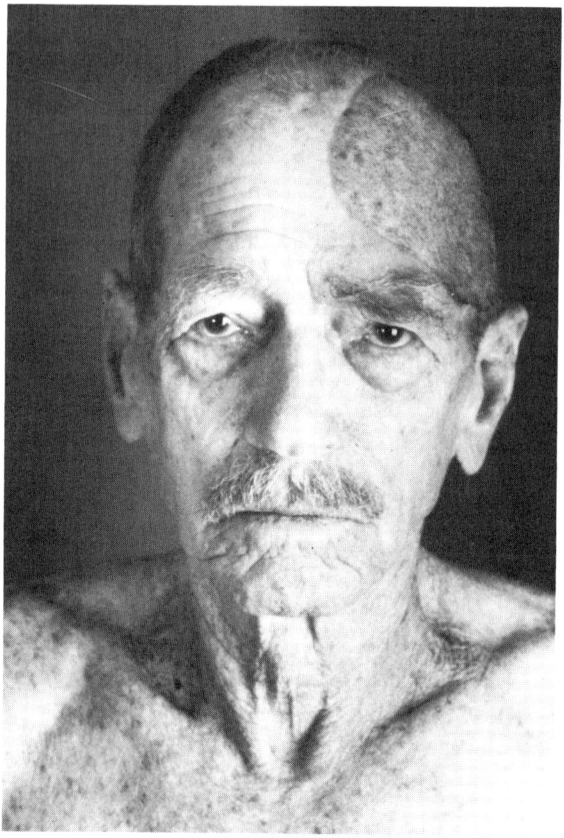

Figure 2. The frontal defect was reconstructed with a parietal scalp flap.

electrons or combination electrons and photons really has no effective alternative [23].

The key to maximizing the therapeutic benefits of radiation therapy while minimizing its long–term effects is understanding the relationship between treatment volume, dose, and fractionation. Although lesions smaller than 1 cm may be treated adequately with only a few fractions, using a high dose with each treatment, the same regimen applied to a larger lesion would result in unacceptable cosmetic changes and possible complications [24].

Lesions of up to about 3 cm can frequently be treated with doses in the range of about 55 Gy over a period of four weeks, while lesions smaller than 1 cm may be treated effectively with doses of about 45 Gy during three weeks. In elderly patients for whom cosmesis may not be as important, effective tumor control may be obtained with several large dose fractions, such as 11 Gy × 3 or 4 Gy × 10. Lesions of 3 to 4 cm or more require higher

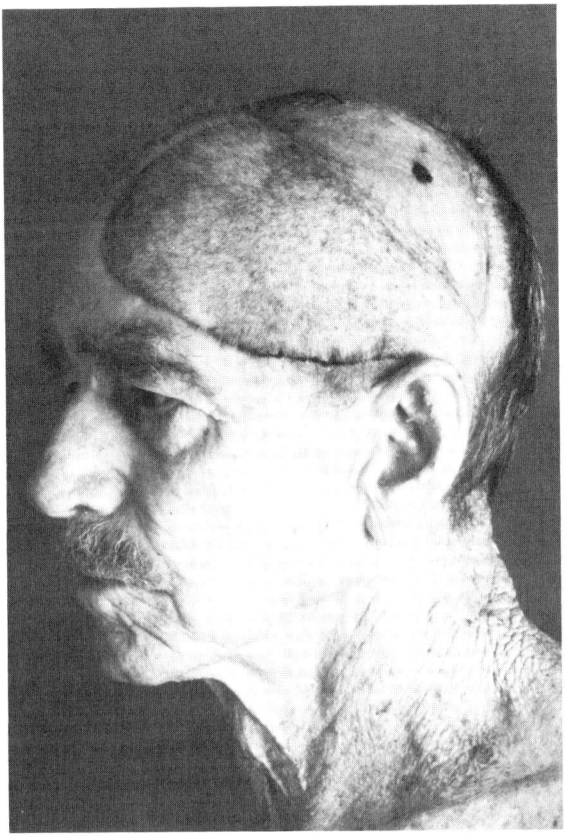

Figure 3. Lateral view demonstrates the donor site of the scalp flap, which was resurfaced with a skin graft.

doses, in the range of 60 to 75 Gy over six to seven weeks, with a field reduction at 50 Gy. However, the best cosmetic results are obtained by protracting the treatment over several weeks and by treating daily, five fractions per week. Patients who have recurrences after surgery also generally receive 60 to 65 Gy in five and a half to six weeks.

Because surgery frequently causes cosmetic and functional defects, for skin cancer of the eyelid, radiation therapy may be preferable (figures 4–6). According to a recent review of 54 patients with squamous and basal cell lesions of the eyelids treated with the electron beam in our institution between 1963 and 1981, 46 (85%) had basal cell carcinomas and 8 (15%) had squamous cell carcinomas [25]. A mean maximum dose of 56.8 Gy in 22 fractions was delivered, although the dose range varied from 45 to 72.5 Gy, with daily fraction sizes ranging from 2.12 to 4.0 Gy. Most patients were treated with 6- or 7-MeV electrons. Tumor size ranged from 0.3 to 4.0 cm,

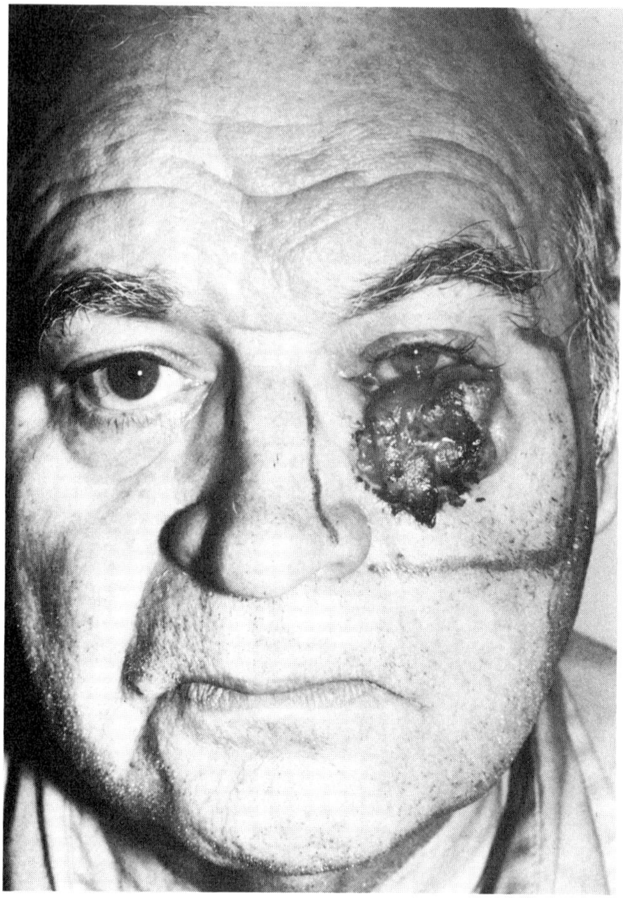

Figure 4. A 64–year–old man with an extensive basal cell carcinoma of the lower eyelid measuring 3 by 3.5 cm. Reproduced with permission from *The Cancer Bulletin*, 38(2), 1986.

with a mean of 1.5 cm. The follow–up period ranged from 27 months to 238 months, the mean follow–up lasting 67 months. Six patients, one with squamous cell and five with basal cell carcinomas (10.9%), had recurrences, three in the treatment field and three at the treatment margin. Of these six patients with recurrences, five had positive margins at biopsy and two had undergone previous surgery. Time to failure ranged from 7 to 182 months with a mean of 56 months. In four of the six patients, the recurrences were subsequently controlled by local surgery with preservation of the eye, whereas the other two required orbital exenteration. One patient with preexisting glaucoma developed a cataract three years after treatment, and one patient with lacrimal duct involvement required surgical tube insertion to achieve successful recanalization. No other major sequelae were noted.

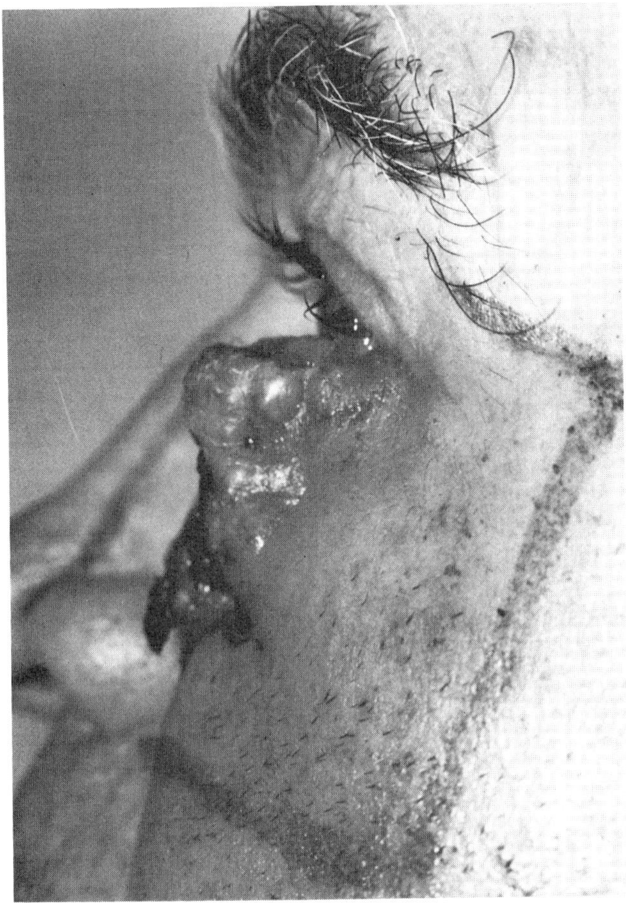

Figure 5. Lateral view of patient (figure 4) demonstrating thickness of lesion. Note the radiotherapy portals allowing an adequate margin. The patient received 68 Gy, beginning with 15 MeV electrons, and the eye was protected with a gold-plated eye shield. Reproduced with permission from *The Cancer Bulletin*, 38(2), 1986.

Carcinoma of the skin of the nasal vestibule is related more to tobacco usage than to sunlight exposure and presents a difficult management problem. The nasal vestibule, which is the anterior entrance to the nasal cavity, is a three–sided cavity. The medial wall of this cavity is the columella. In 1974, Goepfert and colleagues at M.D. Anderson Cancer Center [26] reported that nasal vestibule cancers have a distinctly more aggressive natural history with a worse prognosis than skin cancers of other sites and, therefore require faster and more intensive evaluation and treatment. Unexpected deep extension may occur in the nasal vestibule, upper lip, and other midface regions.

The natural history and treatment of skin tumors of the nasal vestibule

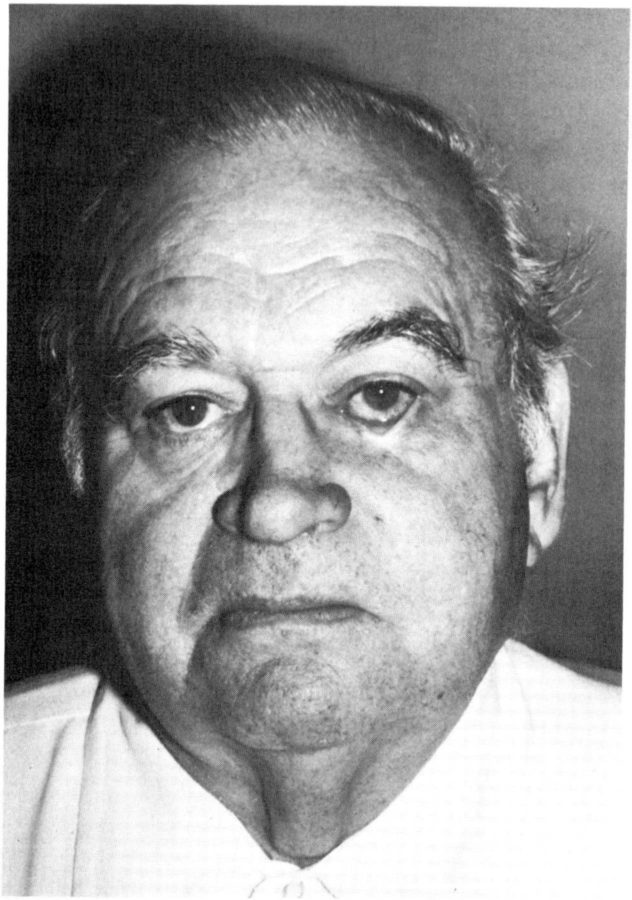

Figure 6. Following therapy, the patient has a mild ectropion but no functional impairment. At three year follow–up, the patient remains disease free. Reproduced with permission from *The Cancer Bulletin*, 38(2), 1986.

have been thoroughly studied and reported in the medical literature [27]. Of nearly 350 patients discussed in 15 reports, only six had regional neck node involvement at presentation. Surgical treatment has an only 10% to 20% recurrence rate but often requires a cosmetically disfiguring operation. According to our recent experience [24] and that of 11 other reported studies of more than 250 patients (who had skin cancer of the nasal vestibule without clinical neck node involvement), radiation therapy alone has a 10% to 20% recurrence rate, with an only 3% recurrence rate for lesions smaller than 2 cm [27]. Radiation therapy is now the favored treatment approach for patients with nasal vestibule cancers without regional node disease because treatment results (recurrence rates and survival data) are as good as or better than those for surgery, the cosmetic outcome is better than for surgery, and the morbidity is low.

Postoperative radiotherapy is generally combined with surgery when the patient has had a previous recurrence, has positive margins, and the lesion has spread to lymph nodes or peripheral nerves. Treatment is usually given five days a week at 2 Gy per fraction for a total dose of 50 Gy, at which time a field reduction is usually done for an additional 10 Gy to the area at highest risk of recurrence. Squamous cell carcinomas involving midline structures such as the nose, nasal vestibule or lip may require radiation to both sides of the neck, but lateralized lesions will generally require treatment only to the ipsilateral neck region.

The addition of interstitial radiation is useful for lesions in certain areas such as the lip. Implants are usually done under general anesthesia and may be used alone or as a boost after external beam irradiation. The needles are left in place for several days, implant time depending on the dose desired.

If postoperative radiotherapy is anticipated, the radiation therapist should examine the patient before surgery so that the treatment fields can be defined with the utmost accuracy. Clinical collaboration will ensure the highest probability for local control and the best cosmetic result.

Pharmacologic Therapy for Advanced Basal and Squamous Cell Carcinomas

Systemic cytotoxic chemotherapy is known to have activity in these cancers, although the data are limited. In an early series from M.D. Anderson Cancer Center [28], 16 patients with advanced head and neck skin squamous cell carcinoma were treated with non–cisplatin–based chemotherapy (bleomycin with various combinations of 5–fluorouracil [5–FU], cyclophosphamide and methotrexate). Seven (44%) responses, with a 25% complete response (CR) rate, were observed. These results were comparable to the overall response rate of 50% for patients with the other (non-skin primary) head and neck SCC sites in this series. More recent studies have focused on cisplatin–based regimens. Guthrie et al. [29] treated 10 patients for advanced nonmelanoma skin cancer (three squamous cell and seven basal cell carcinomas) with cisplatin and doxorubicin. One of the three SCC patients achieved a partial response (PR), while six of the seven BCC patients responded, including four with complete responses. Recently, Rahal et al. [30] from France reported on 19 patients treated with cisplatin, bleomycin, and 5–FU, the latter two drugs given by continuous intravenous infusion for three to five days. All patients had locally advanced, bulky disease which, in general, recurred after surgery or irradiation or both. Of 16 evaluable patients, six CRs were seen among the 15 (94%) patients who responded. Overall, of 35 evaluable patients with head and neck skin SCC in the above three series, 23 (66%) responded to systemic chemotherapy, 10 (29%) responding completely.

Table 5. Activity of retinoids and alpha-interferon in non-melanoma skin cancer.

Neoplasm	Drug	Evaluable patients	Complete response (%)	Partial or mixed response (%)	Total response (%)
Basal cell carcinoma	Retinoic acid[a]	49	16 (33)	32 (65)	98
	Isotretinoin	16	2 (13)	9 (56)	69
	Etretinate	40	3 (8)	14 (35)	43
	alpha-interferon[b]	18	14 (77)	—	77
	alpha-interferon[c]	19	3 (16)	7 (37)	53
Squamous cell carcinoma	Isotretinoin	19	2 (11)	5 (26)	37
	Etretinate	4	1 (25)	1 (25)	50
	Arotinoid	1	0 (0)	1 (100)	100
	alpha-interferon[b]	11	4 (36)	6 (55)	91

a) Topical
b) Intralesional—see text.
c) Listed as 'other skin cancers' (excluding melanoma and cutaneous lymphoma) in ref. 50—details regarding the specific number of squamous and basal cell carcinomas and complete versus partial responses were not available.

Retinoids, the natural derivatives and synthetic analogues of vitamin A, have been shown in preclinical and clinical studies to be active in certain premalignant and malignant squamous epithelial disorders [31]. Retinoic acid inhibits growth and modulates the expression of the squamous phenotype in SCC *in vitro* and *in vivo* [31,32]. Preliminary data suggest that these regulations occur at the transcriptional level after retinoic acid interacts with its recently identified nuclear receptors [33]. In addition to the retinoids' activity in premalignant epithelial lesions [31], their chemopreventive activity in nonmelanoma skin cancer has been elegantly documented in the recent report by Kraemer et al. [34] of high-risk patients with xeroderma pigmentosum.

Retinoids are active as single agents in a limited number of established malignancies [31], and this includes modest activity in advanced cancers of the head and neck [35–37]. The most significant activity of retinoids has been observed in cutaneous malignancies such as cutaneous T-cell lymphoma and nonmelanoma skin cancer [31]. As shown in Table 5, topical treatment with retinoic acid produced 16 complete and 32 partial responses in 49 BCC patients [38–40]. Systemic retinoid therapy has produced an overall response rate of 51%, with a CR rate of 11%, in 57 BCC patients [41–45]. One of these patients had xeroderma pigmentosum with actinic keratoses, in addition to BCC, and had a complete response to etretinate [45]. Although retinoid therapy has been used primarily to treat local disease, one patient with vertebral metastases from BCC achieved a partial response with retinoid therapy, which averted the need for decompressive laminectomy. Cessation of retinoid therapy is generally associated with relapse, especially in patients with multiple lesions [31].

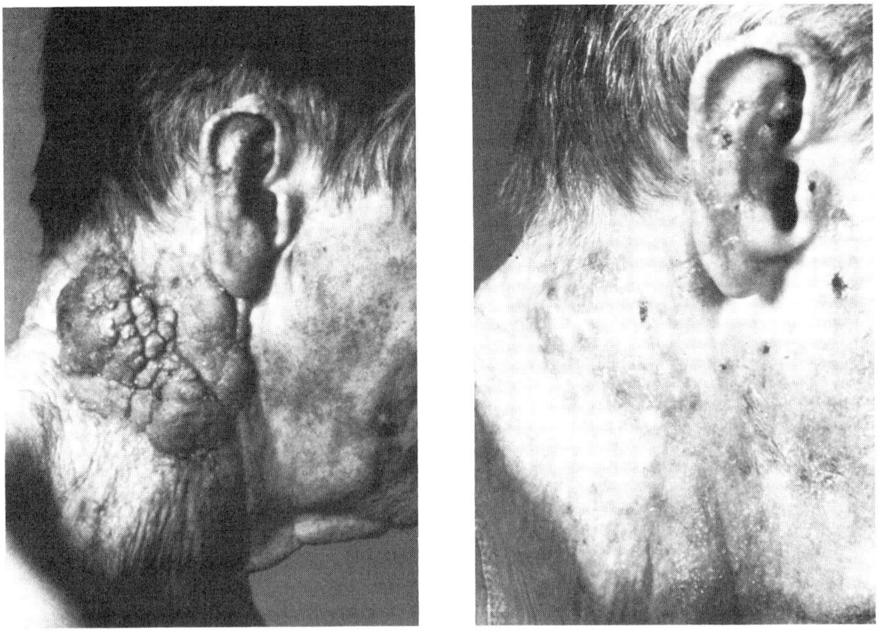

Figure 7. Left panel: Pretreatment photograph showing an exophytic (10 cm by 10 cm) lesion in the right neck. Right panel: Post–treatment photograph of the neck lesion, taken after six months of isotretinoin therapy, shows marked tumor regression. Reprinted with permission from the *Annals of Internal Medicine* 107:499–501, 1987.

Retinoids are active against in situ squamous cell carcinoma of the skin, but their clinical use for invasive cutaneous SCC has been limited [31]. One recent report [46] concerned four patients with far–advanced, moderately–to–well–differentiated cancers that were refractory to local treatment by surgery or irradiation or both. All four patients experienced marked disease regression beginning within three to four weeks of starting isotretinoin therapy. One patient's massive fungating neck lesion showed nearly complete regression, which lasted for 11 months (figure 7). That study has now been extended to a total of 11 evaluable patients—two having complete, two partial, two mixed, and two minor responses. In a recent pilot study at the M.D. Anderson Cancer Center, eight patients with advanced cutaneous SCC were treated with high–dose isotretinoin (2 mg/kg/day). Although objective responses occurred in four patients (one partial and three minor responses), the toxicity was significant, with four of the patients experiencing grade 3 mucocutaneous toxicity. As is summarized in Table 5 [40,44,46–48], 24 patients with SCC of the skin treated with three different synthetic retinoids achieved an overall 42% (10/24) single–agent response rate.

Alpha–interferon has antiproliferative and differentiation–inducing activity *in vitro* and *in vivo* in a number of tumor types, including BCC and SCC

[33–36]. Systemically administered alpha–interferon has produced a 53% response rate in 19 patients with nonmelanoma skin cancer [49]. Although not practical for most patients with advanced disease or multiple lesions, intralesional alpha–interferon in actinic keratoses and nonmelanomatous skin cancer has produced early striking results in localized disease [50–53]. Greenway et al. [51] treated eight basal cell carcinoma patients with intralesional alpha–interferon, and all achieved pathologic CR. In 1981, Ikic and co–workers [52,53] reported four complete and six partial responses in 11 evaluable patients with SCC of the skin and other head and neck sites treated with crude human leukocyte interferon.

Synthetic retinoids and alpha–interferon clearly have antitumor activity in head and neck nonmelanoma skin cancer. Preliminary results using *systemic* retinoid and alpha–interferon single–agent therapy in advanced nonmelanoma skin cancer are promising; as shown in Table 5, however, the overall CR rate with systemic therapy was only 10% (8/80). Based on these drugs' promising single–agent clinical results, different mechanisms of action, combined *in vitro* synergistic activity in certain cell lines, nonoverlapping toxicities, and lack of standard systemic therapy for advanced cutaneous SCC, we designed a prospective clinical trial of combined alpha–interferon (3×10^6 u/day) and isotretinoin (1 mg/kg/day) for patients with advanced, recurrent, or metastatic SCC of the skin. This study was begun six months ago. The major toxicities have been related primarily to alpha–interferon, (for example, cumulative fatigue). Retinoid toxicities have been predictable and mild. This current study in advanced cutaneous SCC has produced promising early results with 10 responses (CR + PR) in the first 11 treated patients. The apparent clinical synergy with these agents in advanced cutaneous SCC and their modest single agent activity [35, 49], provide rationale for the study of this combination in advanced SCC of internal head and neck sites [54].

Conclusion

Skin cancers of the head and neck are an enormous health care problem because of the shear number of patients developing these malignancies every year. Treatment is costly, not only in terms of health care dollars but the psychological impact resulting from cosmetically disfiguring surgical therapy. Only recently has there been an effort to educate the public on the damaging effects of chronic exposure to ultraviolet radiation and the benefit of limiting sun exposure as well as the use of sun screens. Certainly more resources should be spent on reducing the risk factors responsible for the induction of skin cancer.

For patients with advanced skin cancer, the therapy must be individualized. Surgical resection of BCC with clear margins has a high rate of cure. However, for advanced SCC the risk of recurrence even with radical resection is significant when adverse factors such as nerve invasion, lymph node metastases, primary tumors exceeding 2 cm in diameter and bone or muscle invasion are present. In contrast, definitive radiotherapy can result in similar cure rates and superior cosmetic results for lesions of the nasal vestibule, eyelid, and medial canthus. Immediate complex reconstruction following surgical resection is indicated for defects exposing vital structures such as the dura or cornea. Reconstruction should be delayed when the risk of recurrence is high and may be safely performed when the patient is considered cured.

References

1. Haynes HA, Mead KW, Goldwyn RM: Cancers of the skin. In: Devita Jr VT, Helaman S, Rosenberg SA (eds), Cancer: Principles and Practice of Oncology, vol 2. Philadelphia: Lippincott, pp 1343–1369, 1985.
2. Andrade R, Gumport SL, Popkin G, Reese R: Cancer of the skin, vol 2. Philadelphia: WB Saunders, pp 899–949, 1976.
3. Whitaker DC: Clinical evaluation of tumors of the skin. In: Thawley SE, Panje WR (eds), Comprehensive Management of Head and Neck Tumors, vol 2. Philadelphia: WB Saunders, pp 1158–1172, 1987.
4. Silverberg E, Lubera JA: Cancer statistics, 1988. Ca 38:5–22, 1988.
5. Panje WR, Ceilley RI: The influence of embryology of the mid–face on the spread of epithelial malignancies. Laryngoscope 89:1914–1920, 1979.
6. Levine H: Cutaneous carcinoma of the head and neck: management of massive and previously uncontrolled lesions. Laryngoscope 93:87–105, 1983.
7. Hauben DJ, Zirkin H, Mahler D, Sacks M: The biologic behavior of basal cell carcinoma: Part I. Plast Reconstr Surg 69:103–109, 1982.
8. Scanlon EF, Volkmer DD, Oviedo MA, et al.: Metastatic basal cell carcinoma. J. Surg Oncol 15:171–180, 1980.
9. Brownstein MH, Rabinowitz AD: The precursors of cutaneous squamous cell carcinoma. Int J Derm 18:1–16, 1979.
10. Immerman SC, Scanlon EF, Christ M, Knox KL: Recurrent squamous cell carcinoma of the skin. Cancer 51:1537–1540, 1983.
11. Möller R, Reymann F, Hou–Jensen K: Metastases in dermatological patients with squamous cell carcinoma. Arch Dermatol 115:703–705, 1979.
12. Jackson GL, Ballantyne AJ: Role of parotidectomy for skin cancer of the head and neck. Am J Surg 142:464–469, 1981.
13. Cottle WI: Perineural invasion by squamous cell carcinoma. J Dermatol Surg Oncol 8:589–600, 1982.
14. Goepfert HG, Dichtel WJ, Medina JE, Lindberg RD, Luna MD: Perineural invasion in squamous cell skin carcinoma of the head and neck. Am J Surg 148:542–547, 1984.
15. Larson DL, Rodin AE, Roberts DK, O'Steen WK, Rapperport AS, Lewis SR: Perineural lymphatics: myth or fact. Am J Surg 112:448–492, 1966.
16. Jackson RJ, Adams RH: Horrifying basal cell carcinoma: A study of 33 cases and a comparison with 435 non–horror cases and a report on four metastatic cases. J Surg Oncol 5:431–463, 1973.
17. Wolf DJ, Zitelli JA: Surgical margins for basal cell carcinoma. Arch Dermatol 123:340–344, 1987.
18. Koplin L, Zarem HA: Recurrent basal cell carcinoma. Plast Reconstr Surg 65:656–664, 1980.

19. Mohs FE: Chemosurgery microscopically controlled method of cancer excision. Arch Surg 42:279–295, 1941.
20. Hanke CW, Weisberger EC: Invasion of the parotid gland by basal cell carcinoma: Implications for therapy. J Dermatol Surg 12:849–852, 1986.
21. Panje WR, Bumstead RM, Ceilley RI: Secondary intention healing as an adjunct to the reconstruction of the mid–facial defects. Laryngoscope 90:1148–1154, 1980.
22. Hogstrom KR, Fields RS: Use of the CT in electron beam treatment planning: current and future development. In: Ling CC and Morton RJ (eds), Computed Tomography in Radiation Therapy. New York: Raven Press, p 241, 1983.
23. Tapley NduV: Skin and lips. In: Tapley NduV (ed), Clinical Application of Electron Beam, New York: John Wiley, pp 93–122, 1976.
24. Chobe R, McNeese MD, Weber R, Fletcher GH, Kong JP: Radiation therapy for carcinoma of the nasal vestibule. Otolaryngol 98:67–71, 1988.
25. Sinesi C, McNeese MD, Peters LJ, Goepfert H, King J, Mills MD: Electron beam therapy for eyelid carcinomas. Head Neck Surg 10:31–37, 1987.
26. Goepfert H, Guillamondegui OM, Jesse RH, Lindbert RD: Squamous cell carcinoma of nasal vestibule. Arch Otolaryngol Head Neck Surg 10:8–10, 1974.
27. Wong CS, Cummings BJ: The place of radiation therapy in the treatment of squamous cell carcinoma for the nasal vertibule. A review. Acta Oncol 27:203–208, 1988.
28. Holoye PY, Byers RM, Gard DA, Goepfert H, Guillamondegui OM, Jesse RH: Combination chemotherapy of head and neck cancer. Cancer 42:1661–1669, 1978.
29. Guthrie Jr TH, McElveen LJ, Porubsky ES, Harmon JD: Cisplatin and doxorubicin: an effective chemotherapy in the treatment of advanced basal cell and squamous carcinoma of the skin. Cancer 55:1629–1632, 1985.
30. Rahal M, Sadek H, Azli M, Cvitkovic E, Djemma A, Wendling JL, Filali T, Avril JP: Advanced loco–regional skin carcinoma. Primary chemotherapy with cisplatin (CDDP), bleomycin (BLM) and 5 fluorouracil (5 FU). Proc ASCO 8:293, 1989.
31. Lippman SM, Kessler JF, Meyskens Fl: Retinoids as preventive and therapeutic anticancer agents. Cancer Treat Rep 71:391–405, 493–515, 1987.
32. Lotan R: Effects of vitamin A and its analogs (retinoids) on normal and neoplastic cells. Biochim Biophys Acta 605:33–91, 1980.
33. Brand N, Petkovich M, Krust A, Chambon P, de The Hugues, Marchio A, Tiollais P, Dejean A: Identification of a second human retinoic acid receptor. Nature 332:850–853, 1988.
34. Kraemer KH, DiGiovanna JJ, Moshell AN, et al.: Prevention of skin cancer in xeroderma pigmentosum with the use of oral isotretinoin. N Engl J Med 318:1633–1637, 1988.
35. Lippman SM, Kessler JF, Al–Sarraf M, et al.: Treatment of advanced squamous cell carcinoma of the head and neck with isotretinoin: A phase II randomized trial. Invest New Drugs 6:13–17, 1988.
36. Takaku F: Clinical trials and cancer risk in Japan. JNCI 73:1483–1485, 1984.
37. Thatcher N, Blackledge G, Crowther D: Advanced recurrent squamous cell carcinoma of the head and neck: Results of a chemotherapeutic regimen with adriamycin, bleomycin, 5–fluorouracil, methotrexate, and vitamin A. Cancer 46:1324–1328, 1980.
38. Belisario JC: Recent advances in topical cytotoxic therapy of skin cancer and pre–cancer. In: Melanoma and Skin Cancer, Proceeding of the International Cancer Conference. Sydney, pp 349–365, 1972.
39. Bollag W, Ott F: Vitamin A acid in benign and malignant epithelial tumors of the skin. Acta Derm Venereol (Stockh) (suppl) 74:163–166, 1975.
40. Grupper CH, Berretti B: Cutaneous neoplasia and etretinate. In: Spitzy KH, Karrer K (eds), Proceedings of the 13th International Congress of Chemotherapy. Vienna, VH Egermann, pp 201/24–27, 1983.
41. Schumacher A, Stuttgen G: Vitamin A–saure hyperkeratosen epithelialia thumoren und akne. Dtsch Med Wochenschr 40:1547–1551, 1971.

42. Sankowski A, Janik P, Bogacka–Zatorska E: Treatment of basal cell carcinoma with 13–cis retinoic acid. Neoplasma 31:615–618, 1984.
43. Peck GL, Olsen TG, Butkus D, et al.: Treatment of basal cell carcinomas with 13–cis retinoic acid (abstr). Proc Am Assoc Cancer Res 20:56, 1979.
44. Meyskens Jr Fl, Gilmartin E, Albert DS, et al.: Activity of isotretinoin against squamous cell cancers and preneoplastic lesions. Cancer Treat Rep 66:1315–1319, 1982.
45. Braun-Falco O, Galosi A, Dorn M, et al.: Tumor Prophylaxe bei Xeroderma Pigmentosum mit Aromatischem Retinoid (Ro 10–9359). Hautarzt 33:445–448, 1982.
46. Lippman SM, Meyskens F: Treatment of advanced squamous cell carcinoma of the skin with isotretinoin. Ann Intern Med 107:499–501, 1987.
47. Levine N, Miller RC, Meyskens F Jr: Oral isotretinoin therapy: use in a patient with multiple cutaneous squamous cell carcinoma and keratoacanthomas. Arch Dermatol 120:1215–1217, 1984.
48. Kingston T, Gaskell S, Markss R: The effects of a novel potent oral retinoid (Ro13–6298) in the treatment of multiple solar keratoses and squamous cell epithelioma. Eur J Cancer Clin Oncol 19:1201–1205, 1983.
49. Taguchi T: Clinical studies of recombinant interferon alfa–2a (RoferonR–A) in cancer patients. Cancer 57:1705–1708, 1986.
50. Edwards L, Levine N, Weidner M, Piepkorn M, Smiles K: Effect of intralesional a2–interferon on actinic keratoses. Arch Dermatol 122:779–782, 1986.
51. Greenway HT, Cornell RC, Tanner DJ, Peets E, Bordin GM, Nagi C: Treatment of basal cell carcinoma with intralesional interferon. J Am Acad Dermatol 15:437–443, 1986.
52. Ikic D, Padovan I, Brodarec I, Knezevic M, Soos E: Application of human leukocyte interferon in patients with tumors of the head and neck. Lancet 1:1025–1027, 1981.
53. Padovan I, Brodarec I, Ikic D, Knezevic M, Soos E: Effect of interferon in therapy of skin and head and neck tumors. J Cancer Res Clin Oncol 100:295–310, 1981.
54. Lippman SM, Hong WK: Differentiation therapy for head and neck cancer: in Multimodality Therapy for Head and Neck Cancer, Snow G, Clark JR (eds). N.Y.: Springer–Verlag, in press.

6. Interstitial Hyperthermia in Head and Neck Oncology

Patrick L. Welton, Don R. Goffinet and Daniel S. Kapp

New methods of treating locally advanced or recurrent head and neck neoplasms are needed. Surgery, radiation therapy and chemotherapy, alone or in combination, are most commonly used. At present, however, these neoplasms often recur despite the most intense conventional therapy. In an effort to more effectively treat localized malignancies, while at the same time sparing adjacent normal tissues, the interstitial placement of either permanent or removable implants has been used [1–6].

The combined effectiveness of hyperthermia and ionizing radiation in the treatment of malignancies is well documented [7–12]. Since the interstitial implantation of radioactive isotopes delivers a high radiation dose to a limited volume, combining this therapy with hyperthermia may provide an increased local control rate. In addition, interstitial hyperthermia overcomes the inabilities of presently available external heating devices to adequately heat large tumor volumes deeper than 3 cm beneath the skin. This problem is especially difficult in the head and neck region because of the presence of large blood vessels which, by rapidly cooling the intended volume, make adequate heating difficult.

Recent reports of the combined use of interstitial irradiation and hyperthermia in the treatment of locally advanced primary or recurrent malignancies have been encouraging. Because of the potential to spatially limit both the radiation and hyperthermia to the tumor volume, this combination may be more effective than external irradiation and hyperthermia in producing tumor control with less normal tissue morbidity. This chapter will present the biologic basis for adding hyperthermia to interstitial irradiation, the current methods and technology used in interstitial hyperthermia, and the results and toxicities which result when this technique is used clinically.

Biologic Basis for Hyperthermia

The rationale for employing hyperthermia in the treatment of malignancy is multifold. Elevated tumor temperatures greater than 42°C are cytotoxic in murine tumors [13,14]. Additionally, some malignant cells may have a

Jacobs, C. (ed): Carcinomas of the Head and Neck: Evaluation and Management.

greater sensitivity to heat damage than their normal tissue counterparts [15]. When combined with radiation, hyperthermia synergistically enhances radiation mediated cell death [16] and is cytotoxic to the most radioresistant cells, including cells in the S–phase of the cell cycle [17]. Hypoxic cells which may be present within poorly perfused necrotic tumors are also radioresistant, and because these cells may be nutrient deprived and at lower pH, they may be relatively heat sensitive [18,19]. In experimental murine tumor systems, cell killing begins at temperatures of approximately 41°C and increases with increasing temperatures. Cell survival curves for exposure to temperatures greater than 43°C resemble those of radiation–induced cell death. As the heating time is prolonged, cell survival declines exponentially.

The synergistic cytotoxic effect of irradiation and hyperthermia can be demonstrated by comparing survival curves of cells which are either irradiated or heated, compared to those treated by both modalities. The time interval between heat and radiation affects cytotoxicity, and therefore, may have important implications for clinical therapy. The combined effects are greatest when heat and irradiation are administered simultaneously. The extent of interaction may differ between tumor and normal tissues as the time between the two modalities increases [18]. The enhancement of cytotoxicity arises in part because of hyperthermic inhibition of the cellular repair of radiation induced sublethal cell damage [16]. The extent of this enhancement is dose–rate related and is greatest for lower dose rates, providing further support for the clinical use of combined interstitial hyperthemia and brachytherapy.

A theoretically important limitation of effective hyperthermia therapy is the development of transient heat resistance (thermotolerance) following an initial heat treatment or during prolonged heating at temperatures even lower than 43°C [20]. Cell lines vary widely in their inherent heat resistance. Cell lines established from human tumors may be more resistant than murine tumors and may develop thermotolerance during exposures to temperatures of 43°C [21]. Thermotolerance is transient but may persist for 72 to 120 hours. Clinical applications of hyperthermia are, therefore, best applied at least several days apart to avoid the potentially lower cytotoxicity resulting because of thermotolerance.

Interstitial Hyperthermia Methods

It is difficult to deliver controlled heat to deep–seated tumors with presently available external microwave or ultrasound devices [8]. Physical and technological limitations as well as variation in the shape and size of tumors and their location relative to large blood vessels and bone usually limit the use of external heating to tumors no more than 3 cm from the body surface. To overcome this limitation, implantable hyperthermic applicators have been developed. Three general types are presently available: radiofrequency local

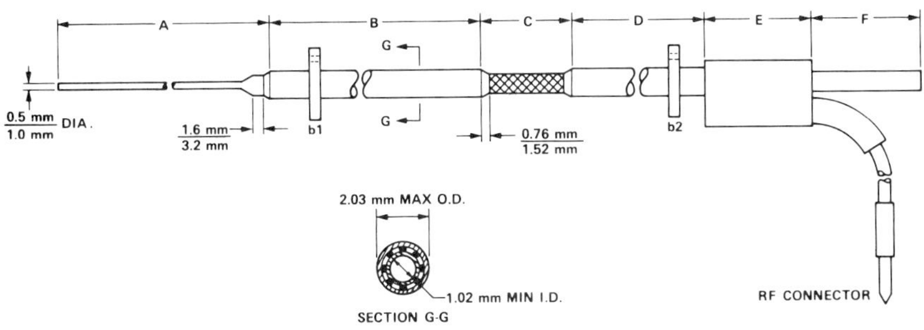

Figure 1. Flexible interstitial hyperthermia/brachytherapy catheter. Leader section (A); Electrically conductive section (single active element) (C).

current field electrodes, microwave antennae, and conduction heating devices such as ferromagnetic seeds and other hot source techniques. These invasive methods can be used to heat localized volumes deep within the body. The advantages and disadvantages of each of these types of hyperthermia devices are discussed below.

Radiofrequency (RF) Electrodes

At Stanford [8] and other centers, implantable electrodes have been designed to permit the induction and maintenance of localized hyperthermia combined with low dose–rate interstitial radiation. The electrodes used may be as simple as hollow steel trocars. Portions of the electrode outside of the treatment volume may be easily insulated to limit the heating of the adjacent normal tissues. More recently, a flexible, partially insulated implantable radiofrequency electrode has been designed in collaboration with Oximetrix, Inc. and is shown in figure 1.

Radiofrequency currents in the range of 0.1 to 10 mHz [22] can be used to produce local heating. An alternating electric current is passed between multiple electrodes placed in the treatment volume. These cause resistive heating in the implanted tissues [22]. Depth of penetration and volume implanted is not limiting in typical electrode arrays, and the frequencies are high enough to prevent nerve polarization and muscle contraction. In practice, power distribution to the electrodes may be multiplexed under computer control using implanted thermocouples for temperature feedback to maintain more uniform heating in the volume of interest.

One advantage of the RF hyperthermia technique is that it is easily combined with standard brachytherapy procedures. Electrode spacing is of critical importance, however. Cold regions result if the electrodes are spaced too widely or if blood flow is too high in the region. Also, since absorbed power decreases inversely with the square of the distance between electrodes, regions of low or high temperatures can be produced if the electrodes diverge or converge, respectively. Thermal burns in normal tissues may be avoided by insulating the portion of the catheter in normal tissues and by avoiding too superficial placement of the electrodes.

Microwave Antennae

Various antenna configurations can be used to deliver microwave energy to implanted tissues. Radiating devices utilizing standard coaxial cables as antennae provide an approximate ellipsoidal heating pattern lateral to the long axis of the antennae. This pattern can be changed by altering the driving microwave frequency [22]. A standard coaxial microwave antenna can be modified by removing the outer layer of coaxial cable for a specified length. This length and the driving frequency of the microwave generator can change the longitudinal and transverse extent of power absorption. The antenna can also be run in coherent modes to permit constructive interference in the tumor between the antennae. The number of antennae and their geometric arrangement are critical considerations in obtaining homogeneous heating when interstitial microwave devices are used. These antennae can also be inserted into afterloading radiation implant tubes, prior to isotope insertion or after removal of the radioactive sources. Major limitations of antennae techniques include cold regions at the tips of the antennae, limited antennae length, limited control of power distribution along the length of the antennae, and dependance of the heating pattern on depth of insertion of the antennae into tissue [23].

Ferromagnetic Seeds

Ferromagnetic seeds are surgically implantable metallic alloys with high–magnetic permeability. These seeds are typically implanted in three dimensional arrays with 1 cm spacing. Tissue heating is accomplished by placing the tumor in an alternating magnetic field. This magnetic field causes heating of the implanted seeds which in turn heat the surrounding tissue by conduction. Heat production is enhanced by having the magnetic field parallel to the long axis of the seeds [24]. Ferromagnetic seeds can also be used in temporary implants by placing the seeds in removable implanted catheters which can also be used for interstitial radioactive implants.

Though ferromagnetic seeds have not been frequently used clinically, such devices have several theoretically attractive properties. The seeds themselves can be constructed to self–regulate temperature distribution throughout the implant volume by the use of special alloys. When heated, these alloys experience a sudden decrease in magnetic permeability at specific temperatures, known as the Curie point, thereby limiting their power absorption and consequently the tissue heating. A wide range of alloys with differing Curie point temperatures have been constructed. Theoretically, even tissues with varying blood flows or inhomogeneous seed arrangements can be heated, since the seeds effectively turn themselves off at their designated temperatures. Because the sources can be permanently implanted, only one procedure is required for multiple treatments. The implantation procedure can be done simultaneously with the placement of afterloading interstitial radiation catheters or the permanent implantation of radioactive sources.

The most prominent disadvantage of this technique is that the temperature distribution during treatment is usually nonuniform, since the heating between seeds is by conduction. In areas of high blood flow, the seeds must be heated to very high temperatures to obtain adequate tissue heating. Also, treatments are usually restricted to one maximum temperature depending on the composition of the alloy used. There is also the risk of seed migration or displacement after implantation, especially if tumor shrinkage occurs.

Other hot source techniques which rely on conduction to heat the implanted tissues have included heating with implanted hot wires or with hot water circulated within implanted plastic catheters. The latter technique is relatively inexpensive, safe, and may produce similar heating patterns as more sophisticated conduction heating techniques [25].

Thermal Dosimetry

In the typical case of interstitial RF or microwave antenna hyperthermia, single temperature readings are obtained for one point on each electrode in the heating array through the use of thermocouple sensors in the case of RF current or fiberoptic sensors with microwave heating [8]. Hollow closed–end catheters can also be placed into the tumor between electrodes or antennae at the time of implantation. These serve as conduits for temperature probes [26], and either manual or mechanical mapping techniques can be used to obtain temperature measurements along the length of these catheters at 0.5 or 1 cm intervals several times during a hyperthermia treatment. These temperature profiles can then be analyzed and compared between different heating methods or treatments [8].

Clinical Results

Very high complete response and local control rates have been achieved with combined interstitial irradiation and hyperthermia in patients with locally advanced tumors or tumors recurrent after primary radiation therapy. Since high local control rates have been reported after interstitial irradiation alone, determination of the additional effect from hyperthermia is difficult without prospective randomized clinical trials. No standard recording or reporting of temperature data has been used which makes comparisons of the uniformity of heating or efficacy of treatment difficult between the various reported clinical series. Such comparisons are further hindered by patient selection, selection of tumors studied, lack of uniform guidelines for brachytherapy, and lack of standardized hyperthermia treatment regimens.

In 1985, Emami described 17 combined interstitial radiation and hyperthermic implants in head and neck sites [27]. All patients had recurrent tumors following extensive surgery and/or radiation therapy. Interstitial radiation doses were between 40 and 60 Gy utilizing ^{192}Iridium seeds, with placements lasting 4 to 7 days. Hyperthermia techniques varied as did their sequencing with the radiation treatment. In approximately one–fourth of the patients, RF heating for 60 minutes was used 4 to 8 hours prior to loading the radioactive sources. In the majority of cases, however, two hyperthermia treatments were given over one hour periods during the course of implant at times during which the ^{192}Iridium sources were temporarily removed. Interstitial heating was produced by coaxial microwave antennae inserted into the afterloading catheters.

With follow–up periods of 16 to 30 months, complete responses were noted in 11 of the 17 patients; partial responses occurred in 5 others, and a single patient had no detectible response. Complications included an orocutaneous fistula in one patient with a floor of mouth primary cancer and prolonged mandibular pain in two other patients.

Puthawala reported [28] on 20 patients with locally advanced head and neck tumors treated by interstitial hyperthermia. All patients had been previously irradiated, and most had been treated surgically as well. Standard afterloading implant techniques were employed to deliver 50 to 55 Gy in 100 to 140 hours using ^{192}Iridium sources. Hyperthermia was delivered through multiple coaxial antennae inserted into the nylon afterloading catheters. Treatments were given just prior to placement and immediately after the removal of the radioactive sources. Temperatures of 41.5°C to 43.5°C for 60 minutes were reported to have been achieved. Seventy–five percent of these patients achieved complete responses, and local control was maintained for a minimum of 12 months in these complete responders. Approximately 20% of the patients had treatment related complications including skin burns and soft tissue necrosis. The authors noted a correlation of complications with focal maximum treatment temperatures above 45°C.

Petrovich et al. [29] have also reported their results on 23 patients with recurrent head and neck cancers treated with interstitial hyperthermic techniques. Interstitial radiation with ^{192}Iridium delivering tumor doses of 40 to 50 Gy accompanied by hyperthermia treatments pre– and post–irradiation was given. Heat was delivered via microwave antennae for 45 to 60 minutes at average temperatures of 42.5°C. Complete responses were noted in 70% of the patients. With a follow–up period of 6 to 30 months, no local recurrences were noted among the complete responders. Complications reported included aspiration pneumonitis in one patient with recurrent carcinoma of the tongue. Skin necrosis also occurred in one patient whose primary cancer involved the buccal mucosa.

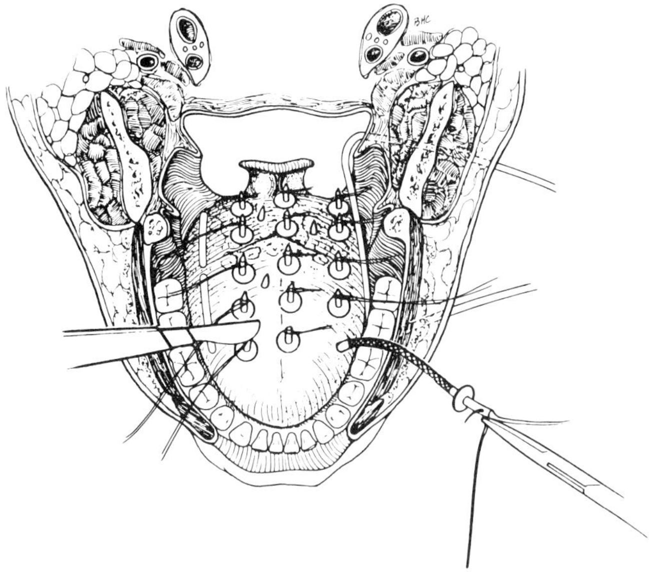

Figure 2. Base tongue interstitial RF hyperthermic implantation technique. Paired trocars, inserted into the tongue through a submental approach, are removed through the mouth and the flexible, specially modified hyperthermic catheters are drawn into position in their place. Traction sutures are positioned for both ease of implant removal and to stabilize the button on the tongue surface. When in position, the catheters are sealed intraorally with a 'Shaw' hemostatic scalpel (Oximetrix, Inc.). Three closed-end probes for temperature mapping are shown in the implant volume. Figure is general, not specific to a patient.

Other series reported by Aristizabal [30], Cosset [31] and Manning [32] revealed similarly high response rates, although each report included primary and recurrent tumors of the cervix, breast, and colon, as well as those from head and neck sites. The data pertaining only to head and neck cancers in these series is difficult to ascertain, although overall complete responses were 60–80% in each of these series.

At Stanford, Goffinet, et al. [33], recently reported on 5 patients with locally advanced or recurrent head and neck carcinomas; four involved the base tongue and one arose in the floor of mouth. Each patient was treated with combined ^{192}Iridium interstitial implantation to doses encompassing tumor volumes of 20 to 42 Gy. RF hyperthermia treatments of 45 minute durations were also given pre– and post–^{192}Iridium loading and removal, respectively. RF heating was temperature modulated with computer–controlled multiplexing and power control between electrodes.

Individual case reports were presented for each patient [33]. Figure 2 demonstrates the base tongue removable after loading hyperthermic interstitial implant technique. All five patients achieved a complete response. Two patients developed local recurrences 8 and 24 months post implantation. Table 1 summarizes treatments for each of the patients. No serious intra-

Table 1. Interstitial ^{192}Ir—RF Hyperthermia Treatment Detail

Patient	Age	Site	Stage	Date of implant	Radiation Ext Beam (cGy)	Dose Implant (cGy)	Implant Volume (cm^3)	^{192}Ir (mgRaEq)	Duration of implant (Hours)	Temperature # (°C)	Duration of Local Control (months)
JN	40	BOT	T_4N_0*	9/83	6000	2500 2000	83.0 125.0	39.2	50.0	40.3 ± 0.7	24**
EK	76	BOT	T_4N_1	2/84	6000	2534 1800	70.0 154.0	54.2	36.3	39.7 ± 1.0	15†
MS††	35	BOT	T_4N_0	5/84	3000	4270	79.8	50.75	61.0	40.1 ± 1.1	16##
BL	60	BOT	T_4N_0	1/85	5000	2420 1760	85.6 146.9	42.2	44.0	39.6 ± 1.2	8**
MT	67	FOM	T_4N_{3C}*	9/84	5940	2013	66.4	39.24	40.25	39.2 ± 1.4	42

Abbreviations: BOT = Base of tongue; FOM = Floor of mouth
* Adenoid cystic carcinoma
** Local recurrence after this time interval
† Died other causes, no evidence of recurrence
†† Prior irradiation for previous malignancy
\# Average temperature ± S.D. (temporal/spatial over tumor maps) maintained during heat treatments
\## Recurrence outside implant volume

operative or postoperative complications were observed directly from the procedure. One patient who had epiglottic involvement required a permanent tracheostomy, however, for persistent epiglottic edema.

Few analyses of thermal and/or radiation parameters predictive of outcome of interstitial hyperthermic implants have been performed due to limited temperature data and small patient numbers. Aristizabal and Oleson [30] in reviewing the literature showed improved complete response rates with higher and more uniform heating of the tumor volumes. Similarly, when criteria for a good implant were defined as minimum temperature in the tumor greater than 42°C, Emani reported increased rates of complete response [27].

Conclusion

Combined interstitial irradiation and hyperthermia have been shown in several small series to produce excellent local control rates in previously irradiated patients or in those with locally advanced neoplasms. The synergistic or complimentary interactions of these modalities, as well as the excellent ability to localize both radiation dose and heat to the tumor volume appear to provide a therapeutic advantage. Because high local control rates have been reported from interstitial irradiation alone, the actual contribution of hyperthermia to these results is unknown. Hampering this effort to discern the effects of each modality is the lack of detailed thermometry data in most series and a lack of standardized performance of both the brachytherapy and hyperthermic components of these treatments. A prospective trial comparing interstitial irradiation with and without hyperthermia has been undertaken by the Radiation Therapy Oncology Group, and its outcome is awaited. Because of the high local control rates from radiation alone and the large number of patient and treatment variables to be considered, such as the extent of prior treatment, the primary site of involvement and the size of the recurrent neoplasm as well as the nonstandardization of hyperthermic dosimetry, interpretation of the results of this trial may be difficult.

Work must continue on quality assurance, standardizing both the hyperthermic and brachytherapy components of the treatment. Ferromagnetic seeds and other hot source techniques, which have had very limited clinical use to date, should be further developed and tested. Technological developments will continue to improve other interstitial techniques making these procedures easier and safer. Segmented RF electrodes will permit longitudinal power modulation [34], and built–in accurate thermometry will allow improved monitoring and better control of heat distribution throughout the implanted tumor volumes. Improved microwave antennae with better heating at the tips [23] and better use of coherently operated microwave electronics are also anticipated. These improvements should allow the highest possible response rates with these techniques while decreasing the risk of complications.

References

1. Emami B, Marks JE: Retreatment of recurrent carcinoma of the head and neck by afterloading interstitial ^{192}Ir implant. Laryngoscopy 93:1345–1347, 1983.
2. Goffinet DR, Fee WE, Wells J, Austin–Seymour M, Clarke D, Mariscal JM, Goode RL: Ir–192 pharyngoepiglottic fold interstitial implants: The key to successful treatment of base tongue carcinoma by radiation therapy. Cancer 55:941–948, 1985.
3. Hilaris BS, Nori D, Beattie EJ, Martini N: Value of perioperative brachytherapy in the management of non–oat cell carcinoma of the lung. Int J Radiat Oncol Biol Phys 9:1161–1166, 1983.
4. Fee WE, Goffinet DR, Paryani S, Goode RL, Levine PA, Hopp ML: Intraoperative Iodine 125 implants. Arch Otolaryngol 109:727–730, 1983.
5. Krithivas G, Feldman MI, Cail DL, Bricout PB, Reyes BL: Interstitial radiotherapy of the base of the tongue: improved non–looping afterloading technique. Radiology 150(2):601–602, 1984.
6. Sandor J, Palos B, Goffinet D, Martinez A, Fessenden P: Dose calculations for planar arrays of ^{192}Ir and ^{125}I seeds for brachytherapy. Applied Radiol 8:41–44, 1979.
7. Bagshaw MA, Taylor MA, Kapp DS, Meyer JL, Samulski TV, Lee ER, Fessenden P: Anatomical site–specific modalities for hyperthermia. Cancer Res 44(Suppl.):4842s–4852s, 1984.
8. Kapp DS, Fessenden P, Samulski TV, Bagshaw MA, Cox RS, Lee ER, Lohrbach AW, Meyer JL, Prionas SD: Stanford University institutional report. Phase I evaluation of equipment for hyperthermia treatment of cancer. Int J Hyperthermia 4(1):75–115, 1988.
9. Oleson JR, Dewhirst MW: Hyperthermia: an overview of current progress and problems. Current Problems in Cancer, (Monograph) 8(6):1–62, 1983.
10. Perez CA, Emami B: A review of current clinical experience with irradiation and hyperthermia. Endocurietherapy/Hyperthermia Oncology 1:265–277, 1985.
11. Samulski TV, Lee ER, Hahn GM: Hyperthermia as a clinical treatment modality. Cancer Treatment Reports 68(1):309–311, 1984.
12. Sapozink MD, Gibbs FA, Gates KS, Stewart JR: Regional hyperthermia in the treatment of clinically advanced, deep–seated malignancy: results of a pilot study employing an annular array applicator. Int J Radiat Oncol Biol Phys 10:775–786, 1984.
13. Crile G Jr: The effects of heat and radiation on cancers implanted in the feet of mice. Cancer Res 25:372–380, 1963.
14. Dewey WC, Westra A, Miller HH, Magasawa H: Heat–induced lethality and chromosomal damage in synchronized Chinese hamster cells treated with 5–bromodeoxyuridine. Int J Radiat Biol 20:505–520, 1971.
15. Cavalrere R, Ciocatto EC, et al.: Selective heat sensitivity of cancer cells. Cancer 20:1351–1354, 1967.
16. Ben–Hur E, Elkind MM, Bronk BV: Thermally enhanced radioresponse of cultured Chinese hamster cells: inhibition of repair of sublethal damage and enhancement of lethal damage. Radiat Res 58:38–51, 1974.
17. Kim SH, Kim JH, Hahn EW: The enhanced killing of irradiated HeLa cells in synchronous culture by hyperthermia. Br J Radiology 48:872–874, 1976.
18. Meyer JL, Kapp DS, Fessenden P, Hahn GH: Hyperthermic Oncology: Current Biology, Physics, and Clinical Results. Pharmac Ther Vol 42:251–288, 1989.
19. Hahn GM: Hyperthermia and Cancer. New York: Plenum, 1982.

20. Gerner EW, Schneider MJ: Induced thermal resistance in Hela cells. Nature 256:500–507, 1975.
21. Hahn GM, Ning SC, Elizaga M, Kapp DS, Anderson RL: A comparison of thermal response of human and rodent cells. Int J Radiat Oncol Biol Phys (in press), 1989.
22. Ali Neyzari MS, Cheung AY: A review of brachyhyperthermic approaches for the treatment of cancer. Endocurietherapy/Hyperthermic Oncology 1:257–264, 1985.
23. Satoh T, Stauffer PR: Implantable helical coil microwave antenna for interstitial hyperthermia. Int J Radiat Oncol Biol Phys 4:497–512, 1988.
24. Brezovich IA, Atkinson WJ, Lilly MB: Local hyperthermia with interstitial techniques. Cancer Research (Suppl) 44:4752–4756, 1984.
25. Wappelmann B, Brezovich IA, Meredith RF, Henderson R, Browner W, Salter MM: Interstitial hyperthermia and hot water perfusion: the influence of catheter spacing. Abstracts of Papers for the Thirty-Seventh Annual meeting of the Radiation Research Society, March 18–23. Seattle, WA 49, 1989.
26. Cetas TC, Connor WG: Thermometry considerations in localized hyperthermia. Med Phys 5(2):79–91, 1978.
27. Emami B, Marks JE, Perez CA, Nussbaum GH, Leybovich L, Von Gerichten D: Interstitial thermoradiotherapy in the treatment of recurrent/residual malignant tumors. Am J Clinical Onc 7:699–704, 1984.
28. Puthawala AA, Syed AMM, Sheikh KMA, Rafie S, McNamara CS: Interstitial hyperthermia in recurrent malignancies. Endocurietherapy/Hyperthermia Oncology 1(2):125–131, 1985.
29. Petrovich Z, Langholz B, Lam K, Lurten G, Cohen D, Jepson J, Astrahan M: Interstitial microwave hyperthermia combined with Iridium-192 radiotherapy for recurrent tumors. Am J Clinical Onc 12(3):264–268, 1989.
30. Aristizabal SA, Oleson JR: Combined interstitial irradiation and localized current field hyperthermia: results and conclusions from clinical studies. Cancer Res 44(Suppl.):4757s–4760s, 1984.
31. Cosset JM, Dutreix J, Dufour J, Janoray P, Damia E, Haie C, Clarke D: Combined interstitial hyperthermia and brachytherapy: Institute Gustave Roussy technique and preliminary results. Int J Radiat Oncol Biol Phys 10:307–312, 1984.
32. Manning MR, Cetas TC, Miller RC, Oleson JR, Connor WG, Gerner EW: Clinical hyperthermia: Results of a phase I trial employing hyperthermia alone or in combination with external beam or interstitial radiotherapy. Cancer 49:205–216, 1982.
33. Goffinet DR, Prionas SD, Kapp DS, Fessenden P, Hahn GM, Lohrbach AW, Mariscal JM, Bagshaw MA: Interstitial ^{192}Ir flexible catheter radiofrequency hyperthermia treatments of head and neck and recurrent pelvic carcinomas. Int J Radiat Oncol Biol Phys (In press), 1989.
34. Prionas SD, Fessenden P, Kapp DS, Goffinet DR, Hahn GM: Interstitial Electrodes Allowing Longitudinal Control of SAR Distributions. *Hyperthermic Oncology* Vol (2), Sugahara T and Saito M (eds). New York: Taylor and Francis, 1989.

7. Photodynamic Therapy in the Management of Head and Neck Cancer

Jack L. Gluckman and Robert P. Zitsch

Photodynamic therapy (PDT) is a relatively new therapeutic modality utilizing a photosensitizing drug, which selectively localizes in tumors and on activation by exposure to light, results in necrosis of the tumor. Like all new therapies directed to cancer, this modality has generated great enthusiasm and initially was heralded as the panacea for this most dreaded of all diseases. Time and experience have tempered this sentiment. However, it does appear to be effective in many situations, although much basic research is required before its exact role in contemporary cancer therapy can be defined. There are two ingredients necessary for this technology to be effective—the photosensitizer and the activating light.

A *photosensitizer*, by definition, is a chemical capable of absorbing light, resulting in an intracellular molecular reaction. It has long been known that many substances have this property, including tetracycline [1], berberine sulphate [2], acridine orange [3], fluorescine [3], rhodamine [4] and various porphyrins [5,6,7]. The first described use of such a photosensitizer in a biologic system occurred at the turn of the century when Raab [8] reported the effect of acridine dye on paramecium incubated and exposed to light. In 1903, Tappenier and Jesionek [9] first utilized this process in the treatment of malignant disease when they treated skin cancers using topical eosin as a photosensitizer, together with white light as the activating light.

Of the photosensitizers, porphyrins have attracted the greatest interest because, in addition to behaving as a photosensitizer, they are retained preferentially by malignant tissue and are detectable by fluorescence. In 1924, Policard [10] first reported a reddish–orange fluorescence in certain malignant tumors which was attributed to the accumulation of endogenous porphyrins as a result of secondary infection by hemolytic bacteria. In 1942, Auler and Banzer [6] injected hematoporphyrin into experimental rats which had been implanted with tumor and observed tumor fluorescence when exposed to ultraviolet light. In 1948, Figge and Weiland [7] studied the uptake of porphyrins in a wide range of tumors and tissue. They demonstrated that porphyrins accumulated not only in tumors, but also in traumatized tissue, lymph nodes and embryonic tissue. This was confirmed by Rasmussen–Taxdall [11] who, however, demonstrated a selective uptake of

Jacobs, C. (ed): Carcinomas of the Head and Neck: Evaluation and Management.

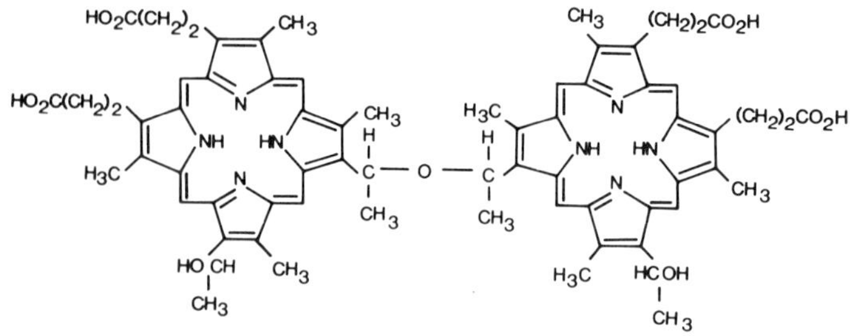

Bis -1-[8-(1-hydroxyethyl) deuteroporphyrin-3-yl] ethyl ether

Figure 1. Structure of dihematoporphyrin ether (DHE).

hematoporphyrin by tumor cells. In 1960, a new preparation called hematoporphyrin derivative (HPD) was first used by Lipson [12]. This contained a mixture of various porphyrins and resulted in red fluorescence in tissues exposed to violet light. Fluorescence in bronchial and esophageal tumors after systemic injection of this substance was noted [13]. Using ultraviolet light, Lipson subsequently demonstrated an 80% correlation between tumor fluorescence and biopsy proven malignancy [14]. Tumors that failed to fluoresce were found to be submucosal or inaccessible to light exposure.

In 1966, hematoporphyrin used as a photosensitizer, together with light from a Xenon lamp, was noted to have a therapeutic effect when Lipson reported partial tumor destruction when using the light to illuminate an ulcerating breast cancer [15]. Since that time multiple animal experiments have confirmed the tumoricidal effect of this treatment [16–18]. Because of dissatisfaction with hematoporphyrin, some work has commenced using other photosensitizers, although mostly this remains at a basic research level.

Drugs

Hematoporphyrin Derivative (HPD); dihematoporphyrin Ether (DHE)

HPD is a mixture of several porphyrins derived from hemoglobin. Some known components of HPD, that is, hematoporphyrin (HP); hydroxyethylvinyldeuteroporphyrin (HVD); and protoporphyrin (PROTO), have been shown not to be effective tumor photosenitizers, and much activity was devoted to isolating the active ingredient [19–23]. In 1981, Dougherty discovered the active photosensitizing component to be Bis–1–[8–(1–hydroxy–ethyl) deuteroporphyrin–3–yl] ethyl ether (figure 1) by using high–performance liquid chromatography, gel exclusion chromatography and nuclear magnetic resonance spectroscopy [24]. This substance (now known as dihematoporphyrin ether—DHE) comprised 45% of hematoporphyrin and was found to reach equivalent tissue levels at half the dose of HPD, resulting in significantly less skin photosensitivity. DHE, therefore, has become the preferred hematoporphyrin derivative for both diagnostic and therapeutic purposes.

While not ideal, DHE appears to fulfill many of the criteria for a satisfactory photosensitizer for use in the diagnosis and treatment of malignant disease in humans: (1) absence of systemic toxicity; (2) activation by light at wavelengths that are transmitted by human tissue; and (3) concentration in malignant tissue generally at a higher level than the surrounding tissue.

1. *Absence of Systemic Toxicity:*

   Both in animals and humans, HPD was found to be nontoxic apart from generalized temporary skin photosensitivity on exposure to light [15,25]. The purified form, DHE, results in even less skin photosensitivity.

2. *Light Activation:*

   When tissue containing DHE is exposed to light, a photochemical reaction occurs resulting in cell necrosis. The degree of necrosis depends on the light penetration through tissue. In general, the longer the light wavelength, the greater the tissue penetration.

   While DHE can be excited by absorption of light over several wavelengths, it is noted that unfortunately the greatest absorption is in the range of 400 nM with smaller peaks at 500 nM, 540 nM, 580 nM and 630 nM (figure 2). Although light at 400 nM would appear ideal, it will only penetrate up to 1 mm. and, therefore, it is not practical for use as an activator for photodynamic therapy. Light at 630 nM, though fairly rapidly dissipated, represents the best available wavelength because it allows tissue penetration of 5–20 mm [26,27].

3. *Tissue Uptake*:

   Initially, DHE was thought to be selectively taken up by neoplastic tissue [6,7,15,25,28,29], however, it is now recognized to be taken up by all tissues, particularly liver, spleen, kidney, lung, skin and muscle [30]. The serum half–life following injection is three hours, and during this period the hematoporphyrin is evenly distributed throughout the stroma and parenchyma of normal tissues. Once the serum level begins to fall, normal parenchymal cells and stroma begin to clear hematoporphyrin, but it is retained in the macrophage cell system and the cells of the reticuloendothelial system for longer periods of time.

   The retention in tumor, however, remains relatively high for several days. The reason for preferential retention in tumors is not clear. Bugelski, et al. [31] theorized that tumors have a high vascular permeability with an inefficient lymphatic clearance. Therefore, protein–bound substances such as DHE are trapped by these tumors. The concentration in tumor is always higher than in muscle and skin. Concentration in liver, kidney and spleen, though, is at all times higher than in tumor.

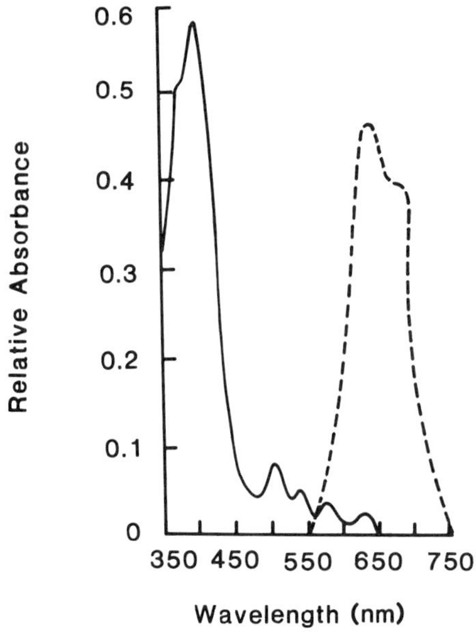

Figure 2. Absorption spectrum (solid line) and red fluorescence spectrum (dotted line) of HPD.

This is because of uptake by reticuloendothelial cells which include macrophages, mast cells and liver Kupfer cells.

Tumors appear to concentrate HPD predominantly in the vascular stroma with the ratio of stroma to tumor cells being approximately 5:1 [31]. After five to seven days, tumor cells demonstrate reduced amounts of hematoporphyrin whereas the stroma continues to demonstrate high levels.

Rhodamine–123

Another photosensitizing agent undergoing comprehensive evaluation is rhodamine–123. More specifically designated methyl o–(6–amino–3′–imino–3H–xanthen–9–yl) benzoate monohydrochloride, it is a cationic, lipophilic mitochondrial dye with a maximal light absorption at a wavelength of 511 nm. Rhodamine–123 is a single member of a group of rhodamine compounds which have been used in the past as histological stains. Certain members of this group, including rhodamine–123, are selectively concentrated in mitochondria of cells. The selective uptake and fluorescent characteristics of rhodamine–123 form a combination of physical properties which have been utilized for the localization of mitochondria in living cells [32].

Rhodamine–123 was first demonstrated by Summerhayes, et al. in 1982 to exhibit a differential in uptake and retention between normal cells and tumor cells [33]. Certain carcinomas were observed to accumulate more rhodamine–123 and retain it for longer periods of time than do most normal cells. A clear reason for this differential in uptake and retention, however, has not yet been elucidated.

The first in vivo investigations on the potential use of rhodamine–123 for cancer chemotherapy were published in 1983 [34], with the selective uptake by tumor cells providing the basis for these investigations. It was shown that in nonlethal doses, rhodamine–123 exhibited significant and measurable antitumor activity in mice. Further toxicity studies, however, demonstrated that the concentrations necessary to produce antitumor effects were also cytotoxic for normal fibroblasts [35]. Therefore, the role of rhodamine–123 strictly as a cancer chemotherapeutic agent appears to be limited.

However, more promising is the potential of rhodamine–123 as a photosensitizer of tumor cells. The first use in this regard, combined with the argon laser was reported in 1986 [36]. The argon laser with an energy wavelength of 514.5 nm can be used to destroy the sensitized tumor cells [35].

These successful in vitro studies have led to further in vivo investigations of the tumoricidal effects of rhodamine–123 photodynamic therapy. Castro et al. [4] demonstrated complete eradication of human squamous cell carcinoma transplanted to nude mice without regrowth using rhodamine–123 photodynamic therapy. The effect occurred with nontoxic doses (1 mg/ml) of the photosensitizer at temperatures as low as 36°C.

Several features of this form of photodynamic therapy are appealing with regard to its future use in humans. The effectiveness of permanent tumor eradication in the animal model is remarkable. The results seem to be purely dependent on a photochemical reaction since they are achieved at nontoxic doses of rhodamine–123 at normal temperatures. Furthermore, there are no known phototoxicity reactions which are commonly observed with hematoporphyrins. However, further studies will be necessary before its use in the treatment of human malignancy can be determined.

Other Photosensitizers

The early clinical successes achieved with the hematoporphyrins has provided the impetus for a search for other photosensitizers. Other promising photochemosensitizers with a potential for clinical use are sulfonated metallophthalocyaines, diaziquone, berberine, N,N′–bis (2–ethyl–1,3–dioxolane)–kryptocyanine (EDKC), nile blue A (NBA), tetra–(4–sulfonatophenyl) porphine (TPPS), silicon naphthalocyanine, hypocrellin A, and prophycenes.

Metals which have been complexed to form sulfonated metallophthalocyaines possessing photochemosensitizing characteristics are zinc, gallium, cerium and aluminum [37,38]. Each of these seem to exhibit preferential uptake by various malignancies in rodent studies leading to selective necrosis of the tumors when exposed to energy from an argon dye laser.

Another compound which has been intensively investigated recently is TPPS. This agent has been used to topically sensitize neoplastic skin lesions in patients, followed by treatment with an argon–pumped dye laser. Patients treated in this fashion had an overall cure rate of 76% [39]. However, other animal studies with the agent suggest a lack of specificity for tumor tissue, prompting a recommendation of caution by the authors [40].

Nile blue A is a cationic dye that exhibits selective localization in experimental tumors in mice [41]. Systemically administered, NBA will facilitate tumor necrosis when melanoma or squamous cell carcinoma tumors in mice are irradiated with an argon–pumped dye laser.

In vitro studies with leukemia cells confirm diaziquone as another photosensitizing agent [42]. Berberine has similarly shown an inhibition of gastric cancer cell growth in vitro when irradiated with light of wavelength 320 nM to 450 nM [43]. Another agent with photosensitizing characteristics which is selective for carcinoma cells is EDKC, a cyanine dye [44].

Finally, other compounds exist which possess physical and chemical properties suggesting a potential for clinical use. These are hypocrellin A [45], silicon naphthalocyanine [46], and prophycenes [47]. The data currently available on the use of these agents is scant, however.

None of these newer photosensitizers has had extensive evaluation either in animals or patients to date. Therefore, the systemic, local and phototoxic reactions which may occur with their use are not known. It is hoped, though, that some of these agents will exhibit better tumor specificity and consequently more complete and selective tumor eradication with less side effects than is currently available with the hematoporphyrins.

Instrumentation

Light Source

The other essential component for photodynamic therapy is the light source. In general, two types of light sources are available, that is, lamps and lasers. Historically, lamps were the light source of choice with both Raab [8] and Tappenier [9] at the turn of the century using white light for their work. Many subsequent workers used blue–violet light to fluoresce and treat tumors [14,25], while others used red light for tumor treatment [15,16].

The major disadvantage of the lamp is that it emits a broad spectrum of light which must be filtered to obtain monochromatic light. As the light is noncoherent and, therefore, of limited brightness, it requires to be focused by a system of mirrors and lenses in order to be effective. The only obvious advantage of a lamp as opposed to a laser is the low cost.

Lasers are the preferred source of light. Since they emit monochromatic coherent light, the power is greater and can be channeled down a single optical fiber. The fiber may then be used for surface illumination or, if necessary, be implanted into the substance of the tumor via a needle. The laser most commonly used for therapy is the Argon ion pumped dye laser.

Types of Lasers Used in PDT

Argon Ion Pumped Dye Laser. This laser consists of a 5 to 20 watt Argon ion laser which pumps a dye laser to produce light at 630 nM. The dyes used in the dye laser include Rhodamine B or Kiton Red. The dye laser converts the wavelength of the blue–green beam (454 nM to 514.5 nM) from the Argon laser to the red–orange range (630 nM). This may produce 1–4 watts when tuned to 630 nM depending on the power emitted by the Argon tube. The light is then coupled to single or multiple optical fibers for delivery.

Gold Vapor Laser. This produces a pulsed beam at 627.8 nM which, therefore, does away with the necessity for a dye laser. It is, at this time, not clear whether this pulsed effect is advantageous by enhancing tumor necrosis, or deliterious by causing damage to surrounding normal tissue. The use of pulsed lasers are being actively investigated with a view to improving the effectiveness of tumor ablation.

Since the gold vapor laser is a relatively new development, and as such is only available in a small number of centers, its effect on a tumor and its surrounding tissue in PDT has not yet been established. It may, however, be potentially more effective than the Argon ion dye laser. Current research is inconclusive [48].

Argon Laser. The argon laser in its own right has been used in animal experiments together with rhodamine–123 as the photosensitizer. This delivers light at 514 nm, but at higher power, output of up to 10 watts [4].

Delivery Systems

A fiberoptic system is used for delivery of the laser energy during photodynamic therapy. The optical fibers are long, flexible rods made of silicone–quartz, covered with a protective coating. The distal end of the optical quartz fiber may be modified in several ways to obtain optimal light delivery. These applicators direct the light to the lesion in a pattern depending on the configuration of the tip. The flat–cut applicator delivers a spot field of light and is used for surface application (figure 3a).

Lenses may be used to improve the light distribution within the spot. Diffusers may be fashioned to produce a distribution pattern depending on the type of diffuser—cylinder diffuser, used to treat a hollow viscus, for example trachea, esophagus, (figure 3b) or point diffusers to illuminate spherical cavities, for example oral cavity (figure 3c).

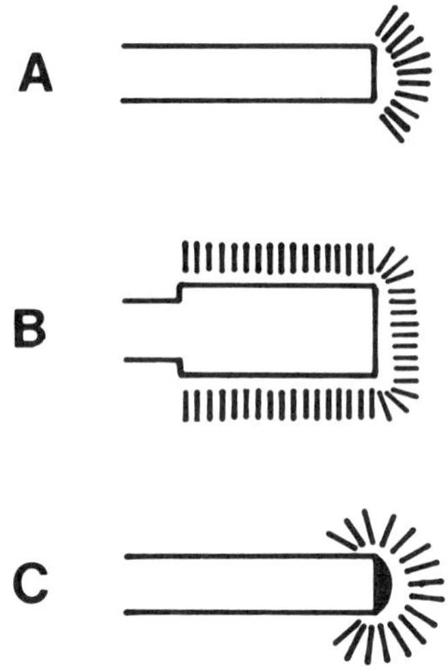

Figure 3. (a) Flat cut applicator, (b) Cylinder diffuser, (c) Point diffuser.

Light Dosimetry

The calculation of the optimal amount of light to be delivered to an affected area is referred to as dosimetry. The required exposure time for tumor ablation is dependent on laser *power output* in watts, *dose rate* measured in watts/cm^2 and *light dose* in Joules/cm^2. This relationship is expressed in the following equation:

$$\text{EXPOSURE TIME (SECONDS)} = \frac{\text{Lightdose (J/cm}^2\text{)}}{\text{Dose rate (W/cm}^2\text{)}}$$

At this stage in the development of this technology, the calculated optimal light dosage is inexact and dependent on many variables. As experience is gained, hopefully this will become easier to calculate.

Photodynamic Therapy (PDT)

In spite of intensive research devoted to this technology, some extremely fundamental problems remain as yet unresolved. Included are an understanding of the exact mode of action, the optimal instrumentation and drug to be used, and the dosimetry of light required in any given patient treatment. As most of the animal and human experience has been gained using DHE and the argon dye–pumped laser, this form of photodynamic therapy will be described, although different drugs and different wavelengths will certainly become available as this technology evolves.

Mode of Action

While the mode of action of PDT is not clear, some understanding of the mechanism at a cellular and subcellular level has resulted from numerous in vitro and in vivo animal experiments. In experimental tumors exposed to PDT, two possible macroscopic reactions may occur, either the tumor may become hemorrhagic or blanched.

The mechanism generally accepted for causing cell necrosis after light exposure is an energy transfer process from the excited triplet state of the hematoporphyrin to oxygen, producing singlet oxygen, which causes irreversible oxidation of some essential cellular components [49]. Oxygen is necessary for this reaction to occur, although there may be a non–oxygen dependent process which may also result in cell necrosis [50].

Another possible mechanism of tumor necrosis is ischemia secondary to an effect on tumor vasculature. After PDT, it has been demonstrated in animal tumors that blood flow becomes sluggish, the red cells coagulate and ultimately the vessels may rupture [31]. Exactly why the tumor vasculature is damaged is unknown, but, as has already been demonstrated, the highest uptake of HPD and DHE is in the vascular stroma. The resultant tumor cell necrosis may, therefore, be on an ischemic basis or due to a direct cytotoxic effect.

There is a striking similarity between the effects produced by PDT and those produced by hyperthermia. However, at the low power produced by the laser, thermal damage does not appear to be a factor. Of interest is that in animal work, both the curability and depth of necrosis produced by PDT can be enhanced by combining heat with PDT [51].

Technique

There are two basic approaches to the administration of PDT: 1) surface illumination; and 2) interstitial implantation. At this stage in the development of this technology, not even the most rudimentary aspects of the ideal therapy have been clearly determined. The following regimen is followed by the authors:

The drug of choice, DHE (2.0 mg/kg body wt), is given intravenously 72 hours prior to the therapy. This is administered I.V. piggyback with 5% dextrose water which is maintained for one hour post–injection while observing for any possible adverse reaction. While 72 hours remains the traditional delay before therapy, in order for clearance of the drug by normal tissue to occur, some physicians have successfully treated three hours after administration of the drug [52]. Precautions should be taken to avoid skin photosensitivity, that is, avoiding sunlight and bright artificial light, protective clothing, and use of sunscreen preparations. This should be continued for 4–6 weeks post–therapy.

If the lesion to be treated is accessible, the procedure is performed without anesthesia, usually with the fiber being held in place using a mechanical holder. If inaccessible, surface illumination is administered via an endoscope, under general anesthesia, if necessary. In treating a bulky lesion, the fiber may be implanted directly into the tumor via a number 15 gauge needle. This will result in circumferential tumor necrosis of approximately 2 cm. The size of the tumor and depth of infiltration will dictate which approach to use.

The Clinical Application of PDT

Background

The efficacy of PDT in the treatment of cancer has long been demonstrated in both animal experiments and the clinical setting. While little work has been done in cancer of the head and neck, the modality has been used in various other areas with varied success.

Dermatology. Basal cell cancer, squamous cell cancer, malignant melanoma, metastatic cancer. Kaposi's sarcoma, Bowen's disease and mycosis fungoides have all been treated with PDT with encouraging results [53–57]. Careful appraisal of the reported results, however, is confusing, as there appears to be little consistency in the type or size of the tumor treated and the technique of application. The following facts are, however, apparent:

Small superficial tumors do extremely well even in areas previously exposed to ionizing radiation. The optimal therapeutic dosage for these superficial tumors appears to be 20 to 35 Joules cm^2 administered 72 hours after injection of HPD. Higher doses appear to affect normal tissue although this may be due to a thermal effect. Larger tumors only benefit if the tumors are localized and even then, if deeply infiltrating, are best treated with a combination of superficial and interstitial implantation of the laser. If the tumors are very large, multiple simultaneous and/or sequential implantations of fibers are necessary to debulk them, but this achieves very little in influencing the course of the disease. Complications other than generalized photosensitivity are rare, but pain and edema may develop in the surrounding tissues, particularly at higher doses of light. Previous ionizing radiation does not appear to be a contraindication to therapy.

Pulmonary. PDT was first used for cancer of the bronchus in 1980 with an excellent result [58]. Since then a number of series have reported predictably varied response. A review of 73 cases by Hayata, et al., revealed that PDT was effective in superficial lesions, but if deep invasion had occurred, it was contraindicated [59]. Reasons for failure included the inability to accurately assess depth of invasion and an inadequate light delivery system. PDT has been also used to palliatively ablate advanced tumors obstructing a mainstem bronchus with excellent results being reported [60]. This was performed using surface illumination, or in the case of large tumors, interstitial implantation. Accumulation of secretions frequently necessitated prophylactic repeat bronchoscopy a few days after therapy to clear the necrotic debris. Severe delayed hemorrhage has also been reported.

Esophagus and Stomach. Early cancers developing in these areas are potentially curable using PDT, however, this would be a most rare scenario. Palliative ablation of larger lesions has been successfully accomplished [61–63].

Urology. It is in this field that PDT has made its most spectacular advances. The lesions which have benefited most are diffuse carcinoma in situ or very superficial bladder cancers, particularly if they are multicentric [52]. Bladder cancer appears to concentrate DHE well, and the normal urothelium shows marked resistance to PDT damage. Larger tumors can undergo palliative ablation with some success [64].

Gynecology. Promising results have been reported following the treatment of vaginal cancers with surface and interstitial application of PDT [65,66]. Its use in recurrent cervical, vaginal and endometrial cancers has also been reported [67].

Neurology. The major thrust in this field appears to be one of adjuvant intraoperative therapy for residual tumor following resection [68]. A major problem has been the development of postoperative cerebral edema.

Ophthalmology. Use of this technology in the management of choroidal malignant melanoma has been described [69]. While the preliminary nature of the reports are stressed, the results have been encouraging. Side effects on the retina have not been observed.

Head and Neck. Review of the literature devoted to the use of PDT in cancer of the head and neck reveals that initially this modality was used predominately in advanced cancer for palliation, particularly in those lesions that are not treatable by, or are refractory to, more conventional therapy [70–73]. While these lesions have frequently demonstrated spectacular response, it is unrealistic to expect this local therapy to influence the course of extensive disease.

This technique has, however, proved reasonably valuable as a palliative procedure. Many treatment failures with local recurrence develop swelling, pain and discomfort, thus severely compromising their quality of life. In most reports where the clear intent was to produce palliation, this was successfully accomplished in a high percentage of cases. In Keller's series [73], where the palliative goals were clearly defined, this was accomplished in two–thirds of the cases, particularly with regard to debulking the tumors, thereby improving swallowing and respiration. Schuller et al. [71] noted marked relief of pain. While many of these responses were transient, a major potential advantage of this therapy is that it can be administered repeatedly. Occasionally complete responses and even isolated cures were achieved. Because of the poor tissue penetration accomplished by surface illumination (maximum of 1–2 cm), the preferred method of administration for palliation of these large tumors is interstitial implantation with multiple fibers.

Another potential use of PDT could be the intraoperative treatment of residual disease after resection. Schuller, et al. [71] attempted this approach; however, in two of three reported cases, this was unsuccessful.

A personal experience in using PDT to treat advanced recurrent head and neck cancer has been somewhat unrewarding, and for this reason a change in philosophy evolved, with the current sentiment being that the true role of PDT in head and neck cancer is the management of superficial mucosal and cutaneous cancers [74,75].

Rationale for the Use of PDT for Treatment of Early Cancers

For the following reasons, PDT may represent the most ideal method of treating superficial cancer of the mucosa of the upper aerodigestive tract:

1. The anatomy of the upper aerodigestive tract frequently allows adequate visualization of the lesion, but renders adequate endoscopic excision or ablation cumbersome and difficult. A technique that only requires visualization and a 'no touch' technique for ablation would potentially be a vast improvement over more conventional means.
2. Theoretically, because of the selective uptake of the drug and, therefore, selective necrosis of the tumor, the anxiety regarding frozen section control would be rendered unnecessary, provided complete exposure to the lesion can be achieved.
3. In most circumstances, this procedure requires no anesthesia and can be performed in an office setting. In certain situations, general anesthesia may be necessary to achieve access to the tumor.
4. Certain lesions may preferentially be treated in this manner, that is, field cancerization with large areas of superficial premalignant and malignant change, and multicentric malignancies. This phenomenon is well documented in the mucosa of the upper aerodigestive tract and is extremely difficult to treat [76,77,78]. This technique allows relatively large areas to be treated with preservation of normal tissue.
5. If recurrent and/or persistent cancer should develop, the lesions may easily be retreated as frequently as necessary to attain ablation. This is in sharp contradistinction to other modalities, for example, radiation therapy.

Many of the above criteria are equally applicable to cutaneous malignancies, and PDT may represent the best therapy for multiple superficial lesions of the skin.

Limitations of PDT in the Management of Head and Neck Cancer

There appears little doubt that PDT causes tumor necrosis, however, the exact role of this therapy in contemporary head and neck cancer management remains ill–defined. The reasons for this include lack of experience with this technique, as well as rather obvious limitations of the technology itself. As experience grows, it appears that large lesions do not respond in a satisfactory manner to PDT and that the ideal lesion is the relatively superficial cancer. Unfortunately, it is impossible at this stage to predict exactly how large a tumor can effectively be treated by this modality as the tumor necrosis is dependent on multiple factors, many of which are poorly understood. These include the following:

1. **Unpredictable tumor ablation due to:**
   a) *Unpredictable Uptake of HPD (DHE) By The Tumor:*
   As has already been demonstrated, the intratumoral distribution of hematoporphyrin in induced animal tumors has only recently been determined. While uptake has been demonstrated in the perivascular stroma, it is still unclear as to whether the tumor cells themselves take up the hematoporphyrin. Whether these findings can be extrapolated to spontaneous tumors occurring in humans has not been established. In addition, it appears that anoxic necrotic tumor may not take up DHE, and this may severely compromise the effectiveness of this therapy. Whether all types of tumor take up the drug equally remains to be determined. An additional problem is that it is still not apparent when the optimal time is to administer the laser therapy following injection of the drug, that is, when the tumor to background tissue levels are optimal for therapy. It is possible that the future development of a more specific and effective photosensitizer would alleviate many of these problems.
   b) *Unpredictable Depth Of Light Penetration:*
   This, in turn, is dependent on multiple factors, including the wavelength of light and instrumentation used to deliver the light. The type of laser used will obviously have an effect on this problem.
   c) *Ability to Expose The Whole Field Of Growth to Light:*
   In the upper aerodigestive tract, the complex nature of the anatomy may render adequate exposure of the tumor to the light extremely difficult. In addition, it is frequently difficult to differentiate grossly what represents benign, premalignant and malignant change. Therefore, in dealing with extensive areas of 'condemned mucosa', a technique will need to be designed to allow treatment of the whole area without compromising normal tissue.

2. **Problems with the technology:**

   The inconveniences of the technique, that is, expense, specialized instrumentation and special training, need to be weighed against the potential advantages, particularly when dealing with superficial lesions which could reasonably be treated by more simple alternative therapies.

   Drug. As has already been presented, hematoporphyrin, even in its purified form, is a less than ideal photosensitizing drug in humans with the most significant drawback being that photosensitivity may last up to thirty days. In addition, the unsatisfactory absorption spectrum and the nonspecific tissue uptake also impair the effectiveness of this technology.

   Laser. The Argon ion pumped dye laser, which is the laser most commonly used, is unfortunately cumbersome, temperamental and is only capable of a low–power output. The Gold Vapor laser ultimately may become the laser of choice to deliver light at this wavelength.

3. **Complications:**

   These include edema, local pain and skin photosensitivity.

   Edema has not been a major problem in our own experience; however, if an extensive area is treated, or if too high a power is used, this may develop. When using high power, a thermal effect may result which would predispose to the edema. Great care should be taken to avoid contact between the applicator tip and the tissue as this may also induce a thermal effect.

   Local pain has not been highlighted in the literature, but has been a constant finding in our experience. The reasons for this are obscure, but it may be due to local fat necrosis or even tumor necrosis.

   In certain situations, these complications have significant implications, with severe laryngeal edema and even permanent laryngeal stenosis resulting.

   By far the most common problem, however, is *skin photosensitivity*. This may last from four to six weeks following the administration of hematoporphyrin. This reaction is usually mild and easily managed by taking appropriate precautions. Occasionally, however, it may be severe and cause considerable discomfort.

Tumor Detection Using Photosensitizers

Although most of the experience with photosensitizing agents has been related to tumor therapy, another potential use is for the detection of early or occult cancers by using the fluorescence exhibited by these agents on exposure to light. The ability to detect cancer which is not readily apparent is an intriguing prospect.

When hematoporphyrin is stimulated by an excitation light, it emits red fluorescence with a peak between 630 and 690 nM (figure 2). The excitation light used may be a lamp or laser. The fluorescence may be apparent to the naked eye, or enhanced by using an image intensifier. The fluorescence signal may also be detected by a frequency modulated audio signal or be quantified on a digital voltmeter.

The optimal method of detecting this fluorescence has been the subject of much research. In 1961, Lipson, et al., demonstrated fluorescence in patients with bronchial and esophageal tumors after systemic administration of HPD using an ultraviolet light source [13]. In a subsequent study, an 80% correlation of tumor fluorescence with biopsy proven malignancy was demonstrated [14]. Tumors that failed to fluoresce were retrospectively found to be submucosal, therefore, being inaccessible to the ultraviolet light, as light at this wavelength will only penetrate to a depth of 1–2 mm. Lack of adequate instrumentation also hindered further progress at that time.

In 1977, Profio and Doiron reported on a more sophisticated system using a mercury arc lamp as their light source, a combination of interference and absorption filters and an image intensifier [79]. This device yielded extremely impressive results, and the addition of the image intensifier made the capability of localizing small bronchogenic tumors a distinct possibility [80]. A disadvantage to this system was that the entire visual field was green, thereby interfering with the endoscopist's ability to recognize clinically abnormal mucosa. Prompted by this, Kinsey, et al. [81], developed a device that enables simultaneous endoscopy with white light and fluorescence detection. This system has been successfully used to detect occult carcinoma in the bladder and bronchi. The evolution of imaging fluorescence endoscopy has been furthered by numerous additions and modifications and will hopefully result in a sophisticated, highly accurate modality for cancer detection.

This approach to the detection of fluorescence is most attractive as it allows direct visualization of the fluorescence which can then be biopsied. Further clinical trials are required to determine its role in the diagnosis of head and neck cancers.

The potential uses of fluorescence detection in the upper aerodigestive tract include:

1. The detection of occult primary tumors in the upper aerodigestive tract which may be developing synchronously with other more obvious primary cancers.
2. The localization of the extent of field cancerization in the upper aerodigestive tract and the identification of premalignant and malignant change in areas of leukoplakia and/or erythroplakia.
3. To aid in the differentiation between radiation change and recurrent tumor following the administration of radiotherapy for cure, particularly where submucosal tumor is suspected.
4. To aid in intraoperative margin control following surgical resection of a tumor. Present approaches relying on clinical impression and multiple frozen sections are most unsatisfactory and potentially hematoporphyrin fluorescence may aid in the more accurate delineation of the extent of the tumor.

While conceptually these diagnostic techniques are exciting, there do exist obvious limitations including inconvenience of the instrumentation and administration of the drug, as well as expense. A clearer appreciation of the reliability of this technology will only become apparent after further animal and clinical experience.

Conclusion

As is hopefully apparent, photodynamic therapy has the potential to be an exciting new advance in the fight against cancer. Unfortunately, at this time, little is known about even the most basic aspects of this technology. We are confident, however, that with time, ultimately PDT will find a role in contemporary cancer management. What exactly this role will be, will depend not only on determining which tumors will ideally respond to this modality, but also rendering this rather complex and expensive therapy 'user friendly'. This will probably require different photosensitizers, lasers and methods of administration. Hopefully, multicenter trials will be instituted that will aid in the evaluation of this technology.

References

1. Rall DD, Loo TL, Lane M, et al.: Appearance and persistance of flourescent material in tumor tissue after tetracylcine administration. J Natl Cancer Inst 19:79–86, 1957.
2. Mellors RC, Glassman A, Papanicolaou GN: A microflourimetric scanning method for the detection of cancer cells in smears of exofoliated cells. Cancer 5:458–468, 1952.
3. Tomson SH, Emmett EA, Fox SH: Photodestruction of mouse epithelial tumors after acridine orange and argon laser. Cancer Research 34:3124–3127, 1974.
4. Castro DJ, Saxton ER, Fetterman H, et al.: Phototherapy with argon lasers and rhodamine–123 for tumor eradication. Otol Head and Neck Surg 98:581–588, 1988.
5. Moore GE: Diagnosis and localization of brain tumors; a clinical and experimental study employing floursecent and radioactive tracer methods. Springfield, Ill: Charles C Thomas, 1953.
6. Auler H, Banzer G: Untersuchungen uber die rolle der prophone beigeschwulstkranken menschen und tieren. Z Krebsforsch 53:65–68, 1942.
7. Figge FHJ, Weiland GS, Manganiello LOJ: Cancer detection and therapy. Affinity of neoplastic embryonic and traumatized regenerating tissues for porphyrins and metalloporphyrins. Proc Soc Exptl Biol Med, 68:640–641, 1948.
8. Raab O: Uber die Wirkung floureszirenden stoffe auf in fusoria. A Biol 39:524–527, 1900.
9. Tappenier H, Jesionek A: Theropeutische reosuche met floureszierenden stoff. Muench Med Wochsder 1:2042–2044, 1903.
10. Policard A: Etudes sue les aspects offerts par des tumeur experimentals examinee a la lumiere de woods. Cr Soc Biol 91:1423–1425, 1924.
11. Rasmussen–Texdall DS, Ward GE, Figge FH: Flourescence of human lymphatic and cancer tissue following high doses of intravenous hematoporphyrin. Cancer 8:78–81, 1955.
12. Lipson RL: The photodynamic and flourescent properties of a particular hematoporphyrin derivative and its use in tumor detection (master's thesis). University of Minnesota, 1960.

13. Lipson RL, Baldes EJ, Olsen AM: Hematoporphyrin derivative: a new aid to endoscopic detection of malignant disease. J Thor Cardiovasc Surg 42:623–629, 1961.
14. Lipson RL, Baldes EJ, Olsen AM: A further evaluation of the use of hematoporphyrin derivative as a new aid for the endoscopic detection of malignant disease. Dis Chest 46:676–679, 1964.
15. Lipson RL, Gray MJ, Baldes EJ: Hematoporphyrin derivative for detection and management of cancer. Proc 9th Internat Cancer Congr, p 398, 1966.
16. Dougherty TJ, Grindey GB, Fiel R, et al.: Photoradiation therapy. II. Cure of animal tumors with hematoporphyrin and light. J Natl Cancer Inst 55:115–119, 1975.
17. Dougherty TJ: Activated dyes as anti-tumor agents. J Natl Cancer Inst 52:1333–1336, 1974.
18. Diamond I, Granelli S, McDonaugh AF, et al.: Photodynamic therapy of malignant tumors. Lancet 2:1175–1177, 1973.
19. Moan J, Evensen JF, Christensen T, et al.: Chemical composition of hematoporphyrin derivative: tumor localizing and photosensitizing properties of its main components. Abstracts of the 10th Annual Meeting of the American Society of Photobiology, pp 173–174, Vancouver, British Columbia, Canada, 1982.
20. Moan J, Christensen R, Sommer S: The main photosensitizing components of hematoporphyrin derivative. Cancer Lett 15:161–166, 1982.
21. Kessel D: Components of hematoporphyrin derivatives and their tumor–localizing capacity. Cancer Res 42:1703–1706, 1982.
22. Berenbaum M, Bonnet R, Scoundes PA: In vivo biological activity of the components of hematoporphyrin derivative. Br J Cancer 45:571–581, 1982.
23. Kessel D: Components of hematoporphyrin derivatives and their tumor–localizing capacity. Cancer Res 42:1703–1706, 1982.
24. Dougherty TJ, Potter WR, Weishaupt KR: The structure of the active component of hematoporphyrin derivative. Porphyrins in Tumor Phototherapy, New York: Plenum, 1984.
25. Lipson RL, Pratt JH, Baldes EJ, et al.: Hematoporphyrin derivative for the detection of cervical cancer. Obstet Gynecol, 24:78–84, 1964.
26. McCaughan JS, Guy JT, Hawley P, et al.: Hematoporphyrin derivative and photoradiation therapy of malignant tumors. Lasers in Surg and Med, 3:199–209, 1983.
27. Doiron DR, Svaasand LO, Profio AE: Light dosimetry in tissue: application to photoradiation therapy. In: Porphyrin Photosensitization, vol 160; Kessel D and Dougherty TJ (eds). New York: Plenum, 1983.
28. Gregorie HB, Horger EO, Ward JL, Green JF, et al.: Hematoporphyrin derivative flourescence in malignant neoplasms. Ann Surg 167:820–827, 1968.
29. Winkelman J, Rasmussen–Taxdal DS: Quantitative determination of porphyrin uptake by tumor tissue following parenteral administration. Bull Johns Hopkins Hosp, 107:228–233, 1960.
30. Gomer CJ, Dougherty TJ: Determination of (3H) and (14C) hematoporphyrin derivative distribution in malignant and normal tissue. Cancer Res 39:146–151, 1979.
31. Bugelski PJ, Porter CW, Dougherty TJ: Autoradiographic distribution of hematoporphyrin derivative in normal and tumor tissue of the mouse. Cancer Res 41:4606–4612, 1981.
32. Johnson LV, Walsh ML, Chen LB: Localization of mitochondria in living cells with rhodamine–123. Proc Natl Acad Sci USA 77:990–994, 1980.
33. Summerhayes IC, Lampidis TJ, Bernal SD, et al.: Unusual retention of rhodamine–123 by mitochondria in muscle and carcinoma cells. Proc Natl Acad Sci USA, 79:5292–5296, 1982.
34. Bernal SC, Lampidis TJ, McIsaac RM: Anticarcinoma activity in vitro of rhodamine–123, a mitochondrial-specific dye. Science 222:169–172, 1983.
35. Castro DJ, Saxton RE, Fetterman HR, et al.: Rhodamine–123 as a new photochemosensitizing agent with the argon laser: 'Non-thermal' and thermal effects on human squamous carcinoma cells in vitro. Laryngoscope 97:554–561, 1987.
36. Marchesini R, Melloni E, Dasdia T, et al.: Photosensitizing properties of rhodamine–123 on different human tumor cell lines. Laser Surg Med 6(2):163, 1986.

37. Van Lier JE, Brasseur N, Ali H, et al.: Sulfonated metallo phthalocyanines: new agents for photodynamic therapy. Lasers Surg Med 6:230–231, 1986 (abstract).
38. Straight RC, Spikes JD, et al.: Phthalocyanine dyes as photodynamic sensitizers in vivo: localization, retention and phototoxicity in a mouse tumor model. Photochem Photobiol, 43(suppl):63S, 1986 (abstract).
39. Sacchini V, Melloni E, Marchesini R, et al.: Topical administration of tetrasodium–meso–tetraphenyl–porphinesulfonate (TPPS) and red light irradiation for the treatment of superficial neoplastic lesions. Tumori 73:19–23, 1987.
40. Jori G, Reddi E, Romandini P, et al.: Studies of the possible utilization of tetra–(4–sulfonatophenyl) porphine in the photodynamic therapy of tumors. Lasers Surg Med 6:231, 1986 (abstract).
41. Oseroff AR, Ohuoha D, Ara G, et al.: Selective photochemotherapy of melanoma and human squamous cell carcinoma using cationic photosensitizers. J Invest Dermatol, 88:510, 1987 (abstract).
42. Kessel D, Thompson P: Photosensitization of leukemia L1210 cells with diaziquone. Cancer Res 46:5587–5588, 1986.
43. Wang MX, Huo LM, Yang HC, et al.: An experimental study of the photodynamic activity of berberine in vitro of cancer cells. J Tradit Chin Med 6:125–127, 1986.
44. Oseroff AR, Ohuoha D, Ara G, et al.: Intramitochondrial dyes allow selective in vitro photolysis of carcinoma cells. Proc Natl Acad Sci USA 83:9729–9733, 1986.
45. Cheng LS, Wang JZ: Photodamage in human erythrocyte membranes, induced by new photosensitizer hypocrellin A. Shin Yen Sheng Wu Hsueh Pao 18:89–97, 1985.
46. Firey PA, Rodgers MAJ: Photo–properties of a silicon naphthalocyanine: a potential photosensitizer for photodynamic therapy. Photochem Photobiol 45:535–538, 1987.
47. Aramendia PF, Redmond RW, Nonell S, et al.: The photophysical properties of porphycenes: potential photodynamic therapy agents. Photochem Photobiol 44:555–559, 1986.
48. Bellnier DA, Lin LW, Parrish JA: Hematoporphyrin derivative and pulse laser photoradiation, prophyrin localization and treatment of tumors. New York: Alan R Liss, pp 533–540, 1984.
49. Weishaupt KR, Gomer CJ, Dougherty TJ: Identification of singlet oxygen as the cytotoxic agent in photoactivation of a murine tumor. Cancer Res 36:2326–2329, 1976.
50. Grossweiner LI, Goyal GG, Richard P: Effects of aggregation and sensitizer binding on liposome membrane photosensitization by hematoporphyrin and hematoporphyrin derivative. (Abstracts) Am Soc Photobiol, p 91, 1982.
51. Waldow SM, Henderson BW, Dougherty TJ: Potentiation of phototherapy by heat. Lasers in Surg and Med 5:83–99, 1985.
52. Benson RC: The Use of hematoporphyrin derivative (HPD) in the localization and treatment of transitional cell carcinoma of the bladder: Porphyrin Localization and Treatment of Tumors. New York: Alan R Liss, pp 795–804, 1984.
53. Forbes I, Cowled A, Leong AS–Y, et al.: Phototherapy of human tumors using hematoporphyrin derivative. Med J Aust 2:489–493, 1980.
54. Kennedy J: HPD photoradiation therapy for cancer at Kingston and Hamilton: porphyrin photosensitization. Kessel D, Dougherty TJ (eds) New York/London: Plenum, 1983.
55. Tokuda Y: Primary skin cancer, lasers and hematoporphyrin derivative in cancer Hayata Y, Dougherty TJ, Igaku-Sloin, (eds) (Tokyo/New York): pp 88, 1983.
56. Wile AG, Dahlman A, Burns RG: Laser photoradiation therapy of cancer following hematoporphyrin sensitization. Lasers in Surg Med 2:163–168, 1982.
57. Tomio L, Calzavara F, Zorat PL, et al.: Photoradiation therapy for cutaneous and subcutaneous malignant tumors using hematoporphyrin: porphyrin localization and treatment of tumors. New York: Alan R Liss, pp 829–840, 1984.
58. Hayata Y, Kato H, Konaka, et al.: Fiberoptic bronchoscopic laser photoradiation for tumor localization in lung cancer. Chest 82:10–14, 1982.
59. Hayata Y, Kato H, Hememiya R, et al.: Indications for photoradiation therapy in early

stage lung cancer on the basis of post–PRT histological findings: porphyrin localization and treatment of tumors. New York: Alan R Liss, pp 747–758, 1984.
60. Balchum O, Doiron DR, Huth G: HPD photodynamic therapy for obstructing lung cancer: porphyrin localization and treatment of tumors. New York: AR Liss, pp 727–745, 1984.
61. Aida M, Hirashima T: Cancer of the esophagus: lasers and hematoporphyrin derivative in cancer Hayata Y, Dougherty TJ (eds). Tokyo/New York: Igaku–Shoin, pp 57–64, 1983
62. Aida M, Kawaguchi M: Gastric cancer, lasers and hematoporphyrin derivative in cancer; Hayata Y, Dougherty TJ (eds). Tokyo/New York: Igaku-Shoin, pp 65–69, 1983.
63. McCaughan JS: Photoradiation of malignant tumors presensitized with hematoporphyrin derivative. In: Porphyrin Localization and Treatment of Tumors. New York: Alan R Liss, pp 805–827, 1984.
64. Hiazumi H, Misaki T, Miyoshi N: Photodynamic therapy of bladder tumors, lasers and hematoporphyrin derivative in cancer Y Hayata, TJ Dougherty (eds.) Tokyo/New York: Igaku–Sloin, pp 85–87, 1983.
65. Ward BG, Forbes IJ, Wowled PA, et al.: The treatment of vaginal recurrences of gynecologic malignancy with phototherapy following hematoporphyrin derivative treatment. Am J Obstet Gynecol 142:(3)356–357, 1982.
66. Soma H, Akiya K, Nutahara S, et al.: Treatment of vaginal carcinoma with laser photoradiation following administration of hematoporphyrin derivative. Report of a Case. Ann Chirvrgiae Gynaecologiae 71:133–136, 1982.
67. Rettenmaier M, Berman M, DiSaia P, et al.: Photoradiation therapy in gynecology. Porphyrin Localization and Treatment of Tumors. DR Doiron (ed) New York: Alan R Liss, 1984.
68. McCulloch GA, Forbes IJ, Lee See K, et al.: Phototherapy in malignant brain tumors. Porphyrin Localization and Treatment of Tumors. New York: Alan R Liss, pp 709–717, 1984.
69. Bruce RA: Photoradiation of choroidal malignant melanoma. Porphyrin localization and treatment of tumors. New York: Alan R Liss, pp 777–784, 1984.
70. Dahlman A, Wile AG, Burns RG, et al.: Laser photoradiation therapy of cancer. Cancer Research 43:430–434, 1983.
71. Schuller DE, McCaughn JS, Rock RP: Photoradiation in head and neck cancer. Arch Otolaryngol 3:351–355, 1985.
72. Wile AG, Novotny J, Mason GR: Photoradiation therapy of head and neck cancer. Am J Clin Oncol 6:39–63, 1984.
73. Keller GS, Doiron DJ: Photodynamic therapy in otolaryngology/head and neck surgery. Presented at the course on PDT at Western Institute for Laser Treatment, Oct 1984.
74. Gluckman JL, Waner M, Shumrick K, et al.: Photodynamic therapy. A viable alternative to conventional therapy for early lesions of the upper aerodigestive tract. Arch Otol Head and Neck Surg 112:949–952, 1986.
75. Gluckman JL, Weissler MC: Role of photodynamic therapy in the management of early cancers of the upper aerodigestive tract. Laser in Med Science 1:217–219, 1986.
76. Gluckman JL, Crissman JD, Donegan JO: Multicentric squamous cell carcinoma of the upper aerodigestive tract. Head and Neck Surg, pp 90–96, 1980.
77. Gluckman JL, Crissman JD: Survival rates in 548 patients with multiple primary neoplasms of the upper aerodigestive tract. Laryngoscope 93:(1)71–74, (Jan.) 1983.
78. Gluckman JL: Synchronous multiple primaries of the upper aero–digestive system. Arch of Otolaryngology 105:597–598, 1979.
79. Profio EA, Doiron DR: A feasibility study for the use of fluorescence bronchoscopy for localization of small lung tumors. Phys Med Biol 22(5):949–957, 1977.
80. Doiron DR, Profio E, Vincent RG, et al.: Fluorescence bronchoscopy for the detection of lung cancer. Chest 76:(1)27–32, 1979.
81. Kinsey TH, Cortese DA, Sanderson DR: Detection of hematoporphyrin fluorescence during fiberoptic endoscopy to localize early bronchogenic carcinoma. Mayo Clin Proc 53:594, 1978.

II

Rehabilitation

8. Mechanisms for Vocal Communication Following Total Laryngectomy

Michael D. Trudeau and David E. Schuller

Effective speech relies on the successful coordination of four motor processes: respiration, phonation, resonation and articulation. Impairment of any of these processes results in decrements in the intelligibility and/or prosody of speech. The obvious communicative sequela to total laryngectomy is aphonia, arising not simply from loss of the phonatory organ, but as well from diversion of respiratory flow (the power source for speech) from the vocal tract. Rehabilitation of speech rests, therefore, on identifying a secondary source of phonation and a means of energizing that source into vibration.

Solutions to these twin problems are best achieved in an interdisciplinary team context. The alaryngeal population is hardly heterogeneous, even with respect to surgery. Various and diverse factors bear on the selection of the optimal means of restoration for any given patient. Among these factors are extent of surgery; the scheduling of nonsurgical treatment, for example, preoperative or postoperative radiation; selection for tracheoesophageal puncture and its timing, that is, concurrent with or subsequent to the laryngectomy; the degree to which the patient can participate in the rehabilitation program; and premorbid patient characteristics, for example, intelligence or drug abuse. The interdisciplinary team must determine the suitability and modifiability of a given method of speech restoration for the individual patient and the patient's communicative needs. Following this determination, the team must implement the rehabilitation plan. In the ideal case, implementation should occur before the total laryngectomy.

This chapter will describe the contributions of the interdisciplinary team members and the three methods of alaryngeal speech restoration with the advantages and limitations of each. Given the long history and available literature concerning speech with artificial devices and esophageal speech, particular emphasis will be given to the more recent advances in surgical–prosthetic voice restoration.

Jacobs, C. (ed): Carcinomas of the Head and Neck: Evaluation and Management.

Interdisciplinary Management

The term 'interdisciplinary' oftentimes is over exploited and currently represents a popular catchword in medicine. The optimal approach to voice rehabilitation, however, truly requires a collaborative, coordinated effort, which allows for the team to utilize the specific skills of the individual team members. The otolaryngologist–head and neck surgeon clearly has a certain realm of expertise not within the domain of the speech pathologist and vice versa. The establishment of an interdisciplinary group enhances not only patient care, but facilitates investigational and educational activities as well. The interdisciplinary voice rehabilitation program at The Ohio State University has been active for the past ten years.

Team management begins in the preoperative period with an emphasis on patient and family education. Information about voice rehabilitation serves to focus the patient beyond the immediate threats of the cancer and major surgery to the prospects of recovery. This decreases patient anxiety and hesitancy about treatment. While the surgeon typically makes the initial contact with the patients, both otolaryngology and speech pathology have special areas of knowledge helpful to the patients. Patients appreciate the opportunity to hear from both professions, particularly when both are present simultaneously. This also fosters the patient's perspective that rehabilitation is a team effort, not the result of isolated individuals. The initial contact by nursing staff is important in this period. Much of the communication between nurse and patient simply reinforces the facts already imparted. Although the patient is not yet prepared for training in the areas of stomal hygiene, diet, or postsurgical activity level, early contact with nursing establishes a ready route for subsequent training and education, as well as reassuring the patient through acquaintanceship with caregivers.

The scope of information provided presurgically is broad, touching on the probable plan of surgery and treatment, the major events of the in–hospital recovery period, possible alterations in lifestyle, and methods of speech rehabilitation. With such a sweeping scope, the depth of information is necessarily limited. Many patients will deluge the team with questions. There are times, however, when the anxiety over the diagnosis of cancer so thoroughly overwhelms the patients that they are unable to focus on the information: the patient's preoccupation with the cancer and its treatment prevents effective education. In this instance, the amount of information provided is contracted, and more extensive postoperative education is planned.

One member of the team should be delegated the responsibility to arrange a visit from a trained laryngectomee visitor. The physical presence of a person with successfully restored speech provides some substance to the patient's education and allows for a clearer perception of the potential for recovery. Training of these visitors is provided through the affiliated chapters of the International Association of Laryngectomees. The American

Cancer Society (ACS) coordinates the activities of these chapters, and arrangements can be made through local ACS units. Timing of this visit or visits depends on the patient's receptivity. Patients can benefit from receiving both a preoperative and a postoperative visit, and from involvement in a local chapter. Due regard must be made to each patient's ability to cope with the diagnosis of cancer. Consequent delay in the visit to the postoperative period may be in some patients' best interests.

Tracheoesophageal Speech

Traditionally alaryngeal speech rehabilitation has been divided into preoperative and post–operative stages. For patient training such a dichotomy holds true; nevertheless, the surgeon can do much to assure the success of the rehabilitation program during the course of the laryngectomy. Much has been made of pharyngoesophageal spasm and associated pharyngeal constrictor myotomy as an adjunct to tracheoesophageal puncture for voice restoration [1–4]. While some disagreement may remain over the need for myotomy, the critical issue is whether or not opposition of the p–e segment to air flow is a legitimate concern in planning vocal rehabilitation. Fluent speakers (that is, speakers able to produce multisyllabic, connected speech without inappropriate pauses) appear to require lower esophageal pressures to produce speech (#14 mm Hg) than do nonfluent speakers (3 15 mm Hg), and tracheoesophageal (TE) voicing is not achieved by individuals where intra–esophageal pressures raise above 20 mm Hg [5]. The otolaryngologist–head and neck surgeon must make some provision for controlling for p–e segment opposition to air flow if TE or esophageal speech are to be rehabilitative options.

The participants in this interdisciplinary program continue to be strongly enthusiastic about primary vocal rehabilitation. The creation of the tracheoesophageal fistula is performed after the larynx has been resected and frozen sections of the margins confirm that the cancer resection has been complete. Prior to closing the hypopharyngeal defect created by the total laryngectomy, the surgeon inserts a right angle hemostat through the hypopharyngeal defect into the cervical esophagus. The tip of the hemostat is used to indent the posterior tracheal wall in the midline at a point usually four to five millimeters below the mucocutaneous junction of the tracheal wall and the neck skin following closure. This location can be modified for a number of reasons, such as partial resection of the upper trachea with the laryngectomy or flap reconstruction of the defect. The assistant incises the tracheal mucosa over the tip with an incision for only three or four millimeters. The tip of the hemostat pushes the esophageal mucosa into this incision. An even smaller opening is made in the esophageal mucosa which permits the hemostat tip to be exposed through the opening in the posterior tracheal wall. The end of a #14 French red rubber catheter is grasped with the hemostat by opening the hemostat just wide enough to grab the red rubber catheter. These incisions are made as small as possible to create a tight fistula in order to prevent aspiration via the fistula. The catheter is then drawn through the TE fistula and into the hypopharyngeal defect. It is pulled through the fistula until just the end of the red rubber catheter is showing at the tracheal end of the fistula. A toothless forceps is used to direct the catheter inferiorly into the esophagus for the entire length of the catheter. The catheter is then sutured in the position to stabilize it, and the end is occluded with an umbilical clamp to prevent drainage of gastric contents into the surgical wound. The total time for creation of the tracheoesophageal fistula and stabilization of the catheter is usually no more than five minutes. The hypopharyngeal defect is closed and the operation is completed.

The immediate postoperative routine involves tube feeding for approximately one week. The placement of the catheter at time of the laryngectomy allows feeding through this tube and precludes the need for a nasogastric tube [6]. This affords the patient greater comfort and, with its larger diameter, provides the nursing staff with greater ease in feeding the patient. Assuming an uncomplicated recovery, seven days following the surgery the patient begins feeding by mouth and is discharged one day later. At discharge the red rubber catheter continues to occupy the fistula.

The surgeon, nursing staff, and speech pathologist in their contacts with the patient reinforce the need to retain this tube in the fistula to prevent aspiration and to maintain patency of the fistula. Although the catheter is secured by sutures, the patients are instructed in how to reinsert the catheter should it become dislodged and to return to the hospital immediately in the event they cannot reinsert the tube. This training directly parallels the training the patients will receive in care and use of the voice prosthesis and, therefore, facilitates this subsequent training and serves to involve the patients in their rehabilitation in the initial stages of recovery.

Early in our experience we replaced the catheter with the voice prosthesis prior to discharge, at about the eighth postoperative day. It was not unusual for patients to achieve some voicing. This certainly had a tremendous psychological benefit for the patients. One patient, however, developed a pharyngocutaneous fistula in the twelfth postoperative day, after beginning voice therapy four days prior. As we could not eliminate the increased intra–esophageal and pharyngeal pressure associated with use of the voice prosthesis as contributory to the development of the delayed fistula, we modified our approach so that fitting of the voice prosthesis occurs immediately following the patient's first postoperative follow–up examination with the surgeon. Fitting of the prosthesis and patient training occur in the Otolaryngology Clinic under the supervision of the speech pathologist. This setting promotes confidence on the patient's part, facilitates communication among the patient, surgeon and speech pathologist, and insures a rapid response to any unforeseen difficulties which may arise.

There are four goals at this stage of rehabilitation: first, to review previous patient education, including the rehabilitation options of esophageal and electrolaryngeal speech; second, to select the proper type and length of voice prosthesis; third, to train the patient in independent care of the prosthesis; and fourth, to train the patient in producing speech of the highest possible quality. Typically the first three goals may be met in one session. Progression through the goals is dependent upon the patient's capabilities at the time. Sometimes the goal is merely to have the patient feel comfortable with the mechanics of caring for the prosthesis. There are those patients who are so challenged by learning how to insert, clean, and reinsert the prosthesis, that they are not capable of comprehending the mechanics of voicing within the initial session. At other times, the speech pathologist will proceed onto voicing and speech instruction. Even when connected, and fluent speech is established in this first session, patients cannot attain optimal vocal quality and speech intelligibility without some additional voice therapy. Frequency of additional therapy sessions is determined by the speed with which the patient learns care and use of the prosthesis and improves speaking skills. Patients who are progressing more slowly through the rehabilitation program require more intensive therapy both to facilitate vocal communication and to insure proper care of the prosthesis and protection against aspiration. When possible, speech therapy is conducted at the Otolaryngology Clinic. If need be, referrals are made to resources in the patients' communities. Even when voice therapy is completed, the speech pathologist makes contact with the patient during at least the first postoperative year's follow–up visits with the otolaryngologist–head and neck surgeon. This contact allows for close monitoring of the patient to insure that a pattern of adequate prosthesis care is followed, that recently learned speech skills are stabilized, and that appropriate referrals for other services, for example social work, may be initiated as needed.

Long–term rehabilitation involves an evaluation by the speech pathologist at a frequency that is dictated by the individual patient's needs. The ability to have close interdisciplinary cooperation enhances the early detection of problems that can be encountered in those patients who have had previous voice rehabilitation. The most common long–term challenge centers on salivary drainage around or through a prosthesis. Drainage through the device indicates either that the valve is worn and the device requires replacement or that the device no longer fits the patient properly. Either problem may be rapidly resolved by the speech pathologist. Drainage around the prosthesis, which occurs rarely, indicates dilation of the TE fistula. This dilation may be due to factors such as improperly fitting prosthesis, or loss of tissue elasticity due to radiation therapy, etc. Because the vast majority of our patients use prostheses which are 16 Fr in diameter, it is tempting to solve the drainage around the device by resorting to a larger diameter prosthesis (20 Fr). This is never our first choice, however, as if it does not prove a satisfactory solution, it results in a larger fistula with inherently greater possibility for aspiration. We first determine if a change in prosthesis design or fitting will solve the problem. Next, we attempt to promote stenosis of the TE fistula by stenting with a 14 Fr catheter for 48 hours. If these approaches are unsuccessful, a larger diameter prosthesis may be advisable in that other solutions will involve some form of surgical intervention. The surgery may range from relatively minor approaches, such as cautery, to total closure of the fistula followed by creation of a new fistula.

Modern approaches to tracheoesophageal speech represent the successful culmination of years of failed attempts to restore speech through the surgical reconnection of the pulmonary system with the speech mechanism [7]. While the vibratory body varied in these early procedures, the power source remained the pulmonary air stream, which was diverted into the esophagus or hypopharynx. In reconnecting the airway with the digestive tract, these early methods of voice restoration solved the problems of power source and vibratory body, but simultaneously created a new problem in that aspiration of food or fluid was again possible. Successful restoration procedures required solutions to the three problems of power source, vibratory body, and prevention of aspiration. Until 1980 these problems proved intractable. These early attempts can be categorized as surgical methods which used body tissues to create valved or unvalved shunts to divert the air stream and protect the airway, or as surgical–prosthetic methods which merged the use of prostheses with surgical technique to accomplish diversion and protection. In the main, body tissue proved inadequate to the task, and prostheses were either ineffective or cumbersome.

This latter point is important in assessing the merit of surgical or surgical–prosthetic methods of voice restoration. In that electrolaryngeal and esophageal speech already pose viable options in vocal rehabilitation, any emerging method should produce speech at least as adequate as speech attainable by existing methods. The emerging method should pose negligible surgical and long–term health risks, including the risk of aspiration. Finally, the method must be relatively easy for the patient to utilize and maintain. Singer and Blom [8] and Panje [9], in introducing their respective procedures and prostheses, proposed that TE speech could meet the above criteria.

In intelligibility of speech, proficient use of an artificial larynges appears to pose an advantage over esophageal or TE speech [10]. This advantage probably derives in part from the consistency of the signal which lacks the wide fluctuations in fundamental frequency and intensity found in esophageal and TE speech [11,12]. This same consistency, however, also contributes to the mechanical quality associated with this vocal mode. Esophageal and TE speech have been shown to be distinct from each other acoustically [13,14], with TE speech subject to different influences of aerodynamic and myoelastic control [15]. Some investigators have speculated that TE speech, by virtue of its pulmonary driving force, would be more similar to laryngeal speech than is esophageal. In the acoustical sense,

TE speech has been shown to be distinct not only from esophageal speech, but from laryngeal speech as well [13]. In the perceptual sense, when speaker proficiency is commensurate, listeners evaluate TE speech as equivalent to esophageal speech in acceptability or pleasantness [14,16]. Thus, the literature indicates that TE speech is different from, but not necessarily superior or inferior to electrolaryngeal or esophageal speech.

With respect to TE puncture (TEP) procedures, the issues of patient care and use and of potential health risks posed by the procedures tend to be closely associated. Failure in proper care of the prosthesis often leads to health problems, for example, aspiration via the fistula or the need for a second surgical procedure to reopen the fistula. Patients who care adequately for the prosthesis can typically make the next step and use the prosthesis to produce speech. The major exception is that patient whose family or significant others assist substantially in prosthesis care. A case in point was a patient with Parkinson's disease and moderate to severe hearing loss whose spouse and daughter accomplished all stoma hygiene and prosthesis care. The patient was noncompliant in following treatment for the Parkinson's disease and in use of amplification for his hearing loss. Although able to produce at least 30 syllables on one intake of air, this patient had great difficulty in consistently and effectively occluding the stoma. This appeared to be due not so much to the motor deficit of the Parkinson's disease as to his inability for auditory monitoring of air leakage around the stoma associated with his refusal to turn on his hearing aid. He eventually abandoned TE speech in favor of electrolaryngeal speech, which he felt he could hear better.

In reviewing 108 cases of surgical–prosthetic voice restoration, 96 with the Singer–Blom procedure, the authors found little indication that TEP presented patients with any increased threat to health in either the long or short–term, or that completion of the TEP at the time of laryngectomy presented any increased risk of complications [17]. This finding was congruent with the success reported by others in supporting primary TEP [6,18–22]. Over the eight year span of our study, no patient developed aspiration pneumonia, indicating the success of the TEP procedure with prosthesis in preventing leakage of esophageal contents into the trachea.

Based on the results of the case review, eight of ten patients with TEP will produce connected TE speech. This estimate is conservative for patients with secondary TEP and is liberal for patients with primary TEP. The factors most affecting both groups' success in using TE speech were patient health and, particularly, recurrence of the disease. Patients who remained healthy enough to care for their prostheses and to participate in voice therapy were highly likely (on the order of nine of ten) to develop useful TE speech. These 80% and 90% success rates indicate that some patients cannot utilize TE speech; however, these proportions compare favorably with the 70% success rate found in esophageal speech.

Other factors have been identified as negative prognostic indicators of successful TE voice restoration [23–25]. These include difficulty in receiving follow–up therapy, drug or alcohol abuse, poor manual dexterity, or limited intellectual capacity. While the presence of such conditions is certainly deleterious to successful TE voice rehabilitation, these conditions are deleterious to all three forms of voice rehabilitation. The alcoholic patient is a poor candidate for any rehabilitation program. Many such patients with the aforementioned negative prognostic indicators will fail to achieve TE, esophageal and electrolaryngeal speech, but not all such patients will fail. We contend that if these patients are to succeed in regaining vocal communication, they require that the maximum number of options be available to them to promote the maximum flexibility in therapeutic planning. They also require incorporation into the interdisciplinary team of social workers, other trained counselors, physical therapists, and occupational therapists to meet their diverse needs.

A major consideration in evaluating the potential health risks associated with TEP is its compatibility with sound oncologic practice. Although the authors favor primary TEP, the procedure as originally described by Singer and Blom was designed to occur post–laryngectomy and to require no modification in the surgery which might interfere with tumor removal. Our experience has been that TEP is a viable technique even for those patients with large tumors which necessitate wide neck dissection and pectoralis flap reconstruction. These patients may require prolonged use of tracheostoma vents to stent the airway because the cartilaginous support of the trachea may not extend to the stoma. This complication need not obviate use of a voice prosthesis. Our practice has been to utilize a separate vent and voice prosthesis, as our experience with devices which incorporate both a vent and a voice prosthesis has been unsatisfactory due to irritation of the airway or dilation of the fistula. A lumen is created in the vent at the site of the TE fistula. This permits the voice prosthesis to protrude slightly into the vented airway, allowing easy movement of air into the prosthesis and subsequently into the esophagus. The use of the vent may actually yield better TE speech for these patients because they frequently have irregularly shaped stomas and the vent presents a more uniform surface for stomal occlusion.

In our series of patients with TEP, 51 of 101 patients received radiation therapy. In the short–term, the effects of this treatment often result in the inability to produce voice using the p–e segment. In these cases we encourage use of an intraoral electrolarynx. The effects of the radiotherapy on voice generally fade with time so that TE speech returns within six months of the termination of the radiation treatments. In the long–term, radiotherapy appears to pose no increase in TEP–related complications such as stomal stenosis, accidental extrusion of the voice prosthesis, or leakage and aspiration due to dilation of the TE fistula.

A final consideration in evaluating the merit of TEP is the acceptance of the procedure by those who use it. Based on the responses of 41 respondents to a survey of the 76 surviving patients with TEP from our case load

[26], we found the most common complaint of these patients was difficulty in swallowing (11 patients), a problem more likely associated with the laryngectomy than with the voice prosthesis. The second most common problem reported was leakage around or through the prosthesis (8 patients). Only two of the patients noted this as a chronic condition; the remainder reported it as intermittent. While intermittent leakage is undesirable for the patients, it is an almost unavoidable consequence of prosthesis. Food particles lodging in the valve, failure to clean the prosthesis properly, and eventual deterioration of the prosthesis will allow leakage through the device. This leakage is easily rectified by cleaning or replacing the prosthesis and should pose no long–term inconvenience or health threat to the patient.

Wetmore, et al. [27] noted that patients who had more recently undergone TEP were more likely to be continuing to use the device. A similar trend appeared in our survey, where 91% of the patients less than 18 months after surgery reported using TE speech as opposed to 37.5% of those patients four to eight years post surgery. Wetmore, et al. [27] attributed their results to improved prostheses, better patient selection and to team management. We concur with these factors; yet we remain unconvinced that they totally account for the differences found in our survey. Sampling bias may be a factor, especially for the patients in the long–term group. Patients four to eight years after surgery typically have little contact with their surgeon or speech pathologist. Those who responded to the survey may have disproportionately represented those with problems or complaints. Another possible explanation is that early exposure to all three forms of alaryngeal speech rehabilitation allows the patients to proceed with training in more than one form of speech. Our patients receive primary TEP and training with electrolarynges while recovering in the hospital. Patients who wish to attempt esophageal speech are enrolled in therapy. They, therefore, are experienced with two and sometimes three forms of speech and have the opportunity to select which form meets their needs most effectively. It may be that in restoring speech early in recovery through TEP, the interdisciplinary team provides the patients with the opportunity to develop proficiency in other forms of alaryngeal speech, which they ultimately elect to use. While this issue is unclear, it is apparent that TE speech is a viable form of speech restoration, that it allows an early return of speech, that it has a high success rate and a relatively low rate of complications.

Artificial Devices

Although often termed artificial or electro 'larynges', such nomenclature is misleading as these devices serve none of the valving or protective functions of the larynx, but provide only a source of phonation through an external sound source. Two mechanisms of vibration are common, electromechanical and vibrating reed, with the former more in evidence in this country than the latter. In either case, body tissue is not utilized for vibration. Typically the sound is produced externally to the body and must be transmitted into the vocal tract.

The primary advantage of artificial devices lies in the speed with which patients may use these. Training is rapid, on average requiring considerably less time to develop intelligible speech than occurs with esophageal speech training [28,29]. Patients may begin using an artificial device prior to hospital discharge, well before entry into esophageal voice therapy or before the patient is ready to receive or use a voice prosthesis.

For most patients the vibration is transmitted through the tissues of the neck into the resonating cavities of the vocal tract by placing the vibrating surface in close contact with the upper neck. This variety of device is often termed 'neck-held'. A second means for delivering the 'voice' to the vocal tract is to convey it to the oral cavity via a short tube. Although only the tip of the tube enters the oral cavity by the mouth, this device is referred to as 'intraoral'. There are a variety of both such devices available, and several different samples should be available for patient demonstrations and training [30].

The major advantage of placement of the vibrating surface on the neck is the lack of interference between the articulators and the voicing source. Positioning the tube within the oral cavity can hamper articulation and, thereby, reduce intelligibility. Similarly, movement of the jaw and tongue during articulation can disturb placement of or occlude the tube leading to loss of voice and reduced intelligibility.

For many patients neck placement is not effective because the remaining tissues conduct sound poorly due to alterations inherent in the surgery, in radiotherapy, or in recurrence of the cancer. The neck–held device is also unacceptable in the immediate post–laryngectomy period while sutures and staples are still in place. The battery–powered intraoral devices possess none of these limitations and, therefore, offer a rapid return to speech for most patients and the only viable rehabilitative option for some patients.

All neck–held devices and the majority of the intraoral devices are electromechanical; the intraoral type, however, may utilize a pneumatically driven vibrating reed. The power source is the patient's expired air. These devices consist of a bell–shaped cover for the stoma which diverts air flow over a reed and then conveys the resultant tone to the oral cavity via a tube. Reports of speech with these instruments generally indicate better acoustical and perceptual quality than is obtained with electrically powered devices [31,32]. Despite superior quality, these devices are infrequently found in the United States perhaps due to an aversion to covering the airway [33] or for aesthetic reasons, since use of the device necessitates exposing the stoma.

An unfortunate bias against the artificial device may be found in the literature, suggesting that speech so produced is inferior in quality to other forms of alaryngeal speech [34], or that reliance on a device will somehow inhibit a patient from succeeding with some other more 'preferable' method of speech [35]. Due to its mechanical sound and the limited capacity (in some devices, the inability) to modulate pitch and loudness, the quality of speech achieved with the artificial device is inferior to laryngeal speech. Comparisons with other forms of alaryngeal speech, however, indicate no clear superiority for any form of vocal restoration [10,16,31,32,36–39]. The literature provides no evidence that use of artificial devices limits training in esophageal or tracheoesophageal speech. On the contrary, early return to speech via artificial devices may serve to promote increased proficiency with other forms of alaryngeal speech [40]. The present authors' position is that the preferred form of speech for laryngectomees is that form or forms which individual patients find most useful for meeting their communicative needs.

Esophageal Speech

Esophageal speech is so named because the speaker utilizes the esophagus as a pseudo–lung by which air is stored and released to energize the sphincter muscles at the boundary between the esophagus and the pharynx to produce voice. To achieve esophageal voice, the speaker must learn to contain air in the esophagus and to release it in a timely fashion. Although many individuals can eruct, very few appear able to use gastric air with adequate coordination to allow functional speech [41]. The successful esophageal speaker, therefore, must learn to trap sufficient air rapidly in the esophagus and to release it in a fashion compatible with the production of connected, intelligible speech. This method places large demands on the motor speech system to allow for normal articulation and resonation while simultaneously substituting the trapping/release of air in the esophagus for respiration and the vibration of the p–e segment for the action of the vocal folds.

The latter two processes entail new learning for the laryngectomee, and some time is required to master these. A realistic expectation is that effective speech will develop over a period of nine to twelve months [29]. Even after such a period of therapy, many patients leave speech therapy before they have attained optimal quality of speech.

In trapping esophageal air for voice, the speaker must create a pressure gradient with esophageal pressure negative to oropharyngeal pressure. Air as a fluid will move from areas of higher pressure to areas of lower pressure. This movement of air for esophageal containment and subsequent expulsion is accomplished in three manners: the inhalation method, the glossopharyngeal injection or tongue pumping method, and the plosive or consonant injection method. In the inhalation method, esophageal pressure parallels thoracic pressure. As the esophagus passes through the thorax, it is susceptible to the same pressure changes which draw air into or force air from the lungs. Assuming that the patient can voluntarily relax the p–e segment or that some iatrogenic flaccidity is present, then air may enter and leave the esophagus as part of the normal respiratory cycle. In the two injection methods, intraoral air is compressed and driven into the esophagus. Glossopharyngeal press corresponds to the compressive action of the tongue and pharynx in swallowing with the important difference that the air must be retained in the esophagus, not delivered to the stomach. In plosive injection, sometimes termed the 'Dutch method' for its thorough description by Damste' [42], the transient intraoral pressure peak characteristic of plosive consonants is exploited to impel air into the esophagus.

The question of which manner of air movement is preferable is moot. Each has advantages and limitations vis a vis the other two, but a consistent finding in the research is that the better speakers employ more than one method, often using all three in their speech [43]. Effective therapy should incorporate training in all three methods in order to offer the patient the greatest opportunity to develop the highest quality speech possible.

Several limitations to vocal rehabilitation with esophageal speech arise. As noted above, the therapeutic period may be extensive. Intelligibility of esophageal speech in noisy environments declines rapidly [10,44]. Two of the three methods of capturing air in the esophagus entail coordinated actions of structures in the vocal tract; however, these actions may be impaired by the cancer surgery. Gastric upset is not uncommon as air escapes the esophagus and enters the stomach [45]. Among the more drastic limitations to esophageal speech is that the recurrence of cancer can result in loss of voice [46]. For this reason, unexplained degradation of speaking skills should be viewed with suspicion. Finally, many laryngectomees seem unable to master esophageal speech. This may be due to psychological or physiological reasons [47]. Albeit there is some disagreement over the proportion of patients involved, an approximate figure would be that one in three laryngectomees fails to develop functional esophageal speech [48].

For decades esophageal speech was the preferred method for restoring vocal communication, advances in electronics or in surgical techniques only recently providing acceptable alternatives to esophageal speech. The most obvious advantage of this method is that it is entirely intrinsic to the speaker and requires no further modification of the speaker's anatomy or physiology than those changes already introduced by the surgery. Use of an artificial device or of tracheoesophageal speech often entails some form of manual movement which attracts attention to the disability and restricts manual dexterity for other tasks that may coincide with speech. For the patient who requires the use of both hands, either vocationally or avocationally, esophageal speech may be the method of choice.

Conclusion

In the end, the type of alaryngeal speech successfully used by a patient will be that type which the patient finds most compatible with the individual's lifestyle and needs. With three viable options for restoration of voice and speech, it should be the very rare patient who does not reachieve vocal communication. The close cooperation among the members of the interdisciplinary team serves to direct the patient is selecting speech via artificial devices, the esophageal or TE methods, to assist the patient in overcoming difficulties in rehabilitation, and to reestablish a satisfactory quality of life. The paramount outcome of the total laryngectomy should be patient survival with an acceptable, and in many cases, a relatively unimpaired quality of life.

References

1. Chodosh P, Giancoarlo H, Goldstein J: Pharyngeal myotomy for vocal rehabilitation postlaryngectomy. Laryngoscope 94:52–57, 1984.
2. McGarvey S, Weinberg B. Esophageal insufflation testing in nonlaryngectomized adults. Journal of Speech and Hearing Disorders 49:272–277, 1984.
3. Singer MI, Blom ED, Hamaker RC: Further experience with voice restoration after total laryngectomy. Annals of Otology, Rhinology, and Laryngology 90:498–502, 1981.
4. Singer MI, Blom ED, Hamaker RC: Pharyngeal plexus neurectomy for alaryngeal speech rehabilitation. Laryngoscope 96:50–53, 1986.
5. Lewin JS, Baugh RF, Baker S: An objective method for prediction of tracheoesophageal speech production. Journal of Speech and Hearing Disorders, 52:212–217, 1987.
6. Shagets FW, Panje WR: Primary tracheoesophageal fistula formation for feeding and voice restoration. Laryngoscope 95:1001–1003, 1985.
7. Singer MI: Vocal rehabilitation after total laryngectomy. Laryngoscope, 93:1454–1465, 1983.
8. Singer MI, Blom ED: An endoscopic technique for restoration of voice after laryngectomy. Annals of Otology, Rhinology, and Laryngololgy 89:529–533, 1980.
9. Panje WR: Prosthetic vocal rehabilitation following laryngectomy: The voice button. Annals of Otology, Rhinology, and Laryngology 90:116–120, 1981.
10. Clark JG, Stemple JC: Assessment of three modes of alaryngeal speech with a synthetic sentence identification task (SSI) in varying message-to-competition ratios. Journal of Speech and Hearing Research 25:333–338, 1982.
11. Robbins J, Fisher H, Blom E, Singer M: A comparative acoustic study of normal, esophageal, and tracheoesophageal speech production. Journal of Speech and Hearing Disorders 49:202–210, 1984.
12. Baggs T, Pine S: Acoustic characteristics: tracheoesophageal speech. Journal of Communication Disorders 16:299–307, 1983.
13. Robbins J: Acoustic differentiation of laryngeal, esophageal, and tracheoesophageal speech. Journal of Speech and Hearing Research 27:577–585, 1984.
14. Sedory SE, Hamlet SL, Connor NP: Comparisons of perceptual and acoustic characteristics of tracheoesophageal and excellent esophageal speech. Journal of Speech and Hearing Disorders 54:209–214, 1989.
15. Moon JB, Weinberg B: Aerodynamic and myoelastic contributions to tracheoesophageal voice production. Journal of Speech and Hearing Research 30:387–395, 1987.
16. Trudeau MD: A comparison of the speech acceptability of good and excellent esophageal and tracheoesophageal speakers. Journal of Comunication Disorders 20:111–119, 1987.
17. Trudeau MD, Schuller DE, Hall DA: The timing of tracheoesophageal puncture for voice restoration: primary vs. secondary. Head & Neck Surgery, Supplement II, S130–134, 1988.
18. Hamaker RC, Singer MI, Blom ED, Daniels HA: Primary voice restoration and laryngectomy. Archives of Otolaryngology–Head Neck Surgery 111:182–186, 1985.

19. Maves MD, Lingeman RE: Primary vocal rehabilitation using the Blom–Singer and Panje voice prostheses. Annals of Otology, Rhinology and Laryngology, 91T, 458–460, 1982.
20. Stiernberg CM, Bailey BF, Calhoun KH, Perex DG: Primary tracheoesophageal fistula procedure for voice restoration: The University of Texas branch experience. Laryngoscope 97:820–824, 1987.
21. Trudeau MD, Hirsch SM, Schuller DE: Vocal restorative surgery: why wait? Laryngoscope 96:975–977, 1986.
22. Wenig BL, Mullooly V, Levy J, Abramson AL: Voice restoration following laryngectomy: the role of primary vs. secondary tracheoesophageal puncture. Annals of Otology, Rhinology, and Laryngology 98:70–73, 1989.
23. Bosone Z: Tracheoesophageal fistulization for voice restoration: presurgical considerations and trouble–shooting procedures. In: Laryngectomee Rehabilitation, Second Edition, F Darley and R Keith (eds). San Diego: College–Hill Press, 1986.
24. Schuller DE, Jarrow JE, Kelly DR, et al.: Prognostic factors affecting the success of duckbill vocal restoration. Otolaryngology–Head Neck Surgery 91:396–398, 1983.
25. Silver FM, Gluckman JL, Donegan JO: Operative complications of tracheoesophageal puncture. Laryngoscope 95:1360–1362, 1985.
26. Hall DA: Complications Reported by Long–term Tracheoesophageal Speakers with the Singer–Blom TEP for Voice Restoration. Unpublished masters thesis, The Ohio State University, 1989.
27. Wetmore SJ, Kruger K, Wesson K, Blessing M: Long–term results of the Blom–Singer speech rehabilitation procedure. Archives of Otolaryngology 111:106–110, 1985.
28. Goldstein LP: The artificial larynx: pro and con. In: The Artificial Larynx Handbook, Salmon S and Goldstein L (eds). New York: Grune & Stratton, 1978.
29. Shanks JC: Developing esophageal communication. In: Laryngectomee Rehabilitation, Second Edition, Darley F and Keith R (eds). San Diego: College–Hill, 1986a.
30. Salmon SJ and Goldstein L: (eds). The Artificial Larynx Handbook, New York: Grune & Stratton, 1978.
31. Bennett S, Weinberg B: Acceptability ratings of normal, esophageal, and artificial larynx speech. Journal of Speech and Hearing Research 16:608–615, 1973.
32. Green G, Hults M: Preferences for three types of alaryngeal speech. Journal of Speech and Hearing Disorders 47:141–145, 1982.
33. Berry WR: Indications for use of artificial larynx devises. In: The Artificial Larynx Handbook, S Salmon and L Goldstein (eds). New York: Grune & Stratton, 1978b.
34. Bangs J, Lierle D, Strother C: Speech after laryngectomy. Journal of Speech and Hearing Disorders 11:171–176, 1946.
35. Berry WR: Attitudes of speech pathologists and otolaryngologists about artificial larynges. In: The Artificial Larynx Handbook, S Salmon and L Goldstein (eds). New York: Grune & Stratton, 1978a.
36. Kalb M, Carpenter M: Individual speaker influence on relative intelligibility of esophageal speech and artificial larynx speech. Journal of Speech and Hearing Disorders 46:77–80, 1981.
37. McCroskey R, Mulligan M: The relative intelligibility of esophageal speech and artificial-larynx speech. Journal of Speech and Hearing Disorders 28:37–41, 1963.
38. Merwin G, Goldstein L, Rothman H: A comparison of speech using artificial larynx and tracheoesophageal puncture with valve in the same speaker. Laryngoscope 95:730–734, 1985.
39. Shames G, Font J, Matthews J: Factors related to speech proficiency of the laryngectomized. Journal of Speech and Hearing Disorders 28:273–287, 1963.
40. Duguay MJ: Why not both? In: The Artificial Larynx Handbook, Shirley Salmon and Lewis Goldstein (eds). New York: Grune & Stratton, 1978.
41. Snidecor JC, Isshiki N: Air volume and air flow relationships of six male esophageal speakers. Journal of Speech and Hearing Disorders 30:205–216, 1965.
42. Damste' PH: Oesophageal Speech after Laryngectomy. Groningen: Hoitsema, 1958.

43. Diedrich WM, Youngstrom KA: Alaryngeal Speech. Springfield, Ill.: Charles C Thomas, 1966.
44. Hyman M: Factors influencing the intelligibility of alaryngeal speech. In Laryngectomee Rehabilitation, Second Edition, Darley F and Keith R (eds). San Diego: College–Hill, 1986.
45. Salmon SJ: Methods of air intake for esophageal speech and their associated problems. In: Laryngectomee Rehabilitation, Second Edition, Darley F and Keith R (eds). San Diego: College–Hill, 1986a.
46. Berlin CI, Zo B, Dean H: Clinical measurement during the acquisition of esophageal speech: II. An unexpected dividend. Journal of Speech and Hearing Disorders 28:389–392, 1963.
47. Shanks JC: Essentials for alaryngeal speech: psychology and physiology. In: Laryngectomee Rehabilitation, Second Edition, Darley F and Keith R (eds). San Diego: College–Hill, 1986b.
48. Salmon SJ: Factors that may interfere with acquiring esophageal speech. In Laryngectomee Rehabilitation, Second Edition, Darley F and Keith R (eds). San Diego: College–Hill, 1986b.

9. Neck Dissection: Morbidity and Rehabilitation

Allen Hillel and Carolynn Patten

The first organized approach to cancer of the cervical nodes was described by Crile [1] in 1906. He recognized the frequent failure of control of head and neck cancer due to recurrence not only at the primary site, but also in the neck. He emphasized the need to control the spread of the cancer to the lymph nodes and proposed 'a block dissection of the regional lymphatic system as well as the primary focus.' In 1928 [2], such cancer operations were referred to as 'neck dissections.' In 1951, Martin [3] presented a large series of patients who had undergone neck dissections which had become the treatment of choice for metastatic cervical nodes.

Since a normal neck can contain as many as 60 or 70 lymph nodes on each side, the attempt to locate and remove each node would be impossible. The concept of a neck dissection is based on the removal of all the node bearing tissue on one side of the neck. The boundaries of this en bloc resection are the mandible superiorly, the clavicle inferiorly, the laryngeal strap muscles anteriorly, and the trapezius muscle posteriorly. The superficial limit is the platysma muscle, and the deep limit is the deep cervical fascia.

The surgical technique relies upon finding the anatomical borders of the resection. First, skin flaps that include the platysma muscle are lifted so that the superficial limit of the resection is exposed. No effort to find individual lymph nodes is attempted. Instead, structures that are important to preserve are isolated at the limits of the resection. Inferiorly, the sternoceidomastiod muscle is transected just above the clavicle. The carotid artery and vagus nerve are located and preserved, but the jugular vein is tied to be removed with the specimen. The deep limit is the deep cervical fascia under which the phrenic nerve can be seen.

The anterior surgical limit is defined by separating the sternocleidomastoid muscle from the strap muscles. The superior limit is found by pulling the contents of the submandibular triangle down from under the mandible. Care is taken to preserve the lingual and hypoglossal nerves.

The posterior border of the neck dissection is defined by the anterior border of the trapezius muscle. The innervation to the trapezius, the eleventh cranial nerve (also known as the accessory nerve), is encountered at this point in the procedure as it courses up through the sternocleidomastoid

Jacobs, C. (ed): Carcinomas of the Head and Neck: Evaluation and Management.

muscle to the jugular foramen at the base of the skull. Since the sternocleidomastoid muscle is routinely removed as part of the en bloc resection, the surgeon must choose either to transect the XI nerve (radical neck dissection—RND) or to preserve it by dissecting it out of the muscle (modified neck dissection—MND). The resulting denervation of the trapezius due to transection of the nerve or due to the trauma of dissecting it free from the sternocleidomastiod muscle leads to the disability usually referred to as the eleventh nerve syndrome.

The Eleventh Nerve Syndrome

The eleventh nerve syndrome was first described by Ewing and Martin [4] in 1952. In their study of 100 patients, they noted that about half of them experienced shoulder pain, shoulder droop, and a reduction in shoulder range of motion during abduction.

Subsequently, other authors further defined the syndrome. Szunyogh [5] described a limited active range of motion of 45 to 80 degrees compared to a normal of 170–180 degrees. The passive range of motion was limited by pain at about 90 degrees. Nahum [6] noted that patients within 5 years of surgery had a range of motion with a mean of 56 degrees, but that patients more than 5 years from their surgery had a mean range of motion of 125 degrees. Carenfelt and Eliasson [7] noted similar restrictions in range of motion and also found that mean strength, measured statically at 70 degrees of abduction, was about half that of the unaffected side.

The eleventh nerve syndrome often remains as the most significant long–term morbidity for a patient who has undergone surgical therapy for head and neck cancer. Months after completion of all treatment, when the other sequelae of therapy have resolved, the shoulder weakness and chronic pain have progressed as muscle atrophy has worsened. Since head and neck cancer patients are often in their 50's or 60's, rehabilitation of musculoskeletal injuries are difficult since both physical activity and motivational levels are not at their peak. The shoulder disability that results from eleventh nerve injury often is insurmountable. For those individuals who had engaged in work requiring manual activity, this disability often means the end of their career.

Anatomy

The shoulder joint consists of a complex, overlapping network of muscles and ligaments attached to three bones: the clavicle, the scapula, and the humerus. The only true skeletal attachment to the thorax is through the sternoclavicular joint. The attachment of the scapula to the thorax is by means of muscular attachments rather than by ligaments. Hence, much of the support of the shoulder/arm complex depends on muscle tone rather than fixed attachments. The trapezius muscle, innervated by the eleventh (accessory) cranial nerve, therefore has a crucial role in static shoulder support as well as in shoulder/arm movement.

The trapezius muscle is a broad fan–shaped muscle that has three parts: the upper, the middle, and the lower bellies. The origin of the muscle is from the external occipital protuberance, the nuchal line of the occipital bone, the ligamentum nuchae, and the spinous processes of C7 through T12 [8,9]. The insertion of the muscle forms a broad sweeping attachment to the clavicle anteriorly and continuing around the acromium, spine, and medial border of the scapula.

The portion designated as the upper belly inserts on the lateral clavicle, the medial margin of the acromium, and the upper part of the spine of the scapula. This upper portion is responsible for the active suspension of the shoulder complex and for scapular–thoracic rotation which accounts for 60–80 degrees of motion during lateral abduction of the shoulder in the coronal plane. Paralysis of the upper belly is felt to be the major cause of the eleventh nerve syndrome.

The middle and lower bellies are responsible for retracting the scapula as the shoulder is drawn backward. They work in concert with the rhomboid muscles which are also adductors of the scapula. Paralyses of these portions of the muscle are not felt to be significant contributors to the shoulder syndrome.

The trapezius muscle, due to its major role as a suspensory support of the shoulder, is involved in most shoulder/arm movements, especially those that involve load carrying. Since complex movements of the arm involve the synergistic action of many muscles, it is difficult to choose a motion that isolates trapezius function. However, the movement that best defines trapezius, and hence eleventh nerve function, is abduction of the arm in the coronal plane. This examination is defined in the next section under range of motion testing.

The eleventh nerve arises as a series of rootlets from the lateral spinal cord [10] and is joined by rootlets from each level including C1. This spinal portion of the nerve then crosses behind the vertebral artery and enters the skull through the foramen magnum. Near the posterior inferior cerebellar artery, the cranial root of the nerve joins the spinal root.

The eleventh nerve then exits the skull through the jugular foramen along with the ninth (glossopharyngeal) and the tenth (vagus) cranial nerves. Just outside the jugular foramen, at the inferior ganglion of the tenth nerve, the cranial portion of the eleventh nerve joins the tenth nerve and supplies motor branches [8] to muscles of the pharynx, the palate, and to all the muscles of the larynx. The remaining extracranial eleventh nerve at this point is then comprised solely of the spinal portion of the nerve which is pure voluntary motor innervation to the sternocleidomastoid and trapezius muscles.

The eleventh nerve then courses over the jugular vein and heads posteriorly and inferiorly as it enters the sternocleidomastoid muscle. One or more branches to the sternocleidomastoid muscle leave the nerve before it exits at the posterior edge of the muscle in the posterior triangle of the neck. As the nerve then courses farther posteriorly, it variably receives contributions from C3 and C4 before entering the trapezius muscle, its final destination.

The contributions of C3 and C4 remain a controversial point of anatomy and physiology. Some animal studies [11,12] indicate that these cervical contributions are sensory (proprioceptive), while others [13,14] have found a variable motor contribution. Although some human studies [6,15,16] have found motor contributions other than the eleventh nerve to the trapezius, the majority of studies [17,18,19] indicate that the cervical branches are sensory, and that the eleventh nerve is the sole motor supply to the sternocleidomastoid and trapezius.

Evaluation

Numerous means of subjective assessment can be devised in the form of questionnaires, but the major symptoms can easily be discovered by simple history taking. Although the actual deficit is present immediately after surgery, patients will not describe symptoms until weeks later when peri–surgical problems resolve and activity levels increase. For formal subjective testing, a questionnaire [20] that uses a preoperative comparison base can be employed.

Evaluation of eleventh nerve function can be done by electromyographical (EMG) testing. Standard needle EMG can demonstrate the presence of fibrillation potentials and membrane instability that indicate denervation. In the case of modified neck dissections, membrane stability and electrical activity with voluntary recruitment can be indicators of partial injury, or many months later, indicators of recovery.

Evoked electromyography (EEMG) is another form of electrical nerve testing that uses a transcutaneous electrical stimulation of the eleventh nerve to evoke a trapezius muscle contraction that can be recorded by surface electrodes [21,22,23] (figure 1). The characteristics of the response are useful to indicate early injury when standard EMG might be interpreted as normal. This technique is also effective in recording neuromuscular function intra–operatively. In addition, EEMG provides the data necessary to calculate nerve conduction velocities, another measure of neural function.

Muscle testing is the most reliable indicator of trapezius function when done by an experienced examiner. There are numerous tests that can be done including visual inspection, active and passive ranges of motion, manual muscle testing, static strength tests, and dynamic strength tests. Unfortunately, the muscle test most frequently used is shoulder 'shrugging,' usually with the patient clothed and with the examiner's hands over the acromia of the clavicles. This exam is entirely misleading since brisk shoulder elevation

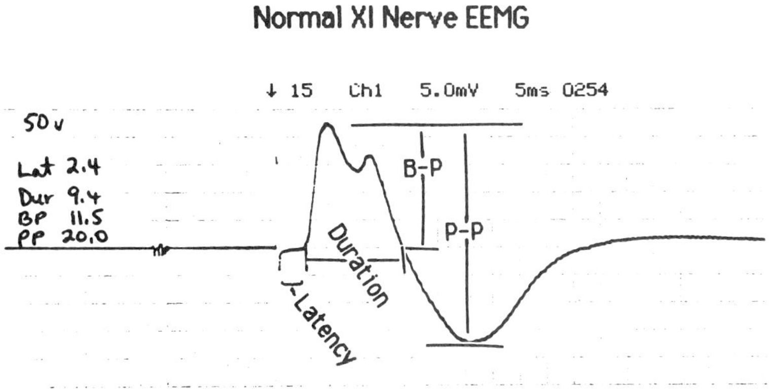

Figure 1. A normal XI nerve EEMG is shown. Latency, duration, baseline–to–peak (B–P), and peak–to–peak (P–P) are indicated. (Reproduced with permission from *Head and Neck Surgery* 10:387–395, 1988).

can be achieved by the levator muscles, even in the complete absence of trapezius function. It is of note that shoulder shrugging has remained an often used exam in spite of its description in Ewing and Martin's hallmark paper [4] on shoulder disability in 1951: 'As a test of the loss of the trapezius it [shoulder shrugging] is worthless.'

Visual inspection of the trapezius muscle mass is performed in the unclothed patient with the hands at the side. If only one neck has undergone surgery, a comparison of sides is useful. With the patient facing away from the examiner, the position of the shoulders can be noted (figure 2a). Usually, any droop of the affected side can be appreciated by inspection, but it is also useful to record the measurement in centimeters from the spinous process of C7 to the acromium on each side. The affected side is usually longer by 2 to 7 cm.

Range of motion (ROM) testing can be done actively (AROM) or passively (PROM). The trapezius muscle is involved with other muscles in supporting the shoulder in almost all shoulder and arm movements. It contributes its most isolated role during lateral abduction in the coronal plane. Lateral abduction is performed by the trapezius in concert with the deltoid and supraspinatus muscles. The deltoid and supraspinatous effect humeral abduction with respect to the scapula, while the trapezius effects scapular rotation with respect to the thorax to complete 180 degrees of abduction. In the eleventh nerve syndrome, the motion cannot be completed beyond 100 degrees due to abnormal scapular rotation (figure 2b) as a result of trapezius dysfunction. If the examiner is careful to prevent the arm from rotating forward out of the coronal plane, substitution with other muscles is prevented, and the deficit of trapezius function can clearly be demonstrated. Measurement is done by means of a hand–held protractor called a goniometer.

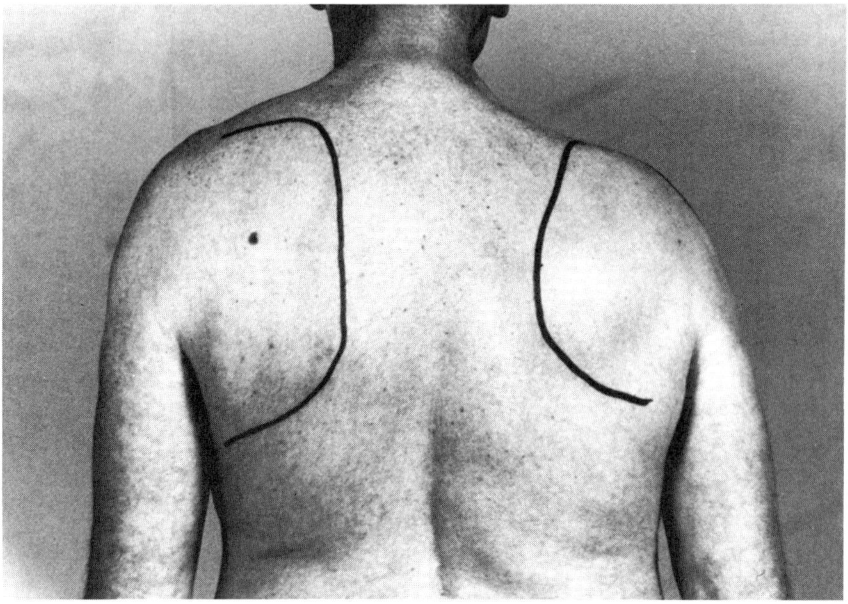

Figure 2a. Posterior view of a patient 2 years after a right modified neck dissection. Note the shoulder droop and trapezius atrophy. In addition, the scapula has been outlined to indicate its abnormal position at rest.

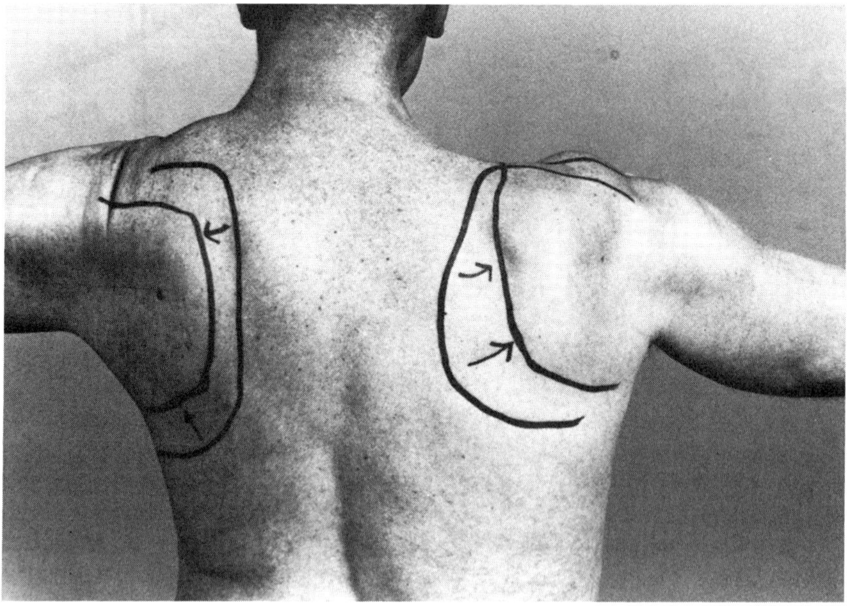

Figure 2b. Compare the scapulo–thoracic motion during active abduction. On the affected right side, the scapula is aberantly displaced upward and laterally as well as distracted from the thoracic wall due to trapezius weakness.

Table 1. Muscle grades: common rating system used during manual muscle tests.

Gradation	Description
5 – Normal	Full range of motion, against gravity, against full resistance
4 – Good	Full range of motion, against gravity, against some resistance
3 – Fair	Full range of motion, against gravity
2 – Poor	Full range of motion, gravity eliminated
1 – Trace	Evidence of contractility, no joint motion
0 – Zero	No evidence of contractility

Normal abduction during AROM is 170 to 180 degrees. If the trapezius is not functioning, or is weak, abduction will be limited to 70 to 130 degrees. AROM is usually performed with the patient standing, but more sensitive measurements can be made in the supine position with a skate supporting the arm. Lateral abduction then occurs in a gravity free plane and a weakened trapezius can be more effective.

With PROM testing the examiner moves the arm through the motion of lateral abduction while asking the patient to relax. This does not test muscle contraction, but instead evaluates joint mobility. Many patients with the eleventh nerve syndrome have restriction of PROM due to changes in the glenohumeral joint and changes in scapular support that allow the scapular rotation necessary for abduction. PROM should also be 180 degrees, and AROM will not be able to exceed PROM.

With manual muscle testing (MMT), the examiner asks the patient to perform an AROM against resistance provided by the examiner. Ratings are from 5 to 0 and are standardized [24] (see Table 1). For evaluation of trapezius function, MMT should be done with lateral abduction at 100 degrees or greater.

Additional evaluation of trapezius function can be accomplished by careful inspection of the patient during simple tasks. Donning or doffing a garment over the head can demonstrate a functional deficit as the patient uses compensatory strategies for overhead shoulder movements. Asking the patient to touch the opposite scapular spine (figure 3) by reaching overhead can demonstrate the slow, intentional, uncomfortable motion of trapezius weakness and also indicates possible joint capsulitis. Asking the patient to lift a two–pound weight overhead as if to place it on a high shelf can demonstrate the need to rotate anteriorly at about 110 degrees of abduction in order to compensate for trapezius weakness.

Strength measurements can be done statically or dynamically. With static measurements the arm is abducted, usually to 90 degrees, while the patient is standing, and the arm attempts to pull against weights or a measuring device (such as a scale) attached to the floor. While this technique does provide numerical data, it cannot be easily interpreted. The ability of a muscle to generate torque varies depending upon the position of the muscle

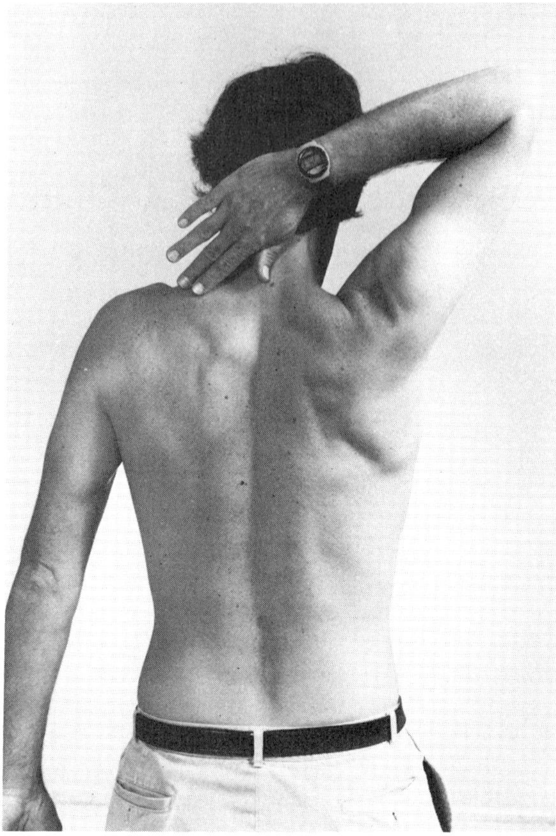

Figure 3a. During a test of joint mobility a normal subject is able to touch the opposite scapular spine overhead during abduction with external rotation.

[25] and, in the case of lateral abduction of the shoulder, has been shown to occur near the midpoint of the AROM [20]. Static strength measurements are by definition at a fixed length–tension and reflect the strength of the muscle only at that position. In addition, static or isometric contraction allows for maximal recruitment of the motor neuron pool [26]. However, maximal recruitment does not occur during functional movement; instead, recruitability declines as a function of increasing speed. Therefore, meaningful measurements of muscle strength are best evaluated during movement.

Dynamic measurements employ a dynamometer to test the torque output of the shoulder/arm during the actual motion of lateral abduction (figure 4). Various dynamometers are available commercially. With these instruments, the patient is stabilized on the examing table and grips the handle on a rotating lever. As the patient performs a vigorous lateral abduction, the dynamometer measures torque production and the position of the arm

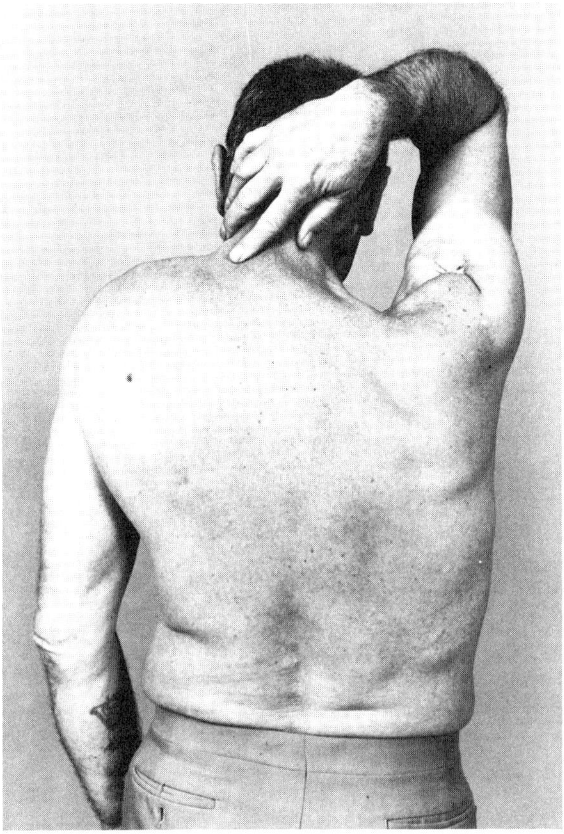

Figure 3b. A patient 2 years after modified neck dissection is limited during abduction with external rotation due to joint capsule involvement.

(figure 5). The peak torque and where it occurs can be measured as well as other important variables such as power, work, and rate of torque generation (torque acceleration energy). In addition, the speed of abduction can be varied to study the decrease in recruitability of the motor neuron pool as speed increases [26]. Although dynamic measurements require expensive equipment and expertise to perform, they provide the most reliable and useful measurements of function.

In addition to the muscular dysfunction secondary to trapezius weakness, examiners should also be aware of specific glenohumeral joint problems that can occur secondary to disuse. It should also be noted that on rare occasions patients with a severe shoulder droop can suffer a brachial plexus traction injury with resultant arm and hand weakness.

Overall, when evaluating shoulder function, it is paramount to consider the 'real world variables' encountered by the patient. The critical factors

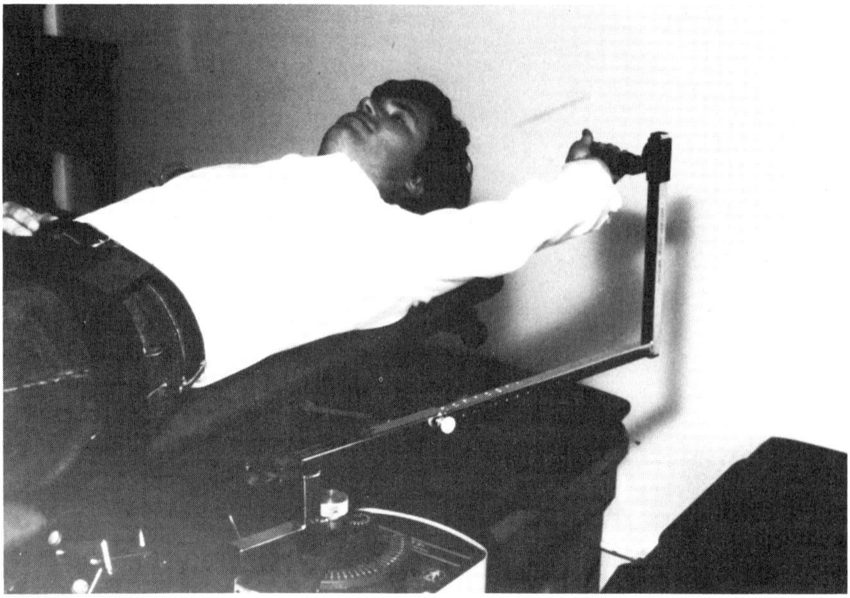

Figure 4. A normal subject undergoing dynamic testing of lateral abduction of the shoulder in a gravity-eliminated position on a Cybex II + Dynamometer. In a vertical testing position, some neck dissection patients are unable to generate torque against the force of gravity.

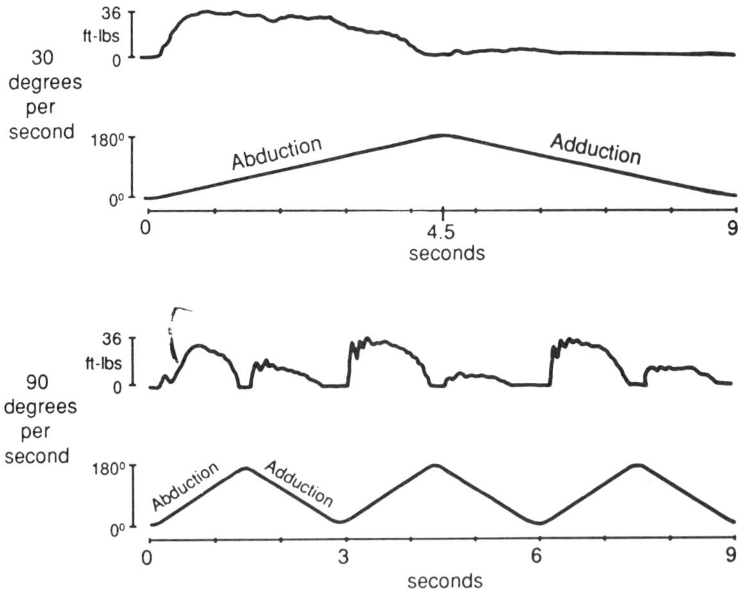

Figure 5. Cybex tracings from a test of lateral abduction in a normal subject examined at test speeds of 30 degrees/second and 90 degrees/second. In each test trial, the upper tracing indicates the torque generated. The lower tracing indicates the corresponding position in the range of motion as well as time.

which prevent normal shoulder motions are gravity, resistance of the task, and the need for movement at functional speeds. The ability to perform lateral abduction in the coronal plane does not in and of itself indicate function. Many individuals with partial deficit are fully able to abduct the involved arm given enough time and no resistance. Many are also able to perform a nearly normal manual muscle test since it is an isometric task. However, to be functional an individual must be able to move in response to the tasks encountered. Inability to move at functional speeds and against functional loads often precludes the patient from returning to work and, in extreme cases, prevents independent living.

Morbidity of Neck Dissection

Since the inception of neck dissection as the surgical treatment for nodal disease of head and neck cancer, controversy has surrounded the many modifications proposed to Crile's classic procedure. The major changes suggested concern the need to remove the eleventh nerve, the sternocleidomastoid muscle, and the internal jugular vein. Alterations from the RND, which removes all three, are called conservative neck dissections. Although nomenclature is inconsistant, the designation of MND implies sacrifice of the internal jugular vein and sternocleidomastoid muscle but preservation of the eleventh nerve. Generally, the most explicit terminology for other variations is to designate an MND with an appropriate descriptor to indicate what was performed (that is an MND with preservation of the internal jugular vein).

The majority of the debate about the various modifications centers about two issues: oncologic efficacy versus morbidity of eleventh nerve syndrome. The oncological issues are many, and numerous investigators have attempted to evaluate the cure rates of the various surgical options. Although a discussion of these issues is beyond the scope of this chapter, the general consensus is that the surgeon must individualize the decision in each case based upon the tumor location, the technical difficulty, and the patient's ability to endure a longer anesthetic.

As caretakers of head and neck cancer patients with advanced life–threatening disease, our focus is understandably centered on survival and cure. We are, therefore, 'in our eagerness to achieve cure,' [4] often unaware of the extent of the disability that we create for our patients. These disabilities, however, ironically become more important as we are more successful with our therapies and 'create' more patients who live many years after our treatments.

To address this quality of life issue, there have been a number of studies that have investigated the morbidity of sacrificing the eleventh nerve during a radical neck dissection. In 1951, Ewing and Martin [4] examined 100 patients and noted pain in 42%, weakness in 10%, loss of motion in 60%, and shoulder droop in 100%. In 1961, Nahum [6] defined the disability as a syndrome after doing a detailed study of seven patients. He noted loss of range of motion, atrophy, shoulder droop, and weakness in all patients. Other authors [27,28,29,30] have noted variable results with significant morbidity ranging from 50 to 100% of patients studied. However, in almost all patients, the physical findings of the eleventh syndrome were present.

Although the intent of preserving the eleventh nerve in an MND is to prevent the eleventh nerve syndrome, it is important to note that this effort is frequently unsuccessful. Carenfelt and Eliasson [7] noted paresis in 21 of 35 (60%) of patients who had eleventh nerve preservation in an MND. Although they noted improvement in all but 6 of these patients, 15 of them were left with a major (6) or minor (9) paresis for an overall morbidity of 43%. Leipzig [29] noted that 50% of patients had objective loss of eleventh nerve innervation to the trapezius.

In spite of the frequent morbidity associated with nerve preservation, all authors have reported that the comparisons of populations of MND and RND patients showed significantly less dysfunction in the MND group. While many of them did have detectable losses, the majority had significantly fewer symptoms than the RND group. It appears that if oncologically permitted, an MND offers the best chance to diminish shoulder dysfunction after neck dissection.

Rehabilitation

Physical therapy has often been recommended for the rehabilitation of patients suffering from the eleventh nerve syndrome. These regimens vary from very simple range of motion exercises to formal physical therapy programs [27,31,32]. However, in spite of attempts to develop standardized therapies, no prospective studies have demonstrated a specific benefit from any particular regimen. Documentation of such benefit is difficult since the extent of disability within any population is so variable. In addition, in those patients who have undergone nerve sparing procedures, recovery due to physical therapy cannot readily be discerned from improvement due to muscle reinnervation. The results of physical therapy are also difficult to evaluate since only those patients with a high degree of motivation are likely to participate successfully in such programs.

Since gravity related traction comprises a portion of the eleventh nerve syndrome, attempts have been made to provide support to the shoulder statically. The use of orthotic devices has been reported, and one device [33,34], designed to provide an upward force on the shoulder utilizing the pelvis for support, is even patented. Other devices, such as simple slings, provide support and can relieve chronic pain in some patients while they are worn. Surgically, a similar effect has been attempted by suspending the scapula from the spine with strips of fascia. In addition, the insertion of the levator scapulae has been moved laterally to more closely mimic the function of the trapezius muscle [17,35]. All authors describe good results but neither the orthotics nor surgery have seen widespread use.

Attempts at nerve grafting primarily during the radical neck dissection have also been used as a means to rehabilitate the shoulder. In 1965, Harris and Dickey [36] presented a preliminary report of eleventh nerve repair using the greater auricular nerve. Subsequent reports described success in 79% of 44 patients [37] and 100% of 19 patients [18]. The means of assessment of function, however, were clinical observation or simple ROM. EMG testing was done only on 4 patients. More recently, Weisberger [38] reported on 10 patients, 8 of whom had EMGs, and found that their function rated generally between the results seen in RND patients and in MND patients.

Conclusion

Neck dissection remains the best surgical treatment for nodal disease of head and neck cancer. Due to its oncological efficacy, the morbidity associated with the procedure has often gone unrecognized. Numerous efforts to reduce shoulder disability have been attempted. The foremost of these is nerve preservation during a modified neck dissection. Another effective treatment is primary nerve grafting. However, in spite of reports of consistently good results, nerve grafting has not yet been adopted by most surgeons as a theraputic measure after sacrifice of the eleventh nerve. It is most important to note, however, that all techniques of neck dissection, even nerve sparing procedures, are frequently associated with significant morbidity.

With the increasing success of treating head and neck cancer patients, more patients will survive with the resulting disabilities that therapy has created. The deficit created by neck dissection is measurable with formal testing. The discomfort and exertional fatigue are more subjective. The disability, therefore, is a combination of the measurable deficit and the individual's outlook, effort, and psychological status. The differing abilities of patients to cope with dysfunction will to a significant degree determine their final outcome. However, even those affected patients that return to work fulltime will have a diminished capacity for lifting, reaching, head turning, and endurance.

As oncologists, we must recognize that when we have cured a patient, we have often left them with dysfunctions that are our responsibility to evaluate. We need to respond to the disabilities our treatment has created, and, in the case of neck dissection, provide compassion, motivation, and support for the patients with resultant shoulder dysfunction.

References

1. Crile GW: Excision of cancer of the head and neck. JAMA 47:1780–1786, 1906.
2. Bartlett El, Callander CL: Dissections of the neck. Arch Surg 16:1214–1231, 1928.
3. Martin H, del Valle B, Ehrlich H, et al.: Neck dissection. Cancer 4:441–490, 1951.
4. Ewing MR, Martin H: Disability following radical neck dissection. An assessment based on the postoperative evaluation of 100 patients. Cancer 5: 873–883, 1952.
5. Szunyogh B: Shoulder disability following neck dissection. Am J Surg 25: 194–198, 1959.
6. Nahum AM, Mullally W, Marmor L: A syndrome resulting from radical neck dissection. Arch Otolarnygol 74:82–86, 1961.
7. Carenfelt C, Eliasson K: Occurrence, duration, and prognosis of unexpected accessory nerve paresis in radical neck dissection. Acta Otolaryngol 90:470–473, 1980.
8. Grant JCB: An Atlas of Anatomy, 6th edition, Baltimore: Williams & Wilkins, 1972.
9. Pansky B, House EL: Review of Gross Anatomy, 2nd edition, London: Macmillan, 1969.
10. Hollinshead WH: Anatomy for Surgeons: Volume 1, 2nd edition, New York: Harper & Row, 1968.
11. Windle WF, Delozier LC: The absence of painful sensation in the cat during stimulation of the spinal accessory nerve. J Comp Neurol 54:97–101, 1931.
12. Corbin KB, Harrison F: The sensory innervation of the spinal accessory and tongue musculature in the rhesus monkey. Brain 62:191–197, 1938.
13. Russell JSR: An experimental investigation of the cervical and thoracic nerve root in relation to the subject of wry neck. Brain 20:35–55, 1897.
14. Weisberger EC: The efferent supply of the trapezius muscle: a neuroanatomic basis for the preservation of shoulder function during neck dissection. Laryngoscope 97:435–445, 1987.
15. Fahrer H, Ludin HP, Mumenthaler M, et al.: The innervation of the trapezius muscle, an electrophysiological study. J Neurol 207:183–188, 1974.
16. Stell PM, Jones TA: Radical neck dissection: preservation of function of the shoulder. J Laryngol Otol 8(Suppl.):106–107, 1983.
17. Hoaglund FT, Duthie RB: Surgical reconstruction for shoulder pain after radical neck dissection. Am J Surg 112:522–526, 1966.
18. Anderson R, Flowers RS: Free grafts of the spinal accessory nerve during radical neck dissection. Am J Surg 118:796–799, 1969.
19. King PS, Lewis FR, Weddle JL, Fowlks W: Effect of radical neck dissection on total rehabilitation of the laryngectomee. Am J Phys Med 52(1):1–17, 1973.
20. Hillel AD, Kroll H, Dormann J, Medieros J: Radical neck dissection: a subjective and objective evaluation of postoperative disability. J Otolaryngol 18(1):53–61, 1989.
21. Hillel AD, Dobie RA, Little J: Evoked electromyography of the eleventh nerve and trapezius muscle. Head & Neck Surgery 10:387–395, 1988.
22. Eisen A, Bertrand G: Isolated accessory nerve palsy of spontaneous origin. A clinical and electromyographic study. Arch Neurol 27:496–502, 1972.
23. Schumm F, Stohr M: Accessory nerve stimulation in the assessment of myasthenia gravis. Muscle Nerve 7:147–151, 1984.
24. Medical Research Council—Aids to Investigation of Peripheral Nerve Injuries, War Memo #7, 2nd edition, revised. His Majesty's Stationery Office, 1943.
25. Lehmkuhl LD, Smith LK: Brunnstrom's Clinical Kinesiology, 4th edition, Philadelphia: Davis, pp 129–146, 1985.
26. Joyce GC, Rack PMH, Westbury DR: The mechanical properties of cat soleus muscle during controlled lengthening and shortening movements. J Physiol 204:461–474, 1969.
27. Saunders WH, Johnson EW: Rehabilitation of the shoulder after radical neck dissection. Ann Otol 84:812–816, 1975.
28. Fialka V, Vinzenz K: Investigations into shoulder function after radical neck dissection. J Cranio-Max-Fac Surg 16:143–147, 1988.

29. Leipzig B, Suen JY, English JL, et al.: Functional evaluation of the spinal accessory nerve after neck dissection. Am J Surg 146:526–530, 1983.
30. Carenfelt C, Eliasson K: Radical neck dissection and permanent sequelae associated with spinal accessory nerve injuries. Acta Otolaryngol 91:155–160, 1981.
31. Herring D, King Al, Connelly M: New rehabilitation concepts in management of radical neck dissection syndrome, a clinical syndrome. Physical Therapy 67:1095–1099, 1987.
32. Johnson EW, Aseff JN, Saunders W: Physical treatment of pain and weakness following radical neck dissection. Ohio State Med J 74:711–714, 1978.
33. Villanueva R: Orthosis to correct shoulder pain and deformity after trapezius palsy. Arch Phys Med Rehab 58:30–34, 1977.
34. Villanueva R, Ajmani C: The role of rehabilitation medicine in physical restoration of patients with head and neck cancer. The Cancer Bulletin 29(2):46–54, 1977.
35. Dewar FP, Rl Harris: Restoration of function of the shoulder following paralysis of the trapezius by fascial sling fixation and transportation of the levator scapulae. Ann Surg 132:1111–1115, 1950.
36. Harris HH, Dickey JR: Nerve grafting to restore function of the trapezius muscle after radical neck dissection (a preliminary report). Ann Otol Rhinol Laryngol 74:880–886, 1965.
37. Ballantyne AJ, Guinn GA: Reduction of shoulder disability after neck dissection. Am J Surg 112:661–665, 1966.
38. Weisberger EC, Lingeman RE: Cable grafting of the spinal accessory nerve for rehabilitation of shoulder function after radical neck dissection. Laryngoscope 97:918–918, 1987.

III

Advances in Medical Management and Chemotherapeutic Approaches

10. Evaluation and Medical Management of Thyroid Cancer

Margaret M. Petersen and I. Ross McDougall

Thyroid cancer is the most common endocrine cancer, yet there are only about 12,100 new cases per year in the U.S. with 1,100 deaths annually. In contrast, clinically significant thyroid nodules are found in 5% of the population and of those evaluated, about 10% have been shown to be malignant. This has been demonstrated by several studies using fine needle aspiration (FNA) which has been found to be more accurate than ultrasound or scintigraphy in predicing malignancy in thyroid nodules. The above figures suggest that the risk of death from a malignant thyroid nodule is very low. Thyroid cancer generally has a good prognosis, particularly in the 70–90% of patients (in the U.S.) who have well–differentiated cancers. There are now numerous retrospective studies on significant numbers of patients who have been followed for a sufficient length of time to enable important conclusions to be drawn regarding management and therapy [1–4]. Major controversies still exist regarding both the extent of surgical resection of the thyroid following diagnosis and the role of radioiodine therapy. There are a small number of patients with aggressive forms of thyroid cancer in whom the prognosis is bleak and the survival rate so low that clinicians have been unable to follow them long enough to judge whether treatments are influencing outcome.

In this chapter, we aim to present a complete review of thyroid cancer, including classification [5] and discussion of the individual cancers with major emphasis on treatment. In particular, controversial issues are addressed and hopefully clarified so that the reader is left with a complete understanding regarding the diagnosis, management, and treatment of these diseases.

Classification

Well–differentiated papillary or follicular cancers comprise the vast majority (70–90%) of thyroid cancers (Table 1). Of these, 55–65% are papillary, including mixed papillary–follicular and papillary variant of follicular cancer. Fifteen to twenty–five percent are follicular, including clear cell and Hurthle

Jacobs, C. (ed): Carcinomas of the Head and Neck: Evaluation and Management.

Table 1. Classification of types of cancer found in the thyroid.

Cell of origin	Type of cancer
Follicular	Papillary*
	Follicular*
	Anaplastic
Parafollicular	Medullary
Lymphoid	Usually Diffuse Histiocytic
Metastases	Usually breast, kidney, melanoma, lung, gastrointentinal tract
	Thyroglossal Tract, Struma Ovarii

* Occasionally found in Ectopic Sites

cell types which will be discussed separately. Five to fifteen percent are anaplastic, comprising both giant and spindle cell types. This last type has a very poor prognosis. Currently in the U.S. there is a trend to less follicular and anaplastic tumors with an increasing proportion of papillary cancers. Data has shown that anaplastic cancer arises from longstanding papillary cancers, and therefore it is conceivable that earlier diagnosis and treatment of papillary cancer may have influenced this trend, although changes in the natural history of the disease cannot be excluded. All of these cancers are more common in women but there is an increasing incidence in men, and this may be related to the association with external radiation. Five to ten percent of thyroid cancers arise in parafollicular cells, giving rise to medullary carcinoma. Twenty percent of these are associated with familial syndromes of multiple endocrine neoplasia (MEN) IIa and IIb and non–MEN types. A very small number of cancers arise in lymphoid and connective tissue, most commonly non–Hodgkin's lymphoma. Finally, metastases to the thyroid are often found at autopsy although usually they are not clinically significant. Primary cancers from the kidney, breast, lung or melanoma can metastasize to thyroid and present as a mass in the thyroid, which if solitary and removed, can significantly prolong the patient's survival.

Differentiated Thyroid Cancers: Papillary/Mixed Papillary–Follicular

Papillary cancer includes pure papillary, papillary–follicular and papillary variant of follicular cancer, all of which have identical biological behavior and similar prognoses. They comprise 55–65% of well–differentiated thyroid cancers.

Etiology

The most important known etiological factor is a history of head and neck irradiation, and there is abundant evidence in humans and experimental animals to support this [6–8]. Of minor significance is Hashimoto's thyroiditis and its association with papillary cancer [9]. This, however, is somewhat controversial because of the high incidence of lymphoid infiltration in papillary cancers, and no causal relationship has been clearly demonstrated.

Pathology

Papillary cancer can occur anywhere in the thyroid gland. Lesions vary from microscopic to lesions several centimeters in diameter, and they are often multifocal [10]. They are classified as intrathyroidal or extrathyroidal depending on whether they have extended through the capsule. They can be solid or cystic. They usually tend to be hard in consistency, and 50% will have microscopic regional lymph node metastases at the time of the first surgery. Histologically, the epithelial cells are cuboidal and arranged in fronds with a vascular core. Cell nuclei have a characteristic ground glass appearance, sometimes termed 'Orphan Annie' cells. Psammoma bodies are typical but not unique to this cancer.

Clinical

Typically, papillary thyroid cancer presents as a solitary thyroid nodule, usually in a woman between 35 and 45 years of age. The incidence is 2 to 3 times more common in women, and although occurring at all ages, the 4th and 5th decades have the highest frequency [1,3]. The nodule is usually asymptomatic, but occasionally in its more sinister form, the cancer will present as a hard mass in the anterior neck with evidence of invasion of the surrounding structures such as the strap muscles, the trachea, recurrent laryngeal nerve and even the esophagus. Enlargement of regional lymph nodes is uncommon, although 50% of patients do have microscopic lymph node metastases when they come to surgery. If papillary cancer is found in a cervical node, thyroid is the most likely primary cancer, and the clinician should make careful examination of the gland, particulary if there is a history of head and neck irradiation. Very rarely papillary cancer presents with distant metastases to lungs, bones, liver, or brain, and invariably careful palpation of the thyroid will reveal the primary lesion. It is extremely rare for a minimal lesion (that is, less than 1.5 cm in diameter) to spread distantly, and if there is difficulty in palpating the primary, an ultrasound of the thyroid is always recommended in these cases. This is one of the few cancers where a reasonable prognosis can occur despite the presence of metastases.

Clinically, all patients with papillary carcinoma, irrespective of stage, are usually euthyroid, in contrast to those with widespread follicular carcinoma who can be hyperthyroid from autonomous secretion of excess thyroid hormones.

Management

The management of papillary carcinoma depends to a great extent on several simple prognostic factors. It has been shown that the risk of dying from the cancer is increased in older patients and in men. The size of the primary is also very important since lesions 2 cm or smaller almost never lead to death. Local invasion or distant metastases especially to brain or bone, give a worse prognosis [1,3,4,11–14].

Surgery

Initial treatment is surgery. The main debate centers around whether to perform total or subtotal thyroidectomy. The protagonists for total thyroidectomy believe that since the cancer is most likely multifocal this operation removes all cancer even if at a microscopic stage [15–18]. They claim that subsequent radioiodine therapy is easier, as there is no normal thyroid tissue to treat and finally advocate this procedure in the belief that removing both lobes in comparison to one does not increase the surgical risk significantly [19]. Those against total thyroidectomy say the risk of complications, principally hypoparathyroidism and recurrent laryngeal nerve damage, is significantly increased, and the risk of recurrence is no greater after lobectomy or subtotal thyroidectomy than for total thyroidectomy [1,20]. They also say that radioiodine treatment can be done quite adequately even if there is some normal thyroid tissue left. There have been several series reviewing these issues. Although all have reported a decreased recurrence rate following total thyroidectomy, in comparison to subtotal thyroidectomy, all have shown an increased rate of complications, primarily hypoparathyroidism and vocal cord paralysis, which have been sufficiently frequent and troublesome to outweigh the benefit of slight reduction in recurrence rate [21–22,23]. As far as affecting subsequent radioiodine treatment, even after total thyroidectomy, normal thyroid tissue can be imaged in most patients and this has to be ablated first.

On occasion, a problem can arise when lobectomy has been performed for a thyroid nodule interpreted as benign on intraoperative frozen section and found later to be malignant on the permanent slides. In this case, the question of a repeat operation is raised and the decision depends on several of the prognostic factors discussed earlier, for example the age and sex of the patient and the extent of disease. If distant metastases are present, then radioiodine initially to ablate the lobe and later for the metastases is one option. However, reoperation is more definitive, and although the risk of complications during the second procedure is increased, this approach is preferable. Because many clinicians use FNA of nodules to determine which patients are referred for operation, this situation should be less common.

Local lymph node involvement has less prognostic significance than age, sex, size of cancer, extrathyroidal spread or distant metastases. When present, modified lymph node dissection is recommended in preference to radical neck dissection which has not been shown to improve the survival, yet causes unnecessarily troublesome complications, particularly when the sternocleidomastoid is sacrificed along with the spinal accessory nerve [24].

Ipsilateral total lobectomy and contralateral subtotal lobectomy is generally accepted as the most appropriate primary surgical treatment of papillary carcinoma [13]. In patients of less than 45 years of age with a single intrathyroidal cancer less than 3 cm in diameter, ipsilateral lobectomy with isthmusectomy is an alternative, but less desirable.

TSH Suppression

Thyroid replacement is necessary as the patient is invariably thyroid deficient following surgery. In addition, because many thyroid cancers are TSH dependant, thyroxine is prescribed in a dose to suppress TSH. Patients treated with thyroxine have been shown to have a statistically better outcome [20,25,26]. Thyroxine is usually administered in a dose of 100–300 ug/day (approximately 2 ug/kg), and the clinician should monitor this with sensitive TSH assay [27]. Metastases can occur despite TSH suppression, and this is one situation when radioiodine therapy should be considered.

Radioiodine

In approaching radioiodine therapy, the clinician should identify those patients who have extracapsular or local invasion at the time of surgery. This group of patients have an increased risk of dying from their cancer, and they should be given ablative therapy with radioiodine ^{131}I. Like inorganic iodine, ^{131}I is trapped and organified in thyroid tissue. The *B* particle which it emits, destroys tissue over a distance of several mm by delivering an intense dose of radiation, up to tens of thousands of rads, without damaging adjacent normal tissue. This should be contrasted with external beam radiation therapy where about 6,000 rads is the limiting dose. Higher doses cause permanent damage to surrounding normal structures such as the spinal cord or esophagus.

Another advantage of ^{131}I is its ability to be imaged scintigraphically using its gamma emission, and diagnostic scintigraphy is required to evaluate the extent of residual thyroid tissue and to localize distant metastases prior to therapy. It is important that the TSH is not suppressed, otherwise there will be no radioiodine uptake, and, therefore, it is recommended that thyroxine be stopped for at least 4 weeks prior to scanning. This has the disadvantage of rendering patients hypothyroid. Some clinicians take advantage of the shorter half life (36 hours) of triiodothyronine (T3) [28]. Thyroxine is replaced by T3 for 4 weeks then the T3 is stopped. However, there is a degree of overlap as the half–life of thyroxine is 7 days, and occasionally patients may become hyperthyroid temporarily. In any case, after discontinuation of T3, the patient becomes clinically hypothyroid for approximately one week prior to the scan. With the former approach, because of the longer half–life of T4, the patient becomes hypothyroid about the third week and remains hypothyroid for about the same length of time as with the T3 method, so there is little gain in switching medications. Most importantly the patient should not be administered any iodine containing contrast medications. Low iodine diet with a reduced intake of seafood and flour products is recommended. Methods of increasing radioiodine trapping such as diuretics or exogenous TSH have been used, but there is an incidence of allergic reactions with the latter, and their use is not encouraged.

In patients who have only had lobectomy, there will be little or no rise in TSH when T4 is stopped. Despite this, the residual normal thyroid will still trap radioiodine, and if treatment is indicated the lobe can be ablated with ^{131}I. However, if distant metastases are present they will not take up radioiodine unless the remaining thyroid tissue is completely destroyed, so a second dose is usually indicated several months later when the TSH will hopefully be elevated. Two mCi of ^{131}I is the usual dose for diagnostic scanning. Scans are performed 48–72 hours after oral administration of the radionuclide [28]. This ensures time for small functioning metastases to trap the radioiodine and takes advantage of the long half–life of ^{131}I (8 days). ^{123}I is not used because its half–life is only 13 hours, and therefore, a substantial dose would have to be given to ensure adequate 48–hour images. Routinely anterior and posterior whole body scans with spot views of the neck and upper chest are performed using a gamma camera with a medium energy collimator. A pinhole collimator can be used for spot views. We routinely measure the uptake in the neck and in distant metastases.

Abnormal sites of uptake distant from the thyroid bed should be considered for treatment as should residual thyroid tissue if it is known by the surgeons and pathologists that there was local invasion into the surrounding tissues. The ablation of normal thyroid tissue left postoperatively is a controversial issue. When the question of radioiodine ablation of presumed normal residual thyroid is raised, it is important to examine the relevant prognostic factors.

There is a trend toward giving 30 mCi (actually 29.9 mCi) as this is the upper limit for treatment as an outpatient. Although there are several studies where this dose was used, there is no uniform opinion as to its success, and much depends on the volume of residual thyroid and its ability to trap iodine [29–35]. Generally 30 mCi is administered if the patient is under 45 years with a cancer 3 cm or greater. If a repeat diagnostic scan 12 months later shows total ablation, then no further radioiodine is required. If neck uptake persists, then a repeat 30 mCi dosage is advised in younger patients (less than 45 years), and 75 to 100 mCi in older patients is preferred because their prognosis is less good.

If there is abnormal uptake in distant sites, an attempt should be made to quantify the tumor volume by other means, for example, by radiographs,

CT scan (note WITHOUT contrast), ultrasound, or NMR [36]. However, therapy to sites with uptake less than 0.3% of the administered dose is unlikely to be successful. The response to ablative therapy varies with site of the metastasis. Diffuse pulmonary lesions which are not evident radiographically are the most responsive, and the usual administered dose is 100 to 150 mCi (37–40). Damage to normal pulmonary epithelium is not supported by local dosimetry and is very rare [41]. Cannonball pulmonary metastases are not easy to ablate even when they concentrate radioiodine. It is important to note that repeat scans may be negative after apparent ablation, in spite of a positive radiograph due to failure of the metastasis to take up radioiodine because of dedifferentiation. Undetectable thyroglobulin levels combined with a benign clinical course are good evidence of successful therapy.

Bone metastases are more problematic. The majority occur in the axial skeleton, more commonly with follicular cancer and rarely with papillary. The lesions can be osteolytic on radiographs and for that reason may not be scintigraphically evident on standard bone scan [42]. Careful inspection of a good quality, high–resolution bone scan looking for subtle abnormalities is recommended. Liver and brain metastases are rare. In treating CNS and verbetral metastases, there is concern when thyroxine is stopped that high levels of TSH may stimulate further growth of the lesions, precipitating rapid neurological damage because of pressure effects. Deleterious effects related to ^{131}I and/or tumor growth have been described [43–46]. In those cases, we advise carefully coordinating the discontinuation of thyroxine and ^{131}I therapy with close collaboration with neurosurgeons and radiation therapists. In certain cases, radioiodine ablation is considered too hazardous, and external beam radiotherapy is the only feasible approach.

Local spread of the cancer to trachea or other neck structurers requires doses of 75 to 150 mCi for ablation. Spread to local lymph nodes is not a major bad prognostic factor. We would recommend treating nodes positive on scan but impalpable with radioiodine, usually with 100 mCi, and surgically resecting those which are clinically palpable.

A repeat whole body scan of the therapy dose at 7 to 10 days is recommended to prove that the treatment localized where desired. On occasion, additional lesions may be demonstrated which were not previously seen with the test dose [47]. It is not certain whether uptake in these lesions will be sufficient to ablate them. Often diffuse uptake in the liver is seen, and this is due to metabolism of radiolabelled hormones in the liver and should not be mistaken for metastases. Ten percent of papillary cancers fail to concentrate radioiodine even when the TSH is high, and these lesions are, therefore, not visualized.

Side Effects of Radioiodine Therapy

Radiation thyroiditis is a rare complication but one about which the patient should be warned. It is due to the intense radiation dose delivered to the thyroid and manifests itself 7–14 days post treatment as pain and tenderness in the region of residual thyroid with referred pain to the teeth, jaw and ear. Simple analgesics such as aspirin usually afford relief; however, in severe cases, stronger analgesics and prednisone in doses of 30 to 40 mg per day may be required for a period of 2 weeks. More commonly patients report a mild change in sense of taste for a short period following therapy, more often after doses of 100 mCi. Approximately 10% of patients will develop sialadenitis as radioiodine is also taken up by the salivary glands [48]. Hypoparathyroidism is not a complication of radioiodine treatment. Because many of the thyroid cancer patients are young with a good prognosis, it is important to consider the theoretical problems related to the long–term complications of radioiodine. These include induction of a more aggressive form of thyroid cancer and of cancers in organs which have been subject to the highest radiation doses from ^{131}I such as the stomach, salivary glands, kidney, bladder and bone marrow. In addition, the potential risk to future offspring of treated young patients should be considered. Several large clinical series showed no increased risk of second malignancies attributable to radioiodine. Pochin's data suggested that acute leukemia was found more often [49]; however, it should be noted that all 3 cases occurred after cumulative doses of 1,050 mCi on protocols where high doses were given at frequent intervals [50]. It is generally accepted now that one or two therapy doses should be sufficient to ablate residual thyroid, and the intervals betwen therapies should be at least 6 months up to one year. Although isolated cases of leukemia, breast and bladder cancer have been reported, the general consensus is that 'the benefits of therapy do not appear to be outweighed by long–term harmful effects' [50]. Prospective studies are required for full evaluation of the genetic risk to offspring, although one series showed no difference in offspring of 33 treated patients [51]. Azospermia has been reported, but infrequently [52].

In summary, although there is a slight risk of long–term complications from radioiodine therapy, those patients with distant metastases are at much greater risk of complications from their cancer than from radioiodine. In younger patients with well–differentiated tumors who have a good prognosis and a relatively good life expectancy, due care should be given to administering the minimum dose of radioiodine which can successfully treat the cancer.

Radiation Safety Aspects of Radioiodine Treatment

Prior to proceeding with radioiodine treatment, it is important to fully discuss all aspects of radiation safety with the patient. All women of child–bearing age should have a negative pregnancy test, preferably with the beta–HCG method. Because of the risk of radiation exposure to family members and the public, National Council on Radiation Protection and

Measurement, (NRCP) regulations dictate whether the patient should be treated as an inpatient or outpatient [53]. Doses of 30 mCi and greater should be administered as an inpatient. The patient should be assigned to a designated room, lead–lined if possible, which has been prepared by radiation safety personnel. To minimize all possibility of contamination either via saliva, sweat or urine, paper plates, cups and utensils should be used. All fixtures, including the telephone and light switches, are sealed in cellophane, and the areas around the toilet are covered with a protective paper to guard against contamination from splashes or spills. All garbage, including food waste and disposable utensils, are placed in a sealed plastic bag and kept until the patient is discharged, when it can then be disposed of by radiation safety personnel. The iodine is administered orally, in either liquid or capsule form, and great care is taken to avoid contamination or spillage during the procedure. The patient is instructed to drink a minimum of 8 ounces of fluid hourly and to micturate at least every 2 hours over the first 8 hours in an effort to speed the excretion of untrapped radioiodine and reduce the radiation dose to the urinary tract. All personnel involved with the patient should wear radiation dosimeters, and the Nuclear Medicine physician or technologist administering the radioiodine must have thyroid counts within 7 days to ensure there has been no inhalation of radioactivity.

The patient can be discharged when the retained dose is 30 mCi or less, or the emitted radiation is 8 mrem/hour at one meter. After discharge, the patient can then follow the same guidelines for outpatients. We generally recommend that they do not share a bed for the next 2 days and continue to use disposable utensils and take precautions with regard to urine, saliva or sweat contamination for that time. All contact with pregnant women, infants and young children should be avoided in the first week after treatment, and this includes prolonged contact with strangers, for example, at the movies or in restaurants, buses or airplanes. After one week all restrictions can be lifted.

Unfortunately 10% of histologically differentiated thyroid cancers do not accumulate ^{131}I even when there is marked TSH stimulus. These cancers can sometimes be detected on whole body ^{201}Thallium scans [54]. Because these cancers can grow under TSH stimulus, thyroxine should be prescribed in a dose sufficient to suppress this. Metastases should be treated by other means such as external beam radiation therapy or systemic chemotherapy.

The role for systemic chemotherapy is very limited as most patients with differentiated thyroid carcinoma have a good prognosis. There are a few studies which have reported some success with this form of treatment in patients with progressive disease considered untreatable with standard therapies. Agents used have included doxorubicin, either alone or in combination with melphalan, vincristine and bleomycin. This form of therapy should only be used if there is evidence of progressive disease, and the decision to treat must be made jointly by oncologist and thyroidologist.

Thyroglobulin as a Tumor Marker

Serum thyroglobulin has been shown to be increased in recurrent or metastatic thyroid cancer and to be absent after successful ablation of all thyroid tissue [55–57]. In our experience, the results depend upon whether the patient is taking thyroxine or not and also on whether a significant amount of normal thyroid is left postoperatively. In patients on suppressive doses of thyroxine, after total thyroidectomy the sensitivity for detecting disease is 97% and specificity 96%. If residual thyroid is present, the specificity falls to 87%, but the sensitivity remains at 97%. When thyroxine is discontinued, both benign and malignant thyroid tissue is stimulated by TSH [59]. The sensitivity in those without thyroid tissue is 75%, in those with residual thyroid tissue 94%, while the respective specificities are 95% and 71%. We have adopted the following approach in patients thought to have had total thyroid ablation either by surgery alone or by surgery and raidioidine: Thyroxine is stopped for 4 weeks. Prior to administering the tracer of ^{131}I, blood is drawn to check serum TSH and thyroglobulin. If the scan is negative and thyroglobulin undetectable, then complete ablation is virtually assured. Thyroxine is restarted, and the disease is monitored with clinical evaluation and thyroglobulin levels while the patient is on thyroxine. Rarely the scan is abnormal but thyroglobulin is undetectable [60]. In this case the tumor is ablated with radioiodine, but thyroglobulin cannot be used reliably to monitor the course of the disease. Also rarely the scan will be negative and thyroglobulin will be detectable which is perplexing. In this case cancer may be detectable on whole body thallium scintigraphy [54]. In patients who have had less extensive thyroid surgery and are on thyroxine suppression, radioiodine scans are not helpful as only residual thyroid shows up. Thyroglobulin levels can be used to monitor the disease, but in these cases, the levels are usually higher, up to 10 ng/ml in our experience.

Prognosis

Prognosis, both recurrence rate and death rate, is dependent on multiple factors, the most important of which include increasing age, male sex, large primary cancer, distant metastases and dedifferentiated pathology [1,3,61,62]. Absence of Hashimoto's thyroiditis and presence of lymph node metastases [63] in some series predict a slightly worse prognosis.

In most large series, it is very unusual for a patient younger than 40 years or with a primary cancer less than 2 cm in diameter to die from papillary cancer. The additive benefit of ^{131}I is not clear in all studies [64–68], and there are no controlled studies comparing matched patients treated with and without ^{131}I. In general the prognosis is excellent. Mazzaferri and Young [25] reported 6 deaths in 576 patients followed for 10 years, Rossi et al. [21] found 7% of 309 patients died after a median follow–up of 13 years, and Hay et al. [23] found only 6.4% of 860 died after 20 years.

Follicular Cancer

There are differences between follicular and papillary thyroid cancers. Prior head and neck irradiation is not an important causal factor. This cancer tends to be found in older patients, and there is a significant association with multinodular goiter, although it is not clear whether it arises de novo or as a result of malignant transformation. Unlike papillary cancer, the incidence of follicular cancer is falling in the U.S., and this may be related to the decreasing incidence of multinodular goiter, possibly due to increased dietary iodine.

Pathology

Typically pink in color, this well–circumscribed cancer can invade both capsule and vessels. Although it can occur anywhere in the thyroid gland, it is rarely found in the isthmus. Mircroscopically, there are no psammona bodies and no papillae [69]. When the classic features of follicular carcinoma are present and the nuclei have a ground glass appearance, the lesion is classified as a follicular variant of papillary cancer. Pure follicular cancer has an increased tendency to metastasize to bone, lung, liver and brain. Regional lymph node spread is less common. Histologic evidence of significant capsular or vascular invasion are prognostically bad features and important in separating an atypical follicular adenoma from a well–differentiated follicular carcinoma.

Clinical

The cancer usually presents as a thyroid nodule in a woman aged 45–55 years. Although most patients are euthyroid, occasionally this type of cancer is associated with hyperthyroidism either due to excess thyroxine secretion from widespread metastases or a large primary lesion [70,71]. Treatment is initially surgical. Near total thyroidectomy is followed by radioiodine ablation of residual thyroid or metastases. Whole body scans should be done 6 to 12 months later to look for functioning metastases, and if found, these should be treated with a second therapeutic dose of ^{131}I. In those patients with hyperthyroidism, pretreatment with antithyroid drugs is recommended to prevent thyroid storm. The usual treatment dose for ablation is 75–100 mCi and for metastases 150 to 200 mCi. As in papillary cancer, the same principles apply, and disease progression can be monitored with thyroglobulin measurements and whole body ^{131}I scans.

Prognosis

There are several factors which make the prognosis of patients with follicular cancer inferior to that in patients with papillary cancer. These factors include extrathyroidal extension, distant metastases, large size of primary tumor and old age of the patient [72,74].

Hurthle Cell Cancer. Hurthle cells are follicular cells with abundant mitochondria and are found in benign forms of thyroid disease such as Hashimoto's thyroiditis or Graves' disease as well as in neoplasia [75]. Hurthle cell cancers are variants of follicular cancer. They tend to occur in older patients, with a female to male ratio of two to one, and are often resistant to radioiodine treatment. Surgical excision of the primary and resection or external beam radiation therapy of distant metastases or recurrences is the usual approach to treatment.

Clear Cell Cancer. Clear cell cancer is a very rare form of thyroid cancer with a bad prognosis [76]. Treatment is near total thyroidectomy followed by radioiodine treatment if functioning metastases are demonstrated on scan. Chemotherapy and/or external radiation therapy are alternatives depending on the site and extent of spread.

Differentiated Cancers in Non–Thyroidal Sites

Thyroglossal Duct or Cyst

Approximately 70 cases of thyroglossal duct cancer are presented in the literature, the vast majority being papillary cancer [77–79]. Metastases to regional nodes are only described in 10% of patients, probably because the surgeon is not operating for thyroid cancer but to remove a thyroglossal cyst. The standard operation for thyroglassal cyst is generally adequate (Sistrunk operation) and the prognosis is excellent. If there is a nodule in the thyroid, thyroidectomy should be considered since there are rare reports of primary thyroid cancer extending directly into thyroglossal duct and cyst.

Malignant Struma Ovarii

In 1983 there were only 19 reports of malignant thyroid tissue in struma ovarii and only 5 with metastases [80–82]. When the cancer is restricted to the ovary, removal of the ovary is sufficient, but when metastases are present and ^{131}I considered, it is necessary to remove normal cervical thyroid prior to treatment.

Anaplastic Cancer

In the U.S. approximately 5–15% of thyroid cancers are anaplastic; the incidence is greater in Europe. Pathologically, it is apparent that many of these cancers arise from pre–existing differentiated cancers [83]. Circumstantial evidence points to radiation therapy, both external and internal as a causal factor, although the presence of long–standing differentiated cancer per se is more important [84,85].

Anaplastic cancers are classified as giant or spindle cell. Sarcomas of the thyroid are usually anaplastic adenocarcinomas. In older classifications small cell anaplastic cancer is now recognized as either lymphoma or medullary cancer by specific monoclonal antibodies and immunoperoxidase stains [86]. Patients are generally more than 60 years. Dysphagia, dysphonia and dyspnea are characteristic [85]. The cancer is quite lethal, with most patients dying within 6 months of diagnosis. At the time of diagnosis 80% have lymph node and 50% distant metastases. Although clinical diagnosis is frequently obvious in an older patient with a rapidly growing thyroid mass that is hard and fixed, it is important to make a pathological diagnosis. Imaging studies of the thyroid are not usually helpful diagnostically, but chest roentgenogram and computed tomography (CT) of neck and chest can help delineate the extent of disease. If the cancer is confined to the thyroid, the prognosis is dramatically improved, but this is rare as shown by the figures quoted above. When there is obvious evidence of metastases or the cancer is unresectable, diagnosis can be established by needle aspirate or limited open biopsy. When the cancer is resectable, near total thyroidectomy is advised. In one series, 3 patients with resectable cancer survived 5.4 years on average, whereas in 81 patients with unresectable cancer, the mean survival was 4.8 months [83]. In an analysis of 420 patients from 10 publications, Casterline et al. [87] reported that only 2.6% survived 2 years.

The clinician is usually faced with an elderly, ill patient with locally invasive cancer plus metastases. After establishing the diagnosis, therapy includes external radiation and chemotherapy. Various fractionations of external radiation have been used, 100 rads (1 Gy) 4 times per day, 160 rads (1.6 Gy) twice daily or 200 rads (2 Gy) daily to a total of 5,000 to 6,000 rads [50–60 Gy]. Chemotherapy should include doxorubicin which is the most effective single agent [88]. Sometimes chemotherapy causes sufficient shrinkage of the cancer to allow surgical resection [89]. Even with combined radiation and chemotherapy the prognosis is dreadful. Radioiodine therapy is of no value.

Medullary Cancer

Medullary cancers arise from the parafollicular cells which secrete calcitonin. The cancer and its metastases secrete calcitonin which can be used as a tumor marker [90,92]. Medullary cancer can be familial or sporadic [93]. Familial medullary cancers are autosomal dominant and occur as one of 3 syndromes—multiple endocrine neoplasia type IIa (MEN IIa) and type IIb (MEN IIb) and non–MEN cancer. In MEN IIa there can be pheochromocytoma and hyperparathyroidism in addition to medullary carcinoma. MEN IIb has these features plus a typical facies, Marfanoid features and mucosal neuromas. The third type has none of the additional features.

In most series this cancer accounts for 5–10% of thyroid cancers, but if familial cases are identified, this proportion can increase due to inclusion of family members with nonclinical disease diagnosed by provocative tests which cause a rise in the tumor marker calcitonin [94].

The cancers are hard, and 90% of familial cases are multifocal. Familial cases often present with bilateral lesions at the lateral margin of the junction of the upper 1/3 and lower 2/3 of each lobe. Cervical lymph node metastases are present in about 50% of patients with clinically evident primary cancer. In contrast to cancers arising from follicular cells, medullary cancers spread to central rather than lateral nodes. At the time of the first surgery, about 25% of patients have mediastinal nodal involvement. Systemic metastases can occur to lung, liver and bone [95]. Histologically a characteristic finding is amyloid.

The sex distribution is equal. Sporadic cases occur most often in the fifth decade, familial cases earlier, in particular in patients diagnosed by provocative tests. In sporadic cases, the original presentation is usually a thyroid nodule; in familial cases there can be symptoms and signs such as diarrhea, hypertension, flushing. Cushing's syndrome can be due to secretory products plus associated lesions. Early familial cases are asymptomatic and diagnosed by significant rise in calcitonin after intravenous calcium (2 mg/Kg injected rapidly, or, 3 mg/Kg infused over 10 minutes) or pentagastrin (0.5 ug/Kg) [94,96,97]. Some investigators recommend combining calcium and pentagastrin infusion with multiple blood samples over 15 minutes [97].

In sporadic cases conventional ^{123}I scintigraphy is not specific, and needle aspiration of the nodule is more accurate diagnostically. There has been interest in radiopharmaceuticals which have shown positive uptake in primary and metastatic lesions. These include thallium-201 [98], metaiodobenzyl-guanidine (MIBG) labeled with ^{131}I [99,100], pentavalent dimercaptosuccinate labeled with ^{99m}Tc [101] and anticalcitonin antibodies [102]. There are to date no large series which allow reliable calculation of sensitivities, specificities and accuracies of those tests.

Total thyroidectomy is the appropriate treatment, and because of frequent involvement of central lymph nodes they should be removed from the hyoid to the innominate. Patients in whom all cancer is removed at the first operation have a better prognosis. In those where there is residual cancer supervoltage radiation therapy to a dose of 4,5000 to 5,000 rads (45 to 50 Gy) is recommended. Although there are a few reports of residual cancer being treated successfully with ^{131}I [103,104], intuitively this does not make sense since the cells do not concentrate iodine. In larger series this treatment does not reduce recurrences or improve prognosis. Prognosis is best when the cancer is restricted to the thyroid, when surgery removes all cancer, in young patients and in those with MEN IIa. As a group, those with MEN IIb do the worst. Ten–year survival is 60–70% [94,105].

Primary Lymphoma of Thyroid

In a series of 4,200 patients with a nodule in the thyroid, Hamburger et al. [106] found 389 cancers of which 30 were lymphomas. The most common type is diffuse histiocytic [107,108]. Pathologically, there is frequently a gradation from the lymphocytic infiltration of Hashimoto's thyroiditis to lymphoma [109–115]. However, Hashimoto's thyroiditis is a very common clinical problem whereas lymphoma is distinctly uncommon. Holm et al. [116] found 4 cases of lymphoma in 829 patients with pathologically proven Hashimoto's thyroiditis whom they were following. This small percentage, 0.2%, was about 70 times the expected frequency.

Clinically a rapid increase in goiter size or a hard thyroid mass arising in a goiter are common presentations. The condition is about 3 times as common in women, and their average age is about 60 years. Most are euthyroid, but hypothyroidism from involvement of the entire gland [106] or hyperthyroidism from release of thyroid hormone from ruptured follicles have been described [117]. Dysphagia and hoarseness are common. Once the diagnosis is established, standard staging procedures are advised. In stage I disease lobectomy can be curative, although in this stage and stage II, local external radiation therapy to a dose of 4,000 rads (40 Gy) is frequently recommended. In stages III or IV, systemic chemotherapy, or combined radiation plus chemotherapy are necessary.

Metastases to the Thyroid

Although metastases to the thyroid are found in autopsies of up to 25% of patients dying of metastatic cancer, they are not a common clinical presentation. Breast, lung, kidney, melanoma and gastrointestinal tract are the primary site in about 80% of cases [118]. If a patient with a known cancer, especially one of these five types, develops a thyroid nodule, the probability of metastasis must be considered [119]. Fine needle aspirate should be used to make the diagnosis, and when the lesion is single, lobectomy is advised [120]. Rarely removal of a solitary thyroid metastasis results in long–term survival; however, most patients will have other metastases.

References

1. Mazzaferri EL: Papillary thyroid carcinoma: Factors influencing prognosis and current therapy. Semin Oncol 14:315–332, 1987.
2. Tubiana M, Schlumberger M, Rougier P, et al.: Long–term results and prognostic factors in patients with differentiated thyroid carcinoma. Cancer 55:794–804, 1985.
3. McConahey WM, Hay ID, Wollner LB, et al.: Papillary thyroid cancer treated at the

Mayo Clinic, 1946 through 1970: Initial manifestations, pathologic findings, therapy and outcome. Mayo Clin Proc 61:978–996, 1987.
4. Rossi RL, Nieroda C, Cady B, et al.: Malignancies of the thyroid gland. The Lahey Clinic experience. Surg Clin N Am 65:211–230, 1985.
5. Werner SC: Classification of thyroid disease. Report of the committee on nomenclature the American Thyroid Association—Part I. J Clin Endocrinol Metab 29:860–862, 1969.
6. Duffy BJ Jr, Fitzgerald PJ: Cancer of the thyroid in children: A report of 28 cases. J Clin Endocrinol Metab 10:1296–1308, 1950.
7. Favus MJ, Schneider AB, Stachura ME, et al.: Thyroid cancer occurring as a late consequence of head-and-neck irradiation: Evaluation of 1056 patients. N Engl J Med 294:1019–1025, 1976.
8. DeGroot L, Paloyan E: Thyroid carcinoma and radiation: A Chicago endemic. JAMA 225:487–491, 1973.
9. Clark OH, Greenspan FS, Dunphy JE: Hashimoto's thyroiditis and thyroid cancer: Indications for operation. Am J Surg 140:65–70, 1980.
10. Black BM, Kirk TA, Woolner LB: Multicentricity of papillary adenocarcinoma of the thyroid: Influence on treatment. J Clin Endocrinol Metab 20:130–135, 1960.
11. Carcangiu ML, Zampi G, Pupi A, et al.: Papillary carcinoma of the thyroid: A clinicopathologic study of 241 cases treated at the University of Florence, Italy. Cancer 55:805–828, 1985.
12. Staunton MD, Skeet RG: Thyroid cancer: Prognosis in 469 patients. Br J Surg 66:643–647, 1979.
13. Simpson WJ, McKinney SE, Carruthers JS, et al.: Papillary and follicular thyroid cancer: Prognostic factors in 1,578 patients. Am J Med 83:479–488, 1987.
14. Heitz P, Mosher H, Staub JJ: Thyroid cancer: A study of 573 thyroid tumors and 161 autopsy cases observed over a thirty-year period. Cancer 37:2329–2337, 1976.
15. Clark RL Jr, White EC, Russel WO: Total thyroidectomy for cancer of the thyroid: Significance of intraglandular dissemination. Ann Surg 149:858–866, 1959.
16. Clark OH: Total thyroidectomy: The treatment of choice for patients with differentiated thyroid cancer. Ann Surg 196:361–370, 1982.
17. Jacobs JK, Aland JW, Ballinger JR, et al.: Total thyroidectomy: A review of 213 patients. Ann Surg 197:542–548, 1983.
18. Attie JN, Moskowitz GW, Margouleff D, et al.: Feasibility of total thyroidectomy in the treatment of thyroid carcinoma: Postoperative radioactive iodine evaluation in 140 cases. Am J Surg 138:555–560, 1979.
19. Harness JK, Fung L, Thompson NW, et al.: Total thyroidectomy: Complications and technique. World J Surg 10:781–786, 1986.
20. Mazzaferri EL, Young RL, Oertel JE, et al.: Papillary thyroid carcinoma: The impact of therapy in 576 patients. Medicine 56:171–195, 1977.
21. Rossi RL, Cady B, Silverman ML, et al.: Current results of conservation surgery for differentiated thyroid carcinoma. World J Surg 10:612–622, 1986.
22. Starnes HF, Brooks DC, Pinkus GS, et al.: Surgery for thyroid carcinoma. Cancer 55:1376–1381, 1985.
23. Hay ID, Grant CS, Taylor WF, et al.: Ipsilateral lobectormy versus bilateral lobar resection in papillary thyroid carcinoma: a retrospective analysis of surgical outcome using a novel prognostic scoring system. Surgery 102:1088–1095, 1987.
24. Sako K, Marchetta FC, Razack MS, et al.: Modified radical neck dissection for metastatic carcinoma of the thyroid: a reappraisal. Am J Surg 150:500–502, 1985.
25. Mazzaferri EL, Young RL: Papillary thyroid carcinoma: A 10 year follow-up report of the impact of therapy in 576 patients. Am J Med 70:511–518, 1981.
26. Crile G Jr, Antunez AR, Esselstyn CB, et al.: The advantages of subtotal thyroidectomy and suppression of TSH in the primary treatment of papillary carcinoma of the thyroid. Cancer 55:2691–2697, 1985.

27. Hilts SV, Hellman D, Anderson J, et al.: Serial TSH determination after T3 withdrawal or thyroidectomy in the therapy of thyroid carcinoma. J Nucl Med 20:928–932, 1979.
28. Beckerman C, Gottschalk A, Hoffer PB: Optimal time for ^{131}I total body imaging to detect metastatic thyroid carcinoma. J Nucl Med 15:477, Abst 1974.
29. McCowen KD, Adler RA, Ghaed N, et al.: Low dose radioiodine thyroid ablation in postsurgical patients with thyroid cancer. Am J Med 61:52–58, 1976.
30. Ryo UY: Low–dose and high–dose radioiodine in thyroid cancer. Am J Med 61:52–58, 1976.
31. Kuni CC, Klingensmith WC: Failure of low doses ^{131}I to ablate residual thyroid tissue following surgery for thyroid cancer. Radiology 137:773–774, 1980.
32. Siddiqui AR, Edmonson J, Wellman HH, et al.: Feasibility of low doses of ^{131}I for thyroid ablation in postsurgical patients with thyroid carcinoma. Clin Nucl Med 6:158–161, 1981.
33. Ramacciotti C, Pretorius HT, Line BR, et al.: Ablation of nonmalignant thyroid remnants with low doses of radioactive iodine: concise communication. J Nucl Med 23:483–489, 1982.
34. DeGroot LJ, Reilly M: Comparison of 30– and 50–mCi doses of iodine–131 for thyroid ablation. Ann Intern Med 96:51–53, 1982.
35. Snyder J, Gorman C, Scanlon P: Thyroid remnant ablation: Questionable pursuit of an ill–defined goal. J Nucl Med 24:659–665, 1983.
36. Maxon HR, Thomas SR, Hertzberg VS, et al.: Relation between effective radiation dose and outcome of radioiodine therapy for thyroid cancer. N Engl J Med 309:937–941, 1983.
37. Freebberg AS, Ureles AL, Lesses MF, et al.: Pulmonary metastatic lesion successfully treated with radioactive iodine. JAMA 144:16–19, 1950.
38. Turner JE, Weir GJ Jr: Pulmonary metastases from thyroid carcinoma detectable only by ^{131}I scan. Treatment and response. J Nucl Med 13:854–855, 1972.
39. Massin JP, Savoie JC, Garnier H, et al.: Pulmonary metastases in differentiated thyroid carcinoma: study of 58 cases with implications for the primary tumor treatment. Cancer 53:982–992, 1984.
40. Samaan NA, Schultz PN, Haynie TP, et al.: Pulmonary metastasis of differentiated thyroid carcinoma: treatment results in 101 patients. J Clin Endocrinol Metab 65:376–380, 1985.
41. Rall JE, Alpers JB, Lewallen CG, et al.: Radiation pneumonitis and fibrosis: A complication of radioiodine treatment of plumonary metastases from cancer of the thyroid. J Clin Endocrinol Metab 17:1263–1276, 1957.
42. Castillo LA, Yeh SDJ, Leeper RD, et al.: Bone scan in bone metastases from functioning thyroid carcinoma. Clin Nucl Med 5:200–209, 1980.
43. Holmquest DI, Lake P: Sudden hemorrhage in metastatic carcinoma of the brain during treatment with iodine–131. J Nucl Med 17:307–309, 1976.
44. Datz FL: Cerebral edema following iodine–131 therapy for thyroid carcinoma metastatic to the brain. J Nucl Med 27:637–640, 1986.
45. Goldberg LD, Ditchek NT: Thyroid carcinoma with spinal cord compression. JAMA 245:953, 1981.
46. Shortliffe EH, Crapo LM: Thyroid carcinoma with spinal cord compression. JAMA 247:2566–1567, 1982.
47. Nemec J, Rohling S, Zamrazil V, et al.: Comparison of the distribution of diagnostic and thyroablative I–131 in the evaluation of differentiated thyroid cancers. J Nucl Med 20:92–97, 1979.
48. Allweiss P, Braunstein GD, Katz A, et al.: Sialadenitis following I–131 therapy for thyroid carcinoma: concise communication. J Nucl Med 25:755–758, 1984.
49. Pochin EE: Long term hazards of radioiodine treatment of thyroid carcinoma. UICC Monograph Series Vol 12 Thyroid Cancer. Hedinger C (ed) Berlin: Springer–Verlag P293–304, 1969.

50. Edmonds CJ, Smith T: The long–term hazards of the treatment of thyroid cancer with radioiodine. Br J Radiol 59:45–51, 1986.
51. Sarkar SD, Beierwaltes WH, Gill SP, et al.: Subsequent fertility and birth histories of children and adolescents treated with ^{131}I for thyroid cancer. J Nucl Med 17:460–464, 1976.
52. Ahmed SR, Shalet SM: Gonadal damage due to radioactive iodine (I^{131}) treatment for thyroid carcinoma. Postgrad Med J 61:361–362, 1985.
53. National Council on Radiation Protection and Measurements. Report No. 37. Precautions in the management of patients who have received therapeutic amounts of radionuclides, 1970.
54. Brendel AJ, Guyot M, LeFort G, et al.: Thallium–201 imaging in the follow–up of differentiated thyroid carcinoma. J Nucl Med 29:1515–1520, 1988.
55. Van Herle AJ, Uller RP: Elevated serum thyroglobulin: A marker of metastases in differentiated thyroid carcinomas. J Clin Invest 56:272–277, 1975.
56. Shlossberg AH, Jacobson JCJ, Ibbertson HK: Serum thyroglobulin in the diagnosis and management of thyroid carcinoma. Clin Endocrinol 10:17–27, 1979.
57. Blahd WH, Drickman MV, Porter CW, et al.: Serum thyroglobulin, a monitor of differentiated thyroid carcinoma in patients receiving thyroid hormone suppression therapy: concise communication. J Nucl Med 25:673–676, 1984.
58. McDougall IR, Bayer MF: Follow–up of patients with differentiated thyroid cancer using serum thyroglobulin measured by an immunoradiometric assay. Comparison with I–131 total body scans. J Nucl Med 21:741–744, 1980.
59. Bayer MF, McDougall IR, Kriss JP: Retrospective study of serum thyroglobulin measurements performed in patients with differentiated thyroid carcinoma at the Stanford University thyroid clinic between 1979 and 1985. In: Thyroglobulin and thyroglobulin antibodies in the follow–up of thyroid cancer and endemic goiter M Hufner and C Reiners (ed) Georg Thieme Verlang Stuttgart, pp 104–111, 1987.
60. Miller JH, Marcus CS: Metastatic papillary thyroid carcinoma with normal serum thyroglobulin level. Clin Nucl Med 13:652–653, 1988.
61. Hay ID, Grant CS, Taylor WF, et al.: Ipsilateral lobectomy versus bilateral lobar resection in papillary thyroid carcinoma. A retrospective analysis of surgical outcome using a novel prognostic scoring system. Surgery 102:1088–1095, 1987.
62. Cady B, Sedgwick CE, Meissner WA, et al.: Risk factor analysis in differentiated thyroid cancer. Cancer 43:810–820, 1979.
63. Harwood J, Clark OH, Dunphy JE: Significance of lymph node metastasis in differentiated thyroid cancer. Am J Surg 136:107–112, 1978.
64. Leeper RD: The effect of ^{131}I therapy on survival of patients with metastatic papillary or follicular thyroid cancer. J Clin Endocrinol 36:1143–1152, 1973.
65. Varma VM, Beierwalte WH, Nofal MM, et al.: Treatment of thyroid cancer: Death rates after surgery and after surgery followed by sodium iodide I 131. JAMA 214:1437–1442, 1970.
66. Leeper RD: Thyroid Cancer. Med Clin N Am 69:1079–1096, 1985.
67. Beierwaltes WH: The treatment of thyroid carcinoma with radioactive iodine. Semin Nucl Med 8:79–94, 1978.
68. Krishnamurthy GT, Blahd WH: Radioiodine I–131 therapy in the management of thyroid carcinoma: a prospective study. Cancer 40:195–202, 1977.
69. LiVolsi VA: Pathology of thyroid cancer. In: Thyroid Cancer, Greenfield LD (ed). West Palm Beach: CRC Press, pp 85–141, 1978.
70. Ober KP, Cowan FR, Sevier RE, et al.: Thyrotoxicosis caused by functioning metastatic thyroid carcinoma. Clin Nucl Med 12:345–348, 1987.
71. Pont A, Spratt D, Shinn JB: T3 toxicosis due to nonmetastatic follicular carcinoma of the thyroid. West J Med 136:255–258, 1982.
72. Harness JK, Thomson NW, McLeod MK, et al.: Follicular carcinoma of the thyroid gland: Trends and treatment. Surgery 96:972–978, 1984.

73. Lang W, Choritz H, Hundeshagen H: Risk factors in follicular thyroid carcinomas. Am J Surg Pthol 10:246–255, 1986.
74. Young RL, Mazzaferri EL, Rahe AJ, et al.: Pure follicular thyroid carcinoma: Impact of therapy on 214 patients. J Nucl Med 21:733–739, 1980.
75. Watson RG, Brennan MD, Goellner JR, et al.: Invasive Hurthle cell carcinoma of the thyroid: Natural history and management. Mayo Clin Proc 59:851–855, 1984.
76. Fisher ER, Kim WS: Primary clear cell thyroid carcinoma with squamous features. Cancer 39:2497–2502, 1977.
77. Jaques DA, Chambers RG, Oertel JE: Thyroglossal tract carcinoma. A review of the literature and addition of eighteen cases. Am J Surg 1230:439–446, 1970.
78. Joseph TJ, Komorowski RA: Thyroglossal duct carcinoma. Hum Pathol 6:717–729, 1975.
79. Roses DR, Snively SL, Cohen N, et al.: Carcinoma of the thyroglossal duct. Am J Surg 145:266–269, 1983.
80. Pardo–Mindan FJ, Vazquez JJ: Malignant struma ovarii: Light and electron microscopic study. Cancer 51:337–343, 1983.
81. Kempers RD, Dockerty MB, Hoffman DL, et al.: Struma ovarii-Ascitic, hyperthyroid, and asymptomatic syndromes. Ann Intern Med 72:883–893, 1970.
82. McDougall IR, Krasne D, Hanberry JW, et al.: Malignant Struma ovarii presenting as paraparesis from a spinal metastasis. J Nucl Med 30:407–411, 1989.
83. Aldinger KA, Samaan NA, Ibanez M, et al.: Anaplastic carcinoma of the thyroid. A review of 84 cases of spindle and giant cell carcinoma of the thyroid. Cancer 41:2267–2275, 1978.
84. Kapp DS, Li Volsi VA, Sanders MM: Anaplastic carcinoma following well–differentiated thyroid carcinoma: etilogical considerations. Yale J Biol Med 55:521–528, 1982.
85. Carcangiu ML, Steeper T, Zampi G, et al.: Anaplastic thyroid carcinoma. A study of 70 cases. Am J Clin Pathl 83:135–158, 1985.
86. Shevro J, Gal R, Avidor I, et al.: Anaplastic thyroid carcinoma. A clinical, histologic and immunochemical study. Cancer 62:319–325, 1984.
87. Casterline PF, Jaques DA, Blom H, et al.: Anaplastic giant and spindle–cell carcinoma of the thyroid. Cancer 45:1689–1692, 1980.
88. Kim JH, Leeper RD: Treatment of anaplastic giant and spindle cell carcinoma of the thyroid with combination Adriamycin and radiation therapy. A new approach. Cancer 52:954–957, 1983.
89. Spanos GA, Wolk D, Desner MR, et al.: Preoperative chemotherapy for giant cell carcinoma of the thyroid. Cancer 50:2252–2256, 1982.
90. Glotzman D, Pott IT Jr, Ridgeway EC, et al.: Calcitonin as a tumor marker: User of a radioimmunoassay for calcitonin in the postoperative evaluation of patients with medullary thyroid carcinoma. N Engl J Med 290:1035–1039, 1974.
91. Rougier P, Calmettes C, Laplanche A, et al.: The values of calcitonin and carcinoembryonic antigen in the treatment and management of nonfamilial medullary thyroid carcinoma. Cancer 51:855–862, 1983.
92. Tashjian AH Jr, Howland BG, Melvin KEW, et al.: Immunoassay of human calcitonin: Clinical measurement, relation to serum calcium and studies in patients with medullary carcinoma. N Engl J Med 283:890–895, 1970.
93. Pont A: Multiple endocrine neoplasic syndromes. West J Med 132:301–312, 1980.
94. Sizemore GW: Medullary cancer of the thyroid gland. Semi Oncol 14:306–314, 1987.
95. Williams ED: Medullary carcinoma and other disorders involving calcitonin. In: Endocrinology Volume 2, DeGroot LJ, et al. (ed). New York: Grune and Stratton, pp 777–792, 1981.
96. Sizemore GW, Go VLM: Stimulation tests for diagnosis of medullary thyroid carcinoma. Mayo Clin Proc 50:53–56, 1975.
97. Wells SA, Dilley WG, Farndon JA, et al.: Early diagnosis and treatment of medullary thyroid carcinoma. Arch Intern Med 145:1248–1252, 1985.

98. Hoefnagel CA, Delprat CC, Zanin D, et al.: New radionuclide tracers for the diagnosis and therapy of medullary thyroid carcinoma. Clin Nucl Med 13:159–165, 1988.
99. Sisson JC, Frager MS, Valk TW, et al.: Scintigraphic localization of pheochromocytoma. N Engl J Med 305:12–17, 1981.
100. Sisson JC, Shapiro B, Beierwaltes WH, et al.: Radiopharmaceutical treatment of maligant pheochromocytoma. J Nucl Med 24:197–206, 1984.
101. Miyauchi A, Endo K, Ohta H, et al.: ^{99m}Tc(v) Dimercaptosuccinic acid scintigraphy for medullary thyroid carcinoma. World J Surg 10:640–645, 1986.
102. Guilloteau D, Baulieu JL, Besnard JC: Medullary–thyroid–carcinoma imaging in an animal model:Use of radiolabeled anticalcitonin $F(ab)_2$ and metaiodobenzylguanidine. Eur J Nucl Med 11:198–200, 1985.
103. Hellman DE, Kartchner M, Van Antiwerp JD, et al.: Radioiodine in the treatment of medullary carcinoma of the thyroid. J Clin Endocrinol Metab 48:451–455, 1979.
104. Deftos LJ, Stein MF: Radioiodine as an adjunct to the surgical treatment of medullary thyroid carcinoma. J Clin Endocrinol Metab 50:967–968, 1980.
105. Saad MF, Ordonez NG, Rashid RK, et al.: Medullary carcinoma of the thyroid: A study of the clinical features and prognostic factors in 161 patients. Medicine 63:319–341, 1984.
106. Hamburger JI, Miller JM, Kini Sr: Lymphoma of the thyroid. Ann Intern Med 99:685–693, 1983.
107. Rappaport H: Tumors of the Hematopoietic System. Atlas of Tumor Pathology, Fascicle 8, Section 3. Armed Forces Institute of Pathology, 1964.
108. Chak LY, Hoppe RT, Burke JS, et al.: Non–Hodgkin's lymphoma presenting as thyroid enlargement. Cancer 48:2712–2716, 1981.
109. Burke JS, Butler JJ, Fuller LM: Malignant lymphomas of the thyroid. A clinical pathologic study of 35 patients including ultrastructure observations. Cancer 39:1587–1602, 1977.
110. Devine RM, Edis AJ, Banks DM: Primary lymphoma of the thyroid: A review of the Mayo Clinic experience. World J Surg 5:33–38, 1981.
111. Grimley RP, Oates GD: The natural history of malignant thyroid lymphomas. Br J Surg 67:475–477, 1980.
112. Maurer R, Taylor CR, Terry R, et al.: Non–Hodgkin's lymphoma of the thyroid gland. Birch Arch A Path Anat Histol 383:293–319, 1979.
113. Schwarze EW, Papadimitriou CS: Non–Hodgkin's lymphoma of the thyroid. Path Res Pract 167:346–362, 1980.
114. Sirota DK, Segal RL: Primary lymphomas of the thyroid gland. JAMA 242:1743–1746, 1979.
115. Souhami L, Simpson J, Carrurthers JS: Malignant lymphoma of the thyroid gland. Int J Rad Onc Biol Phys 6:1143–1147, 1980.
116. Holm LE, Blomgren, Lowhagen T: Cancer risks in patients with chronic lymphocytic thyroiditis. N Engl J Med 312:601–604, 1985.
117. Shimaoka K, Van Herle AJ, Dindogru A: Thyrotoxicosis secondary to involvement of the thyroid with malignant lymphoma. J Clin Endocrinol Metab 43:64–68, 1976.
118. McCabe DP, Farrar WB, Petkov TM, et al.: Clinical and pathologic correlation in disease metastatic to the thyroid. Am J Surg 150:519–523, 1985.
119. Ivy HK: Cancer metastatic to the thyroid: A diagnostic problem. Mayo Clin Proc 59:856–859, 1984.
120. Watts NB: Carcinoma metastatic to the thyroid: prevalence and diagnosis by fine needle aspiration cytology. Am J Med Sci 293:13–17, 1987.

11. Chemotherapy of Patients with Recurrent Head and Neck Cancer

Richard H. Wheeler

The majority of cancers of the upper aerodigestive tract are epithelial in origin and epidermoid in histology. With over 40,000 cases diagnosed each year, these malignancies rank eighth in incidence and comprise 4.2% of all malignancies seen annually in the United States [1]. As a group they occur more frequently than the leukemias, the lymphomas, cancer of the stomach, pancreas and melanoma. They represent 6.1% of the cancers occurring in males, and 2.4% of those seen in women. Approximately 30% of these patients will recur and die of their malignancy.

The prognosis and pattern of recurrence of squamous cell cancers arising in the head and neck depends somewhat upon the primary site and the treatment given [2–15]. In general, 80% or better of patients with early or stage I disease are cured, whereas 75% or more of patients with stage IV disease do not survive. The majority of recurrences are locoregional, with distant metastases said to occur in only 10–15 percent of patients. However, autopsy series show a much higher frequency of tumor dissemination [3,10]. Patients with nasopharyngeal or pyriform sinus primaries have a higher frequency of distant disease, whereas true glottic and paranasal sinus lesions appear to have a lower incidence [3,7,11,13]. The frequency of distant metastases is higher in patients with larger primary tumors and/or more advanced cervical node involvement. The incidence of clinically apparent distant metastases will exceed 50% in patients with advanced lesions when local control has been achieved [3]. The most common sites of distant spread are the lungs, liver and bones [3,10]. Clearly, the initial treatment of advanced stage patients must include strategies to address distant metastases if the cure rate is to improve substantially.

Local or regional recurrences may occur at the primary site, ipsi– or contralateral neck. The frequency of locoregional recurrence increases with increasing T and N stage. Up to one–third of patients may have neck recurrence in an untreated N_0 neck [2]. Approximately 50% of patients with operable stage III or IV tumors and over 75% of inoperable patients will have persistent or recurrent locoregional disease. Pathologic factors that predict disease recurrence include extracapsular nodal spread, vascular, lymphatic or perineural invasion [12–15]. Studies using flow cytometry have

Jacobs, C. (ed): Carcinomas of the Head and Neck: Evaluation and Management.

shown that analysis of tumor DNA content may improve prediction of prognosis. Retrospective and prospective studies have shown that the presence of an aneuploid tumor population correlates with a poorer prognosis for surgically treated patients [16,17].

The majority of locoregional recurrences become apparent within a year of treatment, and median survival of these patients is less than six months [3,9,13]. Although patients who develop metastases in a previously untreated neck may be successfully treated with surgery and/or radiation therapy [18], and up to 50% of patients with an isolated recurrence in a previously irradiated neck may be cured by surgery [19], less than 15% of patients are successfully salvaged after failure from primary treatment. Most distant metastases become clinically evident within 18 months of clinical diagnosis [3]. All these patients are potential candidates for regional or systemic chemotherapy or other treatment approaches.

Therapy given to patients with locoregional or distant recurrence should be considered palliative. Despite the capability of modern chemotherapy to produce objective responses, or the occasional long–term disease–free survival produced with antineoplastic drug treatment [20], the majority of patients face a short survival. Patients with low performance status, poor nutritional state, extensive prior surgery or irradiation are unlikely to respond to chemotherapy [21,22]. Patients who have received previous chemotherapy for recurrent disease rarely respond to additional chemotherapy. Maximum symptomatic support with judicious consideration of the toxic effects of antineoplastic agents should be the focus of treatment for these patients. For patients more capable of benefiting from, and tolerating, systemic therapy, the results obtained with various single agents and combination drug programs are summarized. Additional factors that could influence patients response to treatment include primary site, histologic differentiation, DNA content and dose, schedule or route of drug delivery [23–25]. Sufficient information does not yet exist to permit consideration of the first three factors in treatment planning. The latter factors will be considered with each agent discussed.

Single Agents

The folate antagonist methotrexate was the first agent to demonstrate significant clinical effect in patients with recurrent head and neck cancer. Reviews summarizing older studies suggested overall response rates of 44 to 50% (Table 1) [23,26]. More recent cooperative group studies have demonstrated response rates of 16–35% and represent a more realistic estimate of therapeutic efficacy [27–30]. Weekly drug administration appears to produce a higher response rate than monthly courses [26] and is less toxic than biweekly administration. In patients with adequate renal function, dose rates of 40–60 mg/m^2 weekly are generally well tolerated. The most com-

Table 1. Single agents in recurrent or disseminated squamous cell cancer of the head and neck.

Agent	# Patients	% Response (% CR)	Ref
Methotrexate			
Weekly or Biweekly	100	50 (15)	26
Monthly	107	29 (0)	26
Weekly	81	26 (7)	27
Weekly	21	24 (0)	28
×3d q 3 wk	50	16 (6)	29
Weekly	83	35 (8)	30
Methotrexate + Leucovorin	83	42	26
Cisplatin			
Variable Schecule	108	33	41
day 1 & 8	22	29 (5)	28
day 1 & 8	50	8 (0)	29
24 Hour Infusion	41	18 (8)	42
Carboplatin	29	28 (7)	80
Bleomycin	298	18 (3)	26
5-Fluorouracil	118	15	26
Not Stated	19	31	22
Infusion	7	57	73
Cyclophosphamide	77	36	26
Vinblastine	35	29	26

mon toxicities observed are mucosites and myelosuppression. Unfortunately, complete responses occur in less than 10% of patients, and partial response durations are short, generally 3–5 months [22–30].

As with most solid tumors, effective therapy of head and neck cancer with methotrexate is limited by tumor cell drug resistance and host toxicity. Based on the clinical demonstration that leucovorin (N^5N^{10} formyl tetrahydrofolate) will prevent toxicity in patients, increase the efficacy of methotrexate in L1210 leukemia in mice, and potentially circumvent a known resistance mechanism of reduced carrier mediated drug transport into the neoplastic cell, multiple studies of high-dose methotrexate with leucovorin rescue have been conducted [23,26,31]. Although responses to methotrexate/leucovorin have been reported in standard dose methotrexate resistant patients, randomized trials have failed to document an overall improved therapeutic effect [27,32,33]. When the additional expense is also considered, routine use of methotrexate/leucovorin in patients with recurrent disease is not warranted. Recent studies suggest that methotrexate resistance in aerodigestive squamous cell cancers may be due to decreased polyglutamylation of this agent with reduced cellular retention [34]. The use of leucovorin would not be expected to circumvent this resistance mechanism.

The clinical development of cisplatin in the 1970s not only identified a new agent active in squamous head and neck cancers, but led to the observation that the use of chemotherapy in previously untreated patients improved the quality and quantity of objective responses [21]. The plethora of resulting studies examining the integration of chemotherapy into the primary treatment of patients with head and neck cancer are discussed elsewhere in this book. The initial trials of cisplatin did demonstrate its clinical activity in head and neck cancer [35]. However, significant toxicity including nausea, vomiting, hearing loss and nephrotoxicity limited enthusiasm for the agent [35–37]. Doses of 75–100 mg/m^2 given over 1 to 5 days and repeated every four weeks were generally recommended. Later, clinical studies that documented the value of intravenous hydration with mannitol for the prevention of renal toxicity [38], and produced more effective antiemetic regimens [39,40], established 100 mg/m^2 bolus, or 50 mg/m^2 days 1 and 8, or 20 mg/m^2/day for five days as a generally safe and tolerable dose for clinical use.

Phase II trials of cisplatin in patients with recurrent epidermoid head and neck cancer revealed an objective response rate of 30% using doses of 50–100 mg/m^2 every 3 to 4 weeks [41]. Phase III studies that used single agent cisplatin have shown response rates of 8%, 29% and 18% with durations of response of 1.5 to 7.6 months [28,29,42]. In all studies complete responses are uncommon. Although randomized studies have not been conducted, there is no obvious difference in therapeutic activity when cisplatin is given by bolus injection [43], 24 hour infusion [42] or on days 1 and 8 [29,44]. A randomized trial that compared 60 mg/m^2 with 120 mg/m^2 bolus every 21 days showed no difference in response rate (16.1% and 17.8%, respectively) [43]. The durations of response were 5.4 and 4.2 months, and the median survival of the entire population treated was 7.9 months. A randomized study in squamous cell carcinoma of the cervix has also failed to demonstrate a dose or schedule dependent therapeutic effect for cisplatin [45]. However, toxicity may be less with the infusion schedule or day 1 and 8 programs.

Despite the lack of dose/response effect for conventional dose rates, the possibility that delivery of higher doses would improve therapeutic efficacy exists. Animal studies have shown that dissolving cisplatin in hypertonic saline [46], or pharmacologically inducing a high chloride excretion in the urine [47] protects the kidney from high doses of cisplatin. Clinical application of these observations has led to the demonstration that 180–200 mg/m^2 of cisplatin can be given over five days [48–52], days 1 and 8 [53] or bolus [49,54] with acute dose–limiting toxicity of myelosuppression rather than nephrotoxicity. The possibility of improved response rate in patients with recurrent head and neck cancer is suggested by three of these studies [50–52]. However, the number of patients treated is small and highly selected. In addition to the marked myelosuppression, the occurrence of more severe ototoxicity, peripheral neuropathy [55] and retinal toxicity [56] make this aggressive dose rate unacceptable for patients with recurrent disease. Its use with radiation therapy in previously untreated patients with inoperable disease is being explored [57].

Pharmacologic interventions other than the use of hypertonic saline are under investigation as possible methods of reducing cisplatin toxicity and allowing dose escalation. The simultaneous administration of sulfur–containing compounds, particularly sodium thiosulfate, thiourea or mesna, in murine systems, will ameliorate normal tissue toxicity [58–60]. A phase I study in man has demonstrated that simultaneous administration of sodium thiosulfate permits dose escalation of intravenous cisplatin to 200 mg/m^2 [61]. Since sodium thiosulfate may reduce the antitumor effect of cisplatin [58], its best use may be as a systemic rescue agent during intracavitary or possibly intra–arterial administration of cisplatin [62].

WR–2721, an organic thiophosphate compound that functions as a radioprotector, also reduces cisplatin nephrotoxicity in mice without reducing its antitumor effect [63]. A phase I study established that 150 mg/m^2 bolus cisplatin could be administrated with only mild, reversible renal toxicity [64]. Further studies will be necessary to evaluate the seven of ten responses observed in patients with head and neck cancer. An improved response rate in patients with metastatic melanoma has been reported [65].

Diethyldithiocarbamate (DDTC) is another sulfur–containing compound that has been shown to reduce cisplatin nephrotoxicity, myelosuppression, and GI toxicity in *in vivo* systems without abrogating the antineoplastic effect [66–68]. This compound may be functioning by mechanisms entirely different from other thiol–containing protectors, since the optimum improvement in therapeutic index occurs when DDTC administration follows cisplatin, and it will reduce the myelosuppression of other anticancer drugs [69]. Although initial trials have not documented an improved therapeutic index with combined DDTC and a cisplatin combination [70], further clinical investigation of this fascinating compound is warranted.

As with methotrexate, no pharmacologic intervention has been conclusively shown to increase the therapeutic efficacy of single agent cisplatin given at conventional doses. Two studies have compared single agent methotrexate and cisplatin in patients with recurrent head and neck cancer [28,29]. No statistical difference in objective response rate was demonstrated. It therefore appears that the two most effective agents in recurrent head and neck cancer have equal therapeutic efficacy when given at conventional doses. The spectrum of toxicity observed with each agent differs, but there is no substantial difference in impact on the patient's quality of life when doses that produce moderate side effects are used.

The antitumor antibiotic bleomycin has been extensively evaluated in recurrent head and neck cancer. As summarized by Carter, the 50% or better regression rate observed in U.S. studies was 18% with an average duration of response of three months [26]. The lack of myelosuppression observed with bleomycin should make it attractive for use in combination regimens. However, acute dose–limiting mucositis makes it difficult to combine full dose bleomycin with full dose methotrexate or irradiation; and the potentially fatal pulmonary toxicity seen with the drug used alone or in combination dampens enthusiasm for its use [71].

Despite its considerable use in other malignancies, 5–fluorouracil (5–FU) was not evaluated as a single agent in head and neck cancer until its successful incorporation into combination therapy with cisplatin [72]. A review of 11 studies of 5–FU given by different schedules for multiple different tumors revealed a 15% objective response rate in 118 patients with recurrent head and neck cancer [26]. Retrospective reviews of patients treated at Wayne State University prior to 1976 revealed an objective response rate of 31% in 19 patients [22]. A subsequent review at the same institution after 1980 uncovered seven patients with recurrent disease who received a 96 hour infusion at 1.0 gm/m^2/day. Four patients achieved an objective response [73]. Although the number of patients treated is too small to precisely establish the single agent activity or allow comparison of the different schedules, the agent clearly has activity in this disease. A study that evaluated the use of infusion or bolus 5–FU in combination with cisplatin, primarily in previously treated patients, showed an advantage to the infusion schedule [74].

Other conventional drugs, including the alkylating agents, vinblastine, and adriamycin have been administered to patients with recurrent head and neck cancer [23,26]. The response rates are generally less than 30% and the number of patients treated small. Interestingly, the response rate to adriamycin also appears to double when it is employed in previously untreated patients [75]. Although these various agents have been employed in combination, they see little use as single agent treatment.

With the modest clinical activity of currently available drugs, discovery of new active agents is a high priority. To date, there are no new compounds of novel structure or mechanism of action with activity in head and neck cancer. The only recent addition to our therapeutic armamentarium is the cisplatin analog carboplatin. The development of less toxic and potentially more active analogs of cisplatin has been a major goal for over a decade [76]. Early clinical testing of carboplatin confirmed its reduced renal toxic and emetic properties [77]. The agent can be administered conveniently in an outpatient setting without cisplatin's requirement for intravenous hydration and high–dose antiemetics. Ototoxicity and neurotoxicity also appear reduced [78]. However, carboplatin is considerably more myelosuppressive than cisplatin given at conventional doses. Bone marrow toxicity, particularly thrombocytopenia, is dose–limiting.

Although randomized, single agent, head to head comparisons of cisplatin and carboplatin are not available, randomized studies in ovarian cancer have demonstrated equivalent efficacy with better patient tolerance to carboplatin [79]. Phase II studies in recurrent head and neck cancer have demonstrated objective response rates of 24% and 26% [80], similar to cisplatin. Therefore, the drugs may be equally active as single agents. However, a recent randomized comparison of cisplatin + 5–FU, carboplatin + 5–FU, and methotrexate demonstrated a higher response rate for cisplatin + 5–FU compared to methotrexate, but no statistical difference between

Table 2. Drug combinations in recurrent or disseminated squamous cell cancer of the head and neck.

Agent*	# Patients	% Response (% CR)
VCR/BLM[88]	9	33 (0)
CTX/VCR/MeCCNU/BLM[82]	31	35 (0)
CTX/ADR/MTX/BLM[83]	26	35 (0)
CCNU/VIB/MTX/BLM[84]	38	50 (3)
CTX/FU/MTX/BLM[85]	39	54 (18)
ADR/VCR/FU/HU/MTX + LV/BLM[86]	24	79 (0)
ADR/VCR/FU/HU/MTX + LV/BLM[87]	39	13 (3)
BLM/VCR/MTC/MTX ± CTX/ADR/CP[20,71]	45	69 (28)
CP/BLM[21]	12	33 (0)
CP/VCR/BLM[89]	22	50 (0)
CP/VIB/BLM[90]	42	45 (14)
CP/ADR/CTX[91,92]	35	43 (9)
CP/FU[93]	30	89 (27)
CP/FU[94]	30	60 (17)
CP/FU[95]	30	53 (13)
CP/FU[96]	30	50 (17)
CP/FU/LV[97]	18	56 (6)
MTX/BLM/CP[98]	31	61 (23)

* Abbreviations: VCR = vincristine; BLM = bleomycin; CTX = cyclophosphamide; MeCCNU = semustine; ADR = doxorubicin; VIB = vinblastine; MTX = methotrexate; CCNU = lomustine; HU = hydroxurea; LV = leucovorin; MTC = mitomycin C; CP = cisplatin; FU = 5–fluorouracil

methotrexate and carboplatin + 5–FU [81]. The dose of carboplatin used had to be decreased from the phase II dose used in single agent studies, and this may have been responsible for reduced effectiveness. Despite the lack of conclusive evidence of single agent equivalence to cisplatin, the absence of mucositis, nausea, vomiting, or a requirement for weekly treatment or intravenous hydration that attend the use of methotrexate or cisplatin, make carboplatin an attractive alternative for patients best treated with single agent therapy. Its place in combination drug therapy requires further study.

Combination Chemotherapy

Numerous multidrug regimens have been used in patients with recurrent head and neck cancer in an attempt to improve therapeutic efficacy. Table 2 lists a representative sampling of these studies [20,21,71,82–98]. Prior to the mid–1970s, the majority of combinations used methotrexate, frequently with bleomycin [20,71,82–87]. Although an occasional publication reported a response rate of 50% or better, there was no obvious therapeutic advantage over single agent therapy, and the toxicity observed was generally greater. The durations of response reported were usually 3–5 months in duration. Combination regimens are employed to increase tumor response by circumventing drug resistance and/or to capitalize on synergistic schedules or drug interactions [99,100]. Ideally, the agents used should have different mechanisms of action, separate spectrums of toxicity to permit each agent to be used at its maximum tolerated dose, and be therapeutically and/or biochemically active in the malignancy under treatment. Since all of the agents in these regimens are myelosuppressive and/or produce mucositis, doses must be frequently attenuated when they are used in combination. This may, in part, explain the lack of increased efficacy. Some of these combinations were designed to manipulate tumor cell kinetics for therapeutic benefit [20,85–88]. There is no convincing clinical evidence that the kinetic design is successful, although this concept may be useful to avoid myelosuppression [101]. Sequential use of active drugs or combinations has also not improved therapeutic efficacy [20,102], and primary head and neck cancers have been resistant to biochemical modulation approaches [103].

Over the past decade, the focus has shifted, and the majority of drug combinations studied have used cisplatin [21,89–98]. Many of these studies have combined cisplatin with bleomycin or 5–FU. Although the reported response rates for these two combinations are not markedly different, 5–FU has become the favored agent based on laboratory evidence of the synergy of this combination [104] as well as a markedly reduced potential for serious pulmonary toxicity. The majority of publications reporting the results of cisplatin/5–FU therapy in patients with recurrent or disseminated disease have reported response rates of 50% or greater with 13–27% complete responses [74,93–96]. This has not been a universal finding with response rates as low as 25% noted in small series [105]. The cisplatin has been given by bolus injection, infusion or over five days with no apparent variation in effectiveness. The 5–FU has generally been administered by infusion, and a small randomized trial has suggested that bolus administration on days 1 and 8 is inferior to continuous infusion [74]. However, five day bolus treatment appears to have equal activity in non–comparative trials [95]. The cumulative laboratory results and recent clinical evidence in colorectal and breast cancer demonstrating improved therapeutic effect of concomitant 5–FU and leucovorin has stimulated evaluation of this approach in head and neck cancer [97]. The 56% response rate recently reported in heavily pretreated patients is encouraging and further evaluation of this combination is warranted.

Despite the optimistic reports of phase II trials, any convincing demonstration of improved tumor response, and the only mechanism that will assess effect on patient survival, is the randomized trial. Table 3 summarizes the phase III studies that have addressed the therapeutic impact of combination drug therapy in recurrent head and neck cancer [27,30,42,81,106–112]. Overall, the impact has been small. Many studies show no improvement in response or survival when combinations are compared to single agent treatment [27,42,106,107,109,112]. Three studies show a statistically significant

Table 3. Randomized studies of chemotherapy in recurrent head and neck cancer.

Regimen*	# Patients	% Response (% CR)	Survival (Mos)	Ref
CP*		11 (3)		
versus	57			106
CP/MTX/BLM		11 (0)		
MTX		26 (7)	5.1	
versus				
MTX + LV	237	24 (2)	4.4	27
versus				
MTX + LV/CTX/ARA-C		18 (3)	3.3	
CP		18 (8)	6.3	
versus	79			42
CP/MTX + LV		33 (15)	6.9	
MTX		33 (8)	5.6	
versus	51			107
CP/VCR/BLM		41 (11)	4.0	
CP		24 (5)	4.2†	
versus				
BLM	117	14 (0)	2.8	108
versus				
CP/BLM		13 (3)	4.0†	
versus				
No Chemotherapy		—	2.1†	
MTX		35 (8)	5.6	
versus	163			30
MTX/CP/BLM		48 (16)†	5.6	
MTX		16 (0)	7.2	
versus	190			109
CP/VLB/BLM		22 (1)	6.8	
ld.				
MTX		19 (0)	2.7†	
versus				
CP		40 (0)	8.7†	
versus				
CP/MTX	124	31 (0)	5.3	110
versus				
CP/FU		33 (4)	6.7†	
MTX/VCR/BLM		28 (5)	7.2	
versus	185			111
CP/MTX/VCR/BLM		51 (16)†	8.4	
CP/FU		30 (5)†	6.6	
versus				
CBP/FU	242	18 (2)	5.2	81
versus				
MTX		11 (1)	5.6	
MTX		25 (5)	6.0	
versus	40			112
CBP/MTX		25 (0)	6.0	

* Abbreviations: VCR = vincristine; BLM = bleomycin; CTX = cyclophosphamide; MeCC-NU = semustine; ADR = doxorubicin; VIB = vinblastine; MTX = methotrexate; CCNU = lomustine; HU = hydroxurea; LV = leucovorin; MTC = mitomycin C; CP = cisplatin; FU = 5–fluorouracil; CBP = carboplatin

† Statistically significant difference

increase in response rate, but at the cost of increased toxicity and with no improvement in survival [30,81,111]. A multi–armed study reported by Campbell did show a significantly longer survival for patients treated with single agent cisplatin compared to methotrexate alone [110]. However, the number of patients in each arm is small, a larger percentage of recurrent disease as opposed to advanced untreated patients was present in the methotrexate arm, no improvement was seen in the drug combination arms, and the patient survival in the methotrexate only arm is distressingly short compared to other studies. Morton et al. [108] reported longer survival in patients who received cisplatin or cisplatin plus bleomycin, but not bleomycin, compared to untreated patients. The untreated control arm again had the largest fraction of patients with recurrent disease, the number of patients is small, and the survival in the control arm is short (two months). The frequency of visits and quality of care for patients in the control arm is not defined.

Many of these randomized studies have small numbers of patients in each arm, low–performance status patients were included, and important prognostic variables were not always well balanced. All of these factors serve to reduce confidence in the conclusions proffered. However, taken *in toto*, it is clear that selected combinations do increase the response rate, but at a cost of increased toxicity and with no improvement in median survival compared to single agents. Treatment in general, and possibly the attainment of a response, may improve median survival. But this conclusion is tenuous, and the survival improvement is small.

Methotrexate and cisplatin, the two most effective agents for head and neck cancer, have different mechanisms of action, dissimilar spectrums of toxicity and should be an ideal combination for head and neck cancer. However, methotrexate is excreted by the kidney in man, and the nephrotoxicity of cisplatin could delay its excretion and substantially increase toxicity. Therefore, combinations of these two agents have had to use reduced doses or less than optimal schedules. The combination of cisplatin, methotrexate and bleomycin developed by Vogl and Kaplan did produce a higher response rate than methotrexate alone [30]. Cavel et al. [111] found that the addition of cisplatin to methotrexate + bleomycin + vincristine improved the objective response rate. Other reports of the cisplatin + methotrexate combination have generally not shown similar results [42,106,110]. Carboplatin is less nephrotoxic than cisplatin and can be combined with full dose weekly methotrexate [112]. Despite increased myelosuppression, this combination is also no more effective than single agent methotrexate. Dichloromethotrexate is metabolized by the liver, has the same clinical activity spectrum as methotrexate and can be given at full dose weekly with cisplatin [113]. Although the combination is clearly active in head and neck cancer, there is no substantial increase in response rate compared to single agent therapy [114]. An *in vitro* study using cultured squamous cell carcinoma cells from a patient with head and neck cancer demonstrated that cisplatin resistant cells are also methotrexate resistant [115] and could explain why better results are not obtained with this two drug combination.

The preponderance of locoregional recurrence, its adverse effect on quality of life, and the marginal benefit of systemic chemotherapy suggest that treatment focusing on local disease could provide significant patient benefit. The use of intra–arterial chemotherapy will be discussed. Another alternative is the use of simultaneous chemotherapy and irradiation. The use and rationale of this approach in untreated patients is discussed elsewhere. Preliminary experience in previously irradiated patients that have used split course radiation, 5–FU and either cisplatin or hydroxyurea have yielded encouraging results that deserve further investigation in the recurrent disease patient [116,117].

Intra–arterial Chemotherapy

The important factors that must be considered when planning a regional approach for drug delivery include (a) a tumor natural history that demonstrates primarily local aggressiveness rather than early widespread metastatic dissemination, (b) a definable and accessible arterial supply that provides selective access to tumor blood supply with minimal normal tissue distribution, and (c) the availability of antineoplastic agents with favorable pharmacokinetic properties and demonstrable antitumor activity against the tumor being treated. The clinical course and anatomic tumor distribution of the majority of patients with primary head and neck cancer fulfill these criteria.

For the majority of anticancer drugs, the dose/response curve is steep [118]. With *in vitro* and animal tumor models, a 2–fold increase in dose can result in a 3– to 10–fold increase in tumor cell kill. The few clinical trials that examined the effect of dose rate on objective tumor response have been hampered by the paucity of highly active agents in many solid tumors and the relatively small dose rate differences employed. In addition, many studies have compared low dose, non–toxic therapy with full dose therapy and do not answer the question of extension of the dose response curve beyond the MTD of systemic therapy. To the extent that regional therapy can achieve a greater than 2– to 3–fold increase in the dose delivered to the tumor, it will provide a mechanism to further evaluate the dose response curve.

The major factors determining drug concentration are the dose rate and the regional blood flow. The higher the dose rate (quantity/unit time) and the lower the regional blood flow (volume/unit time) the greater the drug concentration in the local tumor blood supply [119]. Tumor drug exposure will then be determined by the rate of diffusion or transport of drug across capillary endothelium into the extracellular fluid [120]. Tumor drug exposure can be maximized by increasing the dose rate, infusing into low blood flow regions (or decreasing the blood flow), and using rapidly diffusing antineoplastic agents [121]. However, once drug/blood mixing has occurred, drug delivery becomes proportional to the blood flow rate with greater blood flow providing higher drug delivery. Radionuclide techniques have been used to quantitate regional blood flow to the tumor and a reference normal tissue in patients undergoing intra–arterial chemotherapy for head and neck cancer [122]. These studies show that at least part of the therapeutic advantage of regional chemotherapy in patients with head and neck cancer is due to a tumor/normal tissue blood flow ratio that favors drug delivery to the tumor contained within the infused volume.

The duration of drug exposure is also an important determinant of cytotoxicity. For many agents, particularly drugs which are cytotoxic only during one phase of the cell cycle, the duration of exposure above a critical concentration is more important than the concentration achieved [123,124]. However, agents that are capable of killing resting or cycling cells are primarily concentration dependent and are best administered by intermittent bolus with sufficient time between doses to allow normal tissue recovery [124–126]. Effective chemotherapy, systemic or regional, must take into consideration these important variables of dose and duration. Properly designed infusion treatment regimens should be based on the mechanism of action and the cycle specificity of the drugs used, and on the anticipated growth kinetics of the tumor being treated [124,127].

Ultimately, the tumor drug exposure attained is limited by the toxicity produced, either local or systemic. The amount of systemic toxicity depends upon the systemic drug level and varies with the total body clearance of active drug, the first pass extraction of drug as it goes through the regional capillary bed, and the degree of AV major vessel shunting around the capillary bed. The AV shunting that occurs during head and neck infusion has been determined in patients receiving intra–arterial therapy. The shunt varied from less than 10% to over 40% [122]. The major determinant of local toxicity is the drug sensitivity of the normal tissue within the regional area. Avoidance of agents that characteristically produce toxicity in the infused area would be appropriate. For regional therapy of head and neck cancer, this is difficult since the majority of efficacious drugs (methotrexate, bleomycin, fluoropyrimidines) frequently produce mucositis.

The concept of regional drug delivery is not of recent origin. The rationale for intra–arterial injection of antiseptic substances was elaborated by Parlavecchio at the end of the nineteenth century [128]. Intra–arterial chemotherapy of head and neck cancer was first reported by Klopp, who administered nitrogen mustard by this route and reported tumor regression not obtainable by intravenous administration of therapeutic amounts of the same drug [129]. Methotrexate has been the drug most commonly used intra–arterially. In an early evaluation of the pharmacologic advantage of regional therapy, Clarkson and Lawrence, Jr. [130] demonstrated that a 3– to 4–fold higher concentration of methotrexate was present in the distribution of the external carotid artery compared to the concentration in the systemic circulation. In the majority of studies, concomitant systemic leucovorin has also been administered. The durations of therapy and daily doses administered have varied considerably. The criteria used to judge response were far from uniform, and the regression rates reported have varied from 27 to 76%. The cumulative overall response rate in the series cited is 53% which, as has been noted, is the same as that reported for systemic methotrexate [26].

Other systemically active single agents have been administered intra-arterially for head and neck cancer, including the fluoropyrimidines, bleomycin and cisplatin. Johnson et al. [131] treated 70 patients with head and neck cancer using 5–FU. Most patients received 15 mg/kg/day for four to five days followed by 7.5 mg/kg/day for several more days. Objective response of greater than 50% reduction of tumor size occurred in 25 (36%) of the patients. Bitter [132], using cobalt–57 tagged bleomycin, has demonstrated higher tumor concentrations of the drug following intra–arterial administration compared to the same dose given intravenously. Intra–arterial bleomycin, used as a single agent or in combination with methotrexate, has produced response rates ranging from 18% to 70%[133–136]. The major toxicities observed have been stomatitis and skin rash in the infused region. Pulmonary toxicity has been observed with high cumulative doses. Organ distribution studies in the dog following systemic or intracarotid cisplatin administration have demonstrated 5–fold lower renal cisplatin levels following intra–arterial injection [137]. Higher tumor levels of cisplatin after IA administration have been demonstrated in head and neck cancer patients [138]. Lehane et al. [139] have treated 26 patients with head and neck cancer (19 had no prior therapy) with 100 mg/m^2 of intra–arterial cisplatin infused over one hour and observed responses in 25 patients. No local–regional toxicity was observed. All patients had mild to moderate nausea and vomiting.

In addition to the variable evidence for improved therapeutic results, clinical application of regional chemotherapy in head and neck cancer patients has been retarded by reports of the many complications associated with intra–arterial treatment. Most complications and disadvantages were related to the use of an indwelling catheter. Keeping the catheter in place requires accurate surgical technique, good nursing care and a cooperative patient. Clotting of catheters is an ever present complication. When injections are made, considerable care has to be exercised to prevent air embolism and to avoid dislodging small terminal clots formed in the lumen and around the catheter [140]. Arteritis and infection of the skin around the catheter at the skin level eventually develops in all external catheter systems. Neurologic sequelae may also occur from air embolism or inadvertent dislodgement of an atherosclerotic plaque into the internal carotid system. Migration of the infusion catheter from the external carotid artery into the common or internal carotid artery may expose the brain to direct infusion of antineoplastics, resulting in seizures or neurological impairment [141]. When the side effects of the antineoplastic agents administered are added to the physical complications of catheter insertion and maintenance, complication rates of up to 40% have been reported [142,143].

The recent development of a totally implantable infusion system circumvents many of these technical limitations. The surgical implantation of the pump and delivery catheter has been described in detail [144]. A radionuclide technique has been utilized to assess infusion patterns in head and neck cancer patients treaded with intra–arterial chemotherapy [145]. Following a slow injection of technitium–99 tagged macroaggregated albumin through the pump sideport, computerized tomographic and static post–injection scanning is performed. This allows determination of the infused area and permits detection of CNS infusion that could result from improper catheter placement or collateral circulation.

The therapeutic results obtained in patients treated through the implanted system have been summarized [146,147]. Patients eligible for intra–arterial therapy were defined by (1) histologically demonstrated primary malignancy of the head and neck, (2) tumor confined to the distribution of the external carotid artery and/or the thyrocervical trunk, (3) performance status ≥ 50 Karnofsky, (4) creatinine clearance ≥ 50 ml/minute, WBC $\geq 4{,}000$/ul, platelet count $\geq 150{,}000$/ul, bilirubin < 1.5 mg/ul and (5) no prior radical neck dissection on the side of the tumor unless an accessible vascular supply could be demonstrated by angiography. Patients who had received prior chemotherapy were not excluded.

FUdR, dichloromethotrexate and bleomycin were instilled into the pump chamber for continuous infusion. Cisplatin (1 mg/ml) and mitomycin C (total dose in 30 ml of normal saline) were given by short–term infusion through the sideport of the pump. Cisplatin was infused over 90 minutes and mitomycin C over 30 minutes.

Dichloromethotrexate was used as a single agent in six patients. Therapy was initiated at a dose rate of 1 $mg/m^2/d \times 14$ days and escalated with each subsequent course to toxicity. The maximum tolerated dose (MTD) was limited by local toxicity (mucositis) in five patients. Two of three evaluable patients attained a partial response lasting seven and eight months, respectively. Single agent FUdR was evaluated in six patients. Dose escalation was halted from an initial level of 0.01 mg/kg/day $\times$ 14 days by the development of stomatitis in all patients. No systemic toxicity was observed. One patient had skin toxicity (erythema of the skin overlying the lesion) concomitant with the development of mucositis. One patient attained a partial response lasting four months. Five patients received bleomycin as a continuous seven day infusion. One patient developed stomatitis at a dose rate of 1 unit/day $\times$ 7 days. The other four patients had no toxicity at a dose rate of 4 units/day [146].

The results obtained with the combination of cisplatin + FUdR have been reported [147]. The initial patients were treated with 50 mg/m^2 of cisplatin and dose was escalated to 100 mg/m^2 in later patients. The dose rates of FUdR delivered in combination and the toxicity observed are identical to the results obtained with single agent FUdR. Cisplatin, therefore, appears to have little or no regional toxicity at this dose. Cisplatin was given with systemic hydration and mannitol. Overall, seven of fifteen patients with epidermoid cancers had an objective remission (one CR) for a median of five months. Although these results are similar to those reported for systemic cisplatin + 5–FU, 12 of these 15 patients had received prior chemotherapy often including cisplatin. Previous experience would have predicted virtually no drug activity in this population [22] and supports the concept of a regional advantage. Non–responding patients progressed within the infused region, but most responding patients progressed systemically. Despite this suggestion of improved drug effect, this therapy did not have a major impact on patient survival.

The results observed and the excellent clinical tolerance and performance of the infusion system do encourage further investigation of intra–arterial treatment. These investigations should include evaluation of new agents with appropriate pharmacologic characteristics and exploration of approaches such as regional vasoconstrictors that have the potential to further increase the regional advantage [148]. An additional area of research should be the use of intra–arterial therapy in previously untreated patients. The dose response curve may be steeper in these more drug sensitive tumors, and preliminary results are encouraging [149,150].

Conclusion

Treatment of the patient with recurrent squamous cancer of the head and neck remains frustrating for the physician, not to mention the patient. Despite decades of effort and study, the identification of new active agents, and the development of aggressive drug combinations and sophisticated delivery systems, our ability to significantly affect the survival or quality of life of these patients is small. Frustration should not be allowed to slip into resignation or surrender, however. The information garnered from the treatment of these patients is being applied earlier in the course of disease and may well budge otherwise static cure rates. The fact that currently available treatments are not universally effective means that we must analyze our results critically and apply them cautiously to our patients. Combination chemotherapy will produce higher response rates than single agent treatment, but at a cost of greater toxicity and with no difference in median survival. Patients with poor performance status, or who have received prior chemotherapy for recurrent disease, rarely respond to additional treatment. One interpretation of this information would suggest that patients with a poor chance of response and a high likelihood of toxicity are best managed with aggressive supportive care. Patients with good performance status, who have the best chance for response and tolerance of side effects, may be offered a judiciously employed drug combination. Marginally treatable individuals are probably better approached with single agent therapy with its lower toxicity potential. Most importantly, the opportunity to participate in well conceived clinical trials exploring new therapeutic initiatives should be extended to as many eligible patients as possible. Only then will the treatment options in the future be better than the ones currently in place. Cautious optimism is indeed appropriate [151].

References

1. Silverberg E, Lubera JA: Cancer statistics, 1988, Ca 38:3–20, 1989.
2. Strong EW: Preoperative radiation and radical neck dissection. Surg Clin North 49:271–276, 1969.
3. Probert JC, Thompson RW, Bagshaw MA: Patterns of spread of distant metastases in head and neck cancer. Cancer 33:127–133, 1974.
4. Cachin Y, Eschwege F: Combination of radiotherapy and surgery in the treatment of head and neck cancers. Cancer Treat Rev 2:177–191, 1975.
5. Jesse RH, Fletcher GH: Treatment of the neck in patients with squamous cell carcinoma of the head and neck. Cancer 39:868–872, 1977.
6. Martin SA, Marks JE, Lee JY, et al.: Carcinoma of the pyriform sinus: predictor of TNM relapse and survival. Cancer 46:1974–1981, 1980.
7. Bush SE, Bagshaw MA: Carcinoma of the paranasal sinuses. Cancer 50:154–158, 1982.
8. Perez CA, Purdy JA, Breaux SR, et al: Carcinoma of the tonsillar fossa. Cancer 50:2314–2322, 1982.
9. Tong D, Laramore GE, Griffin TW, et al.: Carcinoma of the tonsillar region. Cancer 49:2009–2014, 1982.
10. Kotwall C, Sako K, Razack MS: Metastatic patterns in squamous cell cancer of the head and neck. Am J Surg 154:439–442, 1987.
11. Schechter GL, Kalafsky JT: Cancer of the hypopharynx and cervical esophagus: management concepts. Oncology 2:17–24, 1988.
12. Brown B, Barnes L, Mazariegos J, et al.: Prognostic factors in mobile tongue and floor of mouth carcinoma. Cancer 64:1195–1202, 1989.
13. Foote RL, Buskirk SJ, Stanley RJ, et al.: Patterns of failure after total laryngectomy for glottic carcinoma. Cancer 64:143–149, 1989.
14. Wang ZH, Million RR, Mendenhall WM, et al.: Treatment with preoperative irradiation and surgery of squamous cell carcinoma of the head and neck. Cancer 64:32–38, 1989.
15. Snyderman NL, Johnson JT, Schramm VL, et al.: Extracapsular spread of carcinoma in cervical lymph nodes: impact upon survival in patients with carcinoma of the supraglottic larynx. Cancer 56:1597–1599, 1985.
16. Haplan AS, Caldarelli DD, Chacho MS, et al.: Retrospective DNA analysis of head and neck squamous cell carcinoma. Arch Otolaryngol Head and Neck Surg 112:1159–1162, 1986.
17. De Braud F, Ensley JF, Hassan M, et al.: Prospective correlation of clinical outcome in patients with advanced, resectable squamous cell carcinomas of the head and neck (SCCHN) with DNA ploidy from fresh specimens. Proc Amer Assoc Cancer Res 30:1046, 1989.
18. Levendag P, Sessions R, Vikram B, et al.: The problem of neck relapse in early stage supraglottic larynx cancer. Cancer 63:345–348, 1989.

19. Marcial VA, Hanley JA, Ydrach A, et al.: Tolerance of surgery after radical radiotherapy of carcinoma of the oropharynx. Cancer 46:1910–1912, 1980.
20. Wheeler RH, Baker SR, Liepman MK, Ensminger WD: Intensive sequential chemotherapy with bleomycin, oncovin, mitomycin C, and methotrexate followed by adriamycin, cisplatin, and cyclophosphamide in squamous cell cancer of the head and neck. Med and Pediatr Oncol 11:12–19, 1983.
21. Randolph VL, Vallejo A, Spiro RH, et al.: Combination therapy of advanced head and neck cancer. Cancer 41:460–467, 1978.
22. Amer MH, Al–Sarraf M, Vaitkevicius VK: Factors that affect response to chemotherapy and survival of patients with advanced head and neck cancer. Cancer 43:2202–2206, 1979.
23. Bertino JR, Boston B, Capizzi RL: The role of chemotherapy in the management of cancer of the head and neck: A review. Cancer 36:752–758, 1975.
24. Mead GM, Jacobs C: Changing role of chemotherapy in the treatment of head and neck cancer. Am J Med 75:582–595, 1982.
25. Ensley J, Maciorowski Z, Hassan M, et al.: Prospective correlation of flow cytometry (FCM) DNA parameters (DNA index and % SPF) and cytotoxic response in previously untreated patients with advanced squamous cell cancers of the head and neck. Proc Amer Assoc Cancer Res 29:105, 1988.
26. Carter SK: The chemotherapy of head and neck cancer. Sem Oncol 4:413–429, 1977.
27. DeConti RC, Schoenfeld D: A randomized prospective comparison of intermittent methotrexate, methotrexate with leucovorin, and a methotrexate combination in head and neck cancer. Cancer 48:1061–1072, 1981.
28. Hong WK, Schaefer S, Issell B, et al.: A prospective randomized trial of methotrexate versus cisplatin in the treatment of recurrent squamous cell carcinoma of the head and neck. Cancer 52:206–210, 1983.
29. Grose WE, Lehane DE, Dixon DO, et al.: Comparison of methotrexate and cisplatin for patients with advanced squamous cell carcinoma of the head and neck region: a southwest oncology group study. Cancer Treat Rep 69:577–581, 1985.
30. Vogl SE, Schoenfeld DA, Kaplan BH, et al.: A randomized prospective comparison of methotrexate with a combination of methotrexate, bleomycin, and cisplatin in head and neck cancer. Cancer 56:432–442, 1985.
31. Kirkwood JM, Canellos GP, Ervin TJ, et al.: Increased therapeutic index using moderate dose methotrexate and leucovorin twice weekly vs weekly high dose methotrexate—leucovorin in patients with advanced squamous carcinoma of the head and neck: A safe new effective regimen. Cancer 47:2414–2421, 1981.
32. Woods RL, Fox RM, Tattersal MHN: Methotrexate treatment of advanced head and neck cancers: A dose response evaluation. Cancer Treat Rep 65(Suppl):155–159, 1981.
33. Taylor SG, McGuire WP, Hauck WW, et al.: A randomized comparison of high–dose infusion methotrexate versus standard–dose weekly therapy in head and neck squamous cancer. J Clin Oncol 2:1006–1011, 1984.
34. Pizzorno G, Chang YM, McGuire JJ, Bertino JR: Inherent resistance of human squamous carcinoma cell lines to methotrexate as a result of decreased polyglutamylation of this drug. Cancer Res 49:5275–5280, 1989.
35. Lippman AJ, Helson C, Helson L, Krakoff IH: Clinical trials of cis–diamminedichloroplatinum (NSC–119875). Cancer Chemother. Rep. 57:191–200, 1973.
36. Higby DJ, Wallace J, Holland JF: Cis–diamminedichloroplatinum (NSC–119875). A phase I study. Cancer Chemother Rep 57:459–463, 1973.
37. Talley RW, O'Bryan RM, Gutterman JU, et al.: Clinical evaluation of toxic effects of cis–diamminedichloroplatinum (NSC–119875)– Phase I clinical study. Cancer Chemother Rep 57:465–471, 1973.
38. Hayes DM, Cvitkovic E, Golbey RB, et al.: High–dose cis–platinum diammine dichloride: amelioration of renal toxicity by mannitol diuresis. Cancer 39:1372–1381, 1977.
39. Gralla RJ, Itri LM, Pisko SE, et al.: Antiemetic efficacy of high–dose metoclopramide:

randomized trials with placebo and prochlorperazine in patients with chemotherapy-induced nausea and vomiting. N Engl J Med 305:905–909, 1981.
40. Kris MG, Gralla RJ, Clark RA, et al.: Consecutive dose–finding trials adding lorazepam to the combination of meloclopramide plus dexamethasone: Improved subjective effectiveness over the combination of diphenhydramine plus metoclopramide plus dexamethasone. Cancer Treat Rep 69:1257–1262, 1985.
41. Loehrer PJ, Einhorn LH: Cisplatin. Ann Int Med 100:704–713, 1984.
42. Jacobs C, Meyers F, Hendickson C, et al.: A randomized phase III study of cisplatin with or without methotrexate for recurrent squamous cell carcinoma of the head and neck. A Northern California Oncology Group Study. Cancer 52:1563–1569, 1983.
43. Veronesi A, Zagonel V, Trielli U, et al.: High–dose versus low–dose cisplatin in advanced head and neck squamous carcinoma: A randomized study. J Clin Oncol 3:1105–1108, 1985.
44. Panettiere FJ, Lehane D, Fletcher WS, et al.: Cis–platinum therapy of previously treated head and neck cancer. The Southwest Oncology Group's two–dose–per–month outpatient regimen. Med Pediatr Oncol 8:221–225, 1980.
45. Bonomi P, Blessing JA, Stehman FB, et al.: Randomized trial of three cisplatin dose schedules in squamous cell carcinoma of the cervix: A Gynecologic Oncology Group study. J Clin Oncol 3:1079–1085, 1985.
46. Litterst CL: Alterations in the toxicity of cis–dichlorodiammine–platinum–II and in tissue localization of platinum as a function of Na Cl concentration in the vehicle of administration. Toxicol Appl Pharmacol 61:99–108, 1981.
47. Earhart RH, Martin PA, Tutsch KD, et al.: Improvement in the therapeutic index of cisplatin (NSC 119875) by pharmacologically induced chloruresis in the rat. Cancer Res 43:1187–1194, 1983.
48. Ozols RF, Corden BJ, Jacob J, et al.: High–dose cisplatin in hypertonic saline. Ann Int Med 100:19–24, 1984.
49. Blumenreich MS, Woodcock TM, Jones M, et al.: High–dose cisplatin in patients with advanced malignancies. Cancer 55:1118–1122, 1985.
50. Forastiere AA, Takasugi BJ, Baker SR, et al.: High–dose cisplatin in advanced head and neck cancer. Cancer Chemother Pharmacol 19:155–158, 1987.
51. Bajorin D, Bosl GJ, Fun R: Phase I trial of escalating doses of cisplatin in hypertonic saline. J Clin Oncol 5:1589–1593, 1987.
52. Havlin KA, Kuhn JG, Myers JW, et al.: High–dose cisplatin for locally advanced or metastatic head and neck cancer: A phase II pilot study. Cancer 63:423–427, 1989.
53. Gandara DR, De Gregorio MW, Wold H, et al.: High–dose cisplatin in hypertonic saline: Reduced toxicity of a modified dose schedule and correlation with plasma pharmacokinetics. A Northern California Oncology Group pilot study in non–small–cell lung cancer. J Clin Oncol 4:1787–1793, 1986.
54. Wheeler RH, Stephens S, Ostroy F: A phase I reappraisal of bolus cisplatin with urinary chloruresis. Proc Amer Assoc Cancer Res 27:171, 1986.
55. Legha SS, Dimery IW: High–dose cisplatin administration without hypertonic saline: Observation of disabling neurotoxicity. J Clin Oncol 3:1373–1378, 1985.
56. Wilding G, Caruso R, Lawrence TS, et al.: Retinal toxicity after high–dose cisplatin therapy. J Clin Oncol 3:1683–1689, 1985.
57. Wheeler RH, Salter M, Stephens S, et al.: Simultaneous therapy with high–dose cisplatin and radiation for unresectable squamous cell cancer of the head and neck: A phase I–II study. NCI Monogr 6:339–341, 1988.
58. Howell SB, Taetle R: The effect of sodium thiosulfate on cis–dichlorodiammine-platinum(II) nephrotoxicity and antitumor activity in L1210 leukemia. Cancer Treat Rep 64:611–616, 1980.
59. Ishizawa M, Taniguchi S, Baba T: Protection by sodium thiosulfate and thiourea against lethal toxicity of cis–diamminedichloroplatinum(II) in bacteria and mice. Japan J Pharmacol 31:883–889, 1981.

60. Allan SG, Smyth JF, Hay FG, et al.: Protective effect of sodium–2–mercaptoethanesulfonate on the gastroentestinal toxicity and lethality of cis–diamminedichloroplatinum. Cancer Res 46:3569–3573, 1986.
61. Pjeifle CE, Howell SB, Felthouse RD, et al.: High–dose cisplatin with sodium thiosulfate protection. J Clin Oncol 3:237–244, 1985.
62. Markman M, Cleary S, Pfiefle CE, Howell SB: High–dose intracavitary cisplatin with intravenous thiosulfate. Cancer 56:2364–2368, 1985.
63. Yuhas JM, Culo F: Selective inhibition of the nephrotoxicity of cisplatinum without altering its antitumor effectiveness. Cancer Treat Rep 64:57–64, 1980.
64. Glover D, Glick JH, Weiber C, et al.: Phase I trials of WR–2721 and cis–platinum. Int J Radiat Oncol Biol Phys 10:1781–1784, 1984.
65. Glover D, Glick JH, Weiber C, et al.: WR–2721 and high–dose cisplatin: An active combination in the treatment of metastatic melanoma. J Clin Oncol 5:574–578, 1987.
66. Borch RF, Pleasants ME: Inhibition of cis–platinum nephrotoxicity by diethyldithiocarbamate rescue in a rat model. Proc Natl Acad Sci USA 76:6611–6614, 1979.
67. Evans RG, Wheatley C, Engle C, et al.: Modification of the bone marrow toxicity of cis–diamminedichloroplatinum(II) in mice by diethyldithiocarbamate. Cancer Res 44:3686–3690, 1984.
68. Bodenner DL, Deglon PC, Keng PC, et al.: Selective protection against cis–diamminedichloroplatinum(II)–induced toxicity in kidney, gut, and bone marrow by dielhyldithiocarbamate. Cancer Res 46:2751–2755, 1986.
69. Schmalbach TK, Borch RF: Myeloprotective effect of diethyldithiocarbamate treatment following 1,3–bis(2–chloroethyl)–i–nitrosourea, adriamycin or mitomycin c in mice. Cancer Res 49:2574–2577, 1989.
70. Paredes J, Hong WK, Felder TB, et al.: Prospective randomized trial of high–dose cisplatin and fluorouracil infusion with or without sodium diethyldithiocarbamate in recurrent and/or metastatic squamous cell carcinoma of the head and neck. J Clin Oncol 6:955–962, 1988.
71. Wheeler RH, Liepman MK, Baker SR, et al.: Bleomycin, vincristine and mitomycin C with or without methotrexate in the treatment of squamous cell carcinoma. Cancer Treat Rep 64:943–949, 1980.
72. Kish J, Drelichman A, Jacobs J, et al.: Clinical trials of cis–platinum and 5–fluorouracil infusion as initial treatment of advanced squamous carcinoma of the head and neck. Cancer Treat Rep 66:471–474, 1982.
73. Tapazoglou E, Kish J, Ensley J, Al–Sarraf M: The activity of a single–agent 5–fluorouracil infusion in advanced and recurrent head and neck cancer. Cancer 57:1105–1109, 1986.
74. Kish, JA, Ensley JF, Jacobs J, et al.: A randomized trial of cisplatin (CACP) + 5–fluorouracil (5–FU) infusion and CACP + 5–FU bolus for recurrent and advanced squamous cell carcinoma of the head and neck. Cancer 56:2740–2744, 1985.
75. Cobleigh MA, Hill JH, Gaflagher PA, et al.: A phase II study of adriamycin in previously untreated squamous cell carcinoma of the head and neck. Cancer 56:2573–2575, 1985.
76. Speer RJ, Ridgway H, Hall LM, et al.: Coordination complexes of platinum as antitumor agents. Cancer Chemother Rep 59:629–641, 1975.
77. Muggia FM: Overview of carboplatin: replacing, complementing, and extending the therapeutic horizons of cisplatin. Semin Oncol 16(Suppl 5):7–13, 1989.
78. Ozols RF: Optimal dosing with carboplatin. Semin Oncol 16(Suppl 5): 14–18, 1989.
79. Alberts DS, Mason–Leddil N: Carboplatin in the treatment of ovarian cancer. Semin Oncol 16(Suppl 5):19–26, 1989.
80. Eisenberger M, Van Echo D, Aisner J: Carboplatin: The experience in head and neck cancer. Semin Oncol 16(Suppl 5):34–41, 1989.
81. Forastiere A, Metch B, Keppen M, et al.: Randomized comparison of cisplatin (CDDP) + 5–fluorouracil (5–FU) vs. carboplatin (CBP) + 5–FU vs. methotrexate (MTX) in advanced squamous cell carcinoma of the head and neck. Proc ASCO 8:168. (And Personal Communication), 1989.

82. Livingston RB, Einhorn LH, Bodey GP, et al.: COMB (cyclophosphamide, oncovin, methyl–CCNU, and bleomycin): a four drug combination in solid tumors. Cancer 36:327–332, 1975.
83. Wittes RE, Spiro RH, Shah J, et al.: Chemotherapy of head and neck cancer: combination treatment with cyclophosphamide, adriamycin, methotrexate, and bleomycin. Med and Pediatr Oncol 3:301–309, 1977.
84. Huang AT, Lucas VS, Baughn SG, Cole TB: A trial of outpatient chemotherapy for recurrent head and neck tumors. Cancer 45:2038–2041, 1980.
85. Cortes EP, Kalra J, Amen VC, et al.: Chemotherapy for head and neck cancer relapsing after radiotherapy. Cancer 47:1966–1970, 1981.
86. Price LA, Hill BT, Calvert AH, et al.: Kinetically–based multiple drug treatment for advanced head and neck cancer. Br Med J 3:10–11, 1975.
87. Tannock I, Sutherland D, Osoba D: Failure of short–course multiple drug chemotherapy to benefit patients with recurrent or metastatic head and neck cancer. Cancer 49:1358–1361, 1982.
88. Livingston RB, Bodey GP, Gottlieb JA, Frei E: Kinetic scheduling of vincristine (NSC–67574) and bleomycin (NSC–125066) in patients with lung cancer and other malignant tumors. Cancer Chemother Rep 57:219–224, 1973.
89. Amer MH, Igbicki RM, Vaitkevicius VK, Al–Sarraf M: Combination chemotherapy with cis–diamminedichloroplatinum, oncovin, and bleomycin (COB) in advanced head and neck cancer. Phase II. Cancer 45:217–223, 1980.
90. Perry DJ, Weltz MD, Brown AW, et al.: Vinblastine, bleomycin and cisplatin for recurrent or metastatic squamous cell carcinoma of the head and neck. Cancer 50:2257–2260, 1982.
91. Creagan ET, Fleming TR, Edmonson JH, et al.: Cyclophosphamide, adriamycin, and cis–diamminedichloroplatinum(II) in the treatment of patients with advanced head and neck cancer. Cancer 47:240–244, 1981.
92. Creagan ET, Fleming TR, Edmonson JH, et al.: Chemotherapy for advanced head and neck cancer with the combination adriamycin, cyclophosphamide, and cis–diamminedichloroplatinum(II): Preliminary assessment of a one–day vs. three–day drug regimen. Cancer 47:2549–2551, 1981.
93. Kish JA, Weaver A, Jacobs J, et al.: Cisplatin and 5–fluorouracil infusion in patients with recurrent and disseminated epidermoid cancer of the head and neck. Cancer 53:1819–1824, 1984.
94. Rowland KM, Taylor SG, Spiers ASD, et al.: Cisplatin and 5–FU infusion chemotherapy in advanced, recurrent cancer of the head and neck: An Eastern Cooperative Oncology Group pilot study. Cancer Treat Rep 70:461–464, 1986.
95. Merlano M, Tatarek R, Grimaldi A, et al.: Phase I–II trial with cisplatin and 5–FU in recurrent head and neck cancer: An effective outpatient schedule. Cancer Treat Rep 69:961–964, 1985.
96. Amrien PC, Weitzman SA: Treatment of squamous cell carcinoma of the head and neck with cisplatin and 5–fluorouracil. J Clin Oncol 3:1632–1639, 1985.
97. Vokes EE, Choi KE, Schilsky RL, et al.: Cisplatin, fluorouracil, and high–dose leucovorin for recurrent or metastatic head and neck cancer. J Clin Oncol 6:618–626, 1988.
98. Vogl SE, and Kaplan BH: Chemotherapy of advanced head and neck cancer with methotrexate, bleomycin, and cis–diamminedichloroplatinum II in an effective outpatient schedule. Cancer 44:26–31, 1979.
99. Frei III E: Combination Chemotherapy: Presidential address. Cancer Res 32:2593–2607, 1972.
100. Martin DS, Stoffi RL, Sawyer RC, Young CW: Application of biochemical modulation with a therapeutically inactive modulating agent in clinical trials of cancer chemotherapy. Cancer Treat Rep 69:421–423, 1985.
101. Wheeler RH, Clauw DJ, O'Toole TE, Ensminger WD: Cytokinetic evaluation of the four–drug combination of bleomycin, vincristine, mitomycin C, and methotrexate

(BOMM) in cultured Burkitt's lymphoma cells and human bone marrow. Cancer 50:1993–1999, 1982.
102. Livingston RB, Einhorn LH, Burgess MA, Gottlieb JA,: Sequential combination chemotherapy for advanced recurrent, squamous carcinoma of the head and neck. Cancer Treat Rep 60:103–105, 1976.
103. Browman GP, Levine MN, Goodyear MD: Methotrexate/fluorouracil scheduling influences normal tissue toxicity but not antitumor effects in patients with squamous cell head and neck cancer: results from a randomized trial. J Clin Oncol 6:963–968, 1988.
104. Schabel FM Jr, Trader MW, Laster WE Jr, et al.: Cis–dichlorodiammineplatinum II combination chemotherapy and cross resistance studies of tumors of mice. Cancer Treat Rep 63:1459–1473, 1979.
105. Creagan E, Ingle J, Schutt A, et al.: A phase II study of cis–diamminedichloroplatinum and 5–fluorouracil in advanced upper aerodigestive neoplasms. Head and Neck Surg 6:1020–1023, 1984.
106. Davis S, Kessler W: Randomized comparison of cis–diamminedichloroplatinum versus cis–diammindichloroplatinum, methotrexate, and bleomycin in recurrent squamous cell carcinoma of the head and neck. Cancer Chemother Pharmacol 3:57–59, 1979.
107. Drelichman A, Cummings G, Al–Sarraf M: A randomized trial of the combination of cis–platinum, oncovin and bleomycin (COB) versus methotrexate in patients with advanced squamous cell carcinoma of the head and neck. Cancer 52:399–403, 1983.
108. Morton RP, Rugman F, Dorman EB, et al.: Cisplatinum and bleomycin for advanced or recurrent squamous cell carcinoma of the head and neck: A randomized factorial phase III controlled trial. Cancer Chemother Pharmacol 15:283–289, 1985.
109. Williams SD, Valez–Garcia E, Essessee I, et al.: Chemotherapy for head and neck cancer: comparison of cisplatin + vinblastine + bleomycin versus methotrexate. Cancer 57:18–23, 1986.
110. Campbell JB, Dorman EB, McCormick M, et al.: A randomized phase III trial of cisplatinum, methotrexate, cisplatin + methotrexate, and cisplatinum + 5–fluorouracil in end–stage head and neck cancer. Acta Otolaryngol 103:519–528, 1987.
111. Cavel M, Cognetti F, Dodion P, et al.: Combination chemotherapy with methotrexate, bleomycin, and vincristine with or without cisplatin in advanced squamous cell carcinoma of the head and neck. Cancer 60:1173–1177, 1987.
112. Eisenberger M, Krasnow S, Ellenberg S, et al.: A comparison of carboplatin plus methotrexate versus methotrexate alone in patients with recurrent and metastatic head and neck cancer. J Clin Oncol 7:1341–1345, 1989.
113. Natale RB, Wheeler RH, Roberts JA: Cisplatin and dichloromethotrexate; A pharmacologically rational combination. NCI Monogr 5:219–223, 1987.
114. Wheeler RH, Natale RB, Roshon SG Baker SR: A phase I–II trial of cisplatin and dichloromethotrexate in squamous cell cancer of the head and neck. J Clin Oncol 2:831–835, 1984.
115. Rosowsky A, Wright JE, Cucchi CA, et al.: Collateral methotrexate resistance in cultured human head and neck carcinoma cells selected for resistance to cis–diamminedichloroplatinum(II). Cancer Res 47:5913–5918, 1987.
116. Taylor SG, Murthy AK, Showel JL, et al.: Improved control in advanced head and neck cancer with simultaneous radiation and cisplatin/5–FU chemotherapy. Cancer Treat Rep 69:933–939, 1985.
117. Vokes EE, Panje WR, Schilsky RL, et al.: Hydroxyurea, fluorouracil, and concomitant radiotherapy in poor prognosis head and neck cancer: a phase I–II study. J Clin Oncol 7:761–768, 1989.
118. Frei E III, Canellos G: Dose: a critical factor in cancer chemotherapy. Am J Med 69:583–594, 1980.
119. Collins JM, Dedrick RL: Pharmacokinetics of anticancer drugs. In: pharmacologic principles of cancer treatment. Chabner B (ed), Philadelphia: WB Saunders, pp 77–99, 1982.

120. Fensmacher J, Gazendam J: Intraarterial infusions of drugs and hyperosomotic solutions as ways of enhancing CNS chemotherapy. Cancer Treat Rep 65(Suppl 2):27–38, 1981.
121. Levin VA, Landahl HD, Patlak CS: Drug delivery to CNS tumors. Cancer Treat Rep 65(Suppl 2):19–26, 1981.
122. Wheeler RH, Ziessman HA, Medvec BR, et al.: Tumor blood flow and systemic shunting in patients receiving, intra–arterial chemotherapy for head and neck cancer. Cancer Res 46:4200–4204, 1986.
123. Bruce WR, Meeker BE, Powers WE, Valeriote FA: Comparison of the dose– and time–survival curves for normal hematopoietic and lymphoma colony–forming cells exposed to vinblastine, vincristine, arabinosylcytosine and amethopterin. J Natl Cancer Inst 42:1015–1023, 1969.
124. Mellett LB: Considerations in design of optimal therapeutic schedules. In: Pharmacology and the Future of Man. Proceedings of the 5th International Congress in Pharmacology, San Francisco, vol 3, Karger, Basal, pp 332–353, 1973.
125. Bruce WR, Meeker BE, Valeriote FA: Comparison of the sensitivity of normal hematopoietic and transplanted lymphoma colony–forming cells to chemotherapeutic agents administered *in vivo*. J Natl Cancer Inst 37:233–245, 1966.
126. Young RC, Rosenoff SA, Myers CE, et al.: Alterations in DNA synthesis induced by chemotherapeutic agents in vivo: Potential applications to clinical treatment schedules. In: Growth Kinetics and Biochemical Regulation of Normal and Malignant Cells. Drewinko B, Humphrey RM, (eds), Baltimore: Williams & Wilkins, pp 787–809, 1977.
127. Jusko WJ: A pharmacodynamic model for cell–cycle–specific chemotherapeutic agents. J Pharmacokin Biopharm 1:175–200, 1973.
128. Parlavecchio G: Sul lavaggio antisettico interstizaile dei tessut dolla vie arteriosa. Policlinico (Sez Prat) 6:667–674, 1899.
129. Klopp CT, Alfordd TC, Bateman J, et al.: Fractionated intraarterial cancer chemotherapy with methyl bis amine hydrochloride: A preliminary report. Ann Surg 132:811–832, 1950.
130. Clarkson B, Lawrence W Jr: Perfusion and infusion techniques in cancer chemotherapy. J Clin North Amer 45:689–710, 1961.
131. Johnson RO, Kisken WA, Curreri AR: A report upon arterial infusion with 5–fluorouracil in 100 patients. Surg Gynec Obste 120:530–636, 1965.
132. Bitter KJ: Pharmacokinetic behavior of bleomycin–cobalt–57 with special regard to intraarterial perfusion of the maxillofacial region. Maxillofac Surg 4:226–231, 1976.
133. Szabo G, Kovacs A: Possibilities of enhancing the effectiveness of intraarterial chemotherapy. Int J Oral Surg 9:33–44, 1980.
134. Burkhardt A, Holtje WJ: Effects of intraarterial bleomycin therapy in squamous cell carcinoma of the oral cavity: biopsy and autopsy examination. Maxillofac Surg 3:217–230, 1975.
135. Richard JM, Sancho H: Intraarterial chemotherapy of head and neck tumors: statistical study of 129 cases treated at the Institute Gustave Roussy. Biomedicine 18:429–435, 1973.
136. Ziekle–Temme BC, Stevens KR Jr, Everts EC, et al.: Combined intraarterial chemotherapy radiation therapy and surgery for advanced squamous cell carcinoma of the head and neck. Cancer 45:1527–1532, 1980.
137. Madajewica S, Kanter P, West C, et al.: Plasma, spinal fluid and organ distribution of cisplatinum (DDP) following intravenous (IV) and intracarotid (IC) infusion. Proc Amer Assoc Cancer Res and ASCO 22:176, 1981.
138. Gouyette A, Apehin A, Foka M, Richard JM: Pharmacokinetics of intra–arterial and intravenous cisplatin in head and neck cancer patients. Eur J Cancer Clin Oncol 22:257–263, 1986.
139. Lehane DE, Sessions R, Johnson P, et al.: Intraarterial cisplatinum administration for advanced squamous cell carcinoma of the head and neck region. International Head and Neck Oncology Research Conference, Rosslyn, VA, Abstract #2.11, 1980.
140. Goldman HL, Bilbao MK, Rosch J, Dotter CT: Complications of indwelling chemotherapy catheters. Cancer 36:1883–1990, 1975.

141. Helsper JT, DeMoss EV: Regional intraarterial infusion of 5–fluorouracil for cancer. Surgery 56:340–348, 1964.
142. Hanna DC, Gaisford JC, Goldwyn RM: Intraarterial nitrogen mustard for control of pain in head and neck cancer. Am J Surg 106:783–785, 1963.
143. Watkins E Jr, Sullivan RD: Cancer chemotherapy by prolonged arterial infusion. SGO 118(1):3–19, 1964.
144. Baker SR, Wheeler RH, Medvec BR: Surgical aspects of intraarterial therapy of outpatients with head and neck cancer. Otolaryngol—Head Neck Surg 93:192–199, 1985.
145. Baker SR, Wheeler RH, Ziesman H, Medvec BR: Radionuclide localization of intra–arterial infusion in head and neck cancer. Cancer Drug Delivery 1:145–156, 1984.
146. Wheeler RH, Baker SR, Medvec BM: Single agent and combination drug regional chemotherapy for head and neck cancer using an implantable infusion pump. Cancer 54:1504–1512, 1984.
147. Forastiere AA, Baker SR, Wheeler RH, Medvec BR: A phase II trial of intra–arterial cisplatin and FUDR in advanced malignancies confined to the head and neck. J Clin Oncol 5:1601–1606, 1987.
148. Ziessman HA, Forastiere AA, Wheeler RH, et al.: The use of a vasoconstrictor to improve tumor blood flow in intra–arterial chemotherapy: A preliminary report. Nuc Med Commun 6:777–786, 1985.
149. Frustaci S, Barzan L, Tumolo S, et al.: Intra–arterial continuous infusion cis–diamminedichloroplatinum in untreated head and neck cancer patients. Cancer 57:1118–1123, 1986.
150. Cheung DK, Regan J, Savin M, et al.: A pilot study of intraarterial chemotherapy with cisplatin in locally advanced head and neck cancers. Cancer 61:903–908, 1988.
151. Jacobs C: Editorial: adjuvant chemotherapy for head and neck cancer. J Clin Oncol 7:823–826, 1989.

12. Combined Chemotherapy and Radiation for Unresectable Head and Neck Cancer

Samuel G. Taylor IV

Use of chemotherapy with radiation therapy, rather than giving the two in sequence, has undergone a resurgence of interest over the last 5 years. 1988 witnessed an approximately equal distribution of publications on combining chemotherapy with radiation and on induction chemotherapy reports in contrast to publications over the previous decade in which reports on induction chemotherapy regimens markedly predominated [1]. This new interest has resulted from several controlled, randomized studies over the years that have demonstrated an advantage to combining chemotherapy with radiation, as well as to the failure of similar controlled studies to find any survival advantage to various induction chemotherapy programs. Reluctance to fully endorse the use of combined chemotherapy and radiation remains widespread, however, due primarily to concern over toxicity.

Normal tissue toxicity is what led investigators during the 1960s and early 1970s away from simultaneous chemotherapy and radiation schedules. Such toxicity remains a real concern, requiring ongoing studies with concomitant treatment to address this important issue. Nevertheless, a sense of improved response rates and, more importantly, an improved durability of response over that previously seen with radiation alone, supported by results of randomized trials, have led investigators using concomitant treatment programs to become increasingly enthusiastic about this approach.

Randomized Studies

Four recent randomized studies have indicated some important directions with combined chemotherapy and radiation. Each of these tested the addition of one drug to radiation therapy.

The best described study was of adding bleomycin to radiation therapy [2]. Several prior studies using this approach were negative including a large European study which was recently updated [3]. The only positive studies in the past had tested the addition of bleomycin to radiation in selected patients with well–differentiated tumors. The study by Fu, et al. [2] selected patients with inoperable stage III and IV cancers from all sites of upper

Jacobs, C. (ed): Carcinomas of the Head and Neck: Evaluation and Management.

aerodigestive tracts. They used an unusually low dose of bleomycin (5 u twice weekly). This was a dose that would hardly be therapeutic by itself, but was sufficient to be synergistic when combined with radiation.

They reported a 3–year relapse–free survival of 15% with radiation and 31% with radiation plus bleomycin in 104 patients treated ($p = 0.02$). Survival was also improved (24% vs. 43%), but this difference was not significant. These differences have become more marked with time. While a more severe normal tissue reaction also occurred, it did not result in interruption of treatment. The authors attributed their positive results to this sensitizing effect. Although a maintenance chemotherapy program was planned, the authors felt this contributed little to the overall chemotherapy benefit with very poor patient compliance (only 27% of patients received 50% of dose).

This study supports a concept that has become well accepted when combining chemotherapy drugs: that the dose of each drug (modality) must be adjusted when combining two treatments with similar organ toxicities but that the combined effects against the cancer can still result in improvement over giving the treatment in sequence at full dose. In the study by Fu, et al., reduction in bleomycin dosage below that which would be considered therapeutic caused a radiation sensitizing effect with improved benefit.

A second trial used a similar approach with methotrexate, a drug that clearly can produce severe mucosal toxicity when combined at full therapeutic dosage with radiation [4]. In this trial only 2 doses were given at the beginning of radiation. Much more intensive methotrexate treatment given as induction chemotherapy prior to radiation has been repeatedly shown to be ineffective.

This trial tested methotrexate–100 mg/m^2 on days 0 and 14 of radiation given as 50 Gy in 15 to 16 fractions over 3 weeks. Folinic acid was given, dependent on 24–hour serum methotrexate levels. Three–hundred and thirteen patients were entered. At a median follow–up of 32 months, survival was 52% with methotrexate and 43% without ($p = 0.075$). Relapse–free survival was significantly improved at the $p = 0.016$ level. As in the previous trial, more acute reactions were noted with combined therapy, but no more frequent treatment interruption or late effects were noted. While the radiation fractionation was not standard, the improved control with this combined therapy is certainly in contrast to the negative results with more intensive methotrexate chemotherapy regimens given sequentially.

Two other randomized trials with chemotherapy and radiation have been reported in abstract form only. One using mitomycin C and radiation noted the ability to give full dose chemotherapy and radiation because of the lack of overlapping toxicities [5]. Benefit was noted in disease–free survival but not survival. It is surprising that a drug with such limited activity in head and neck cancer could cause any measurable benefit when combined with radiation. A detailed analysis of this trial will hopefully be forthcoming.

A second trial tested the addition of low–dose, weekly cisplatin (20 mg/m^2 week) to radiation [6]. This trial found no differences in disease–free or overall survival. Publication of the results of this trial may be delayed by the negative results. This negative study has been a disappointment to many oncologists, but is important in indicating that the dose and schedule of such therapy is very important. The negative results could have been anticipated from the follow–up results of phase II studies with comparable regimens.

Another way to combine radiation with chemotherapy is to alternate treatments. This schedule requires a split course of radiation, usually 2 weeks of radiation and one week of chemotherapy. Such a schedule was developed by O'Connor, et al. [7] but has failed to become widely accepted because of substantial mucosal toxicity and because a split course of interrupted radiation is felt to be inferior treatment by many radiation oncologists.

In fact, in two separate randomized studies, this schedule of treatment has been found to be superior to giving the same chemotherapy separate from an uninterrupted program of conventional radiation. The first was a large cooperative group trial by the South–East Cooperative Oncology Group from England [8]. This trial, with 267 patients, compared 4 cycles of vincristine, methotrexate and bleomycin (±5–fluorouracil) given as 2 cycles before and 2 cycles after uninterrupted radiation or as alternating treatment with one cycle (week) of chemotherapy followed by 2 weeks of radiation for 3 alternating cycles and one additional chemotherapy cycle at the end. Disease–free survival tended to be better with the alternating regimen ($p = 0.07$), but survival was similar between the two treatment arms. While a significant benefit was not identified, clearly the split course fractionation scheduled was *no worse* than standard fractionation schedules when combined with chemotherapy.

The second study was even more definitive. This study by Merlano, et al. [9] compared vinblastine, bleomycin and methotrexate given every 14 days for 4 cycles followed by conventionally fractionated radiation versus the same chemotherapy given for 4 cycles with 3 cycles of radiation (20 Gy over 2 weeks) between each chemotherapy treatment. Median progression–free survival was 26 weeks with 36% of patients disease–free in the sequential arm and 34 weeks with 51% of patients disease–free in the alternating arm ($p = 0.046$). Toxicity was worse in the alternating arm with 31% having severe or worse mucositis compared to 4% in the sequential arm ($p < 0.0001$). Median survival was 41 weeks compared to 54 weeks for alternating therapy. This was not significant in that analysis, but a more recent update [10] was able to show a significant survival benefit as well (38 weeks versus 59 weeks, $p < 0.03$).

These studies, taken together, show that combining chemotherapy with radiation, even with interruptions in the radiation therapy (split course fractionation) is better than sequential treatment. Combined with the studies sited above of radiation versus radiation plus chemotherapy, they give a clear indication that combined chemotherapy and radiation can alter the disease course of head and neck cancer.

Single Drug Chemotherapy

Over the last several years, no drug has received more attention than cisplatin as a radiation potentiator in head and neck cancer. While not always consistent, several reports attest to its radiation sensitizing properties in animal models [11–13]. It has been used in several different schedules in phase II studies in humans. The most common dose–schedule for combining cisplatin with radiation therapy clinically has been administering 15 to 20 mg/m^2 weekly or for 4 to 5 days every 3 to 4 weeks. When given to unresectable stage III or IV patients, the majority of such phase II trials have had complete response rates of less than 50% and median survivals of less than 18 months (Table 1) [14]. These results are not substantially different from those expected with radiation alone in this disease and make the negative results of the randomized Intergroup trial of weekly cisplatin of no surprise.

Cisplatin is tightly protein–bound in the blood stream. The availability of cisplatin during first passage through the tumor vasculature may be very important for tissue uptake. While randomized studies in advanced head and neck cancer have failed to support any importance for a dose–effect relationship, high response rates with intra–arterial chemotherapy would suggest otherwise [15,16]. The availability of free drug for tissue uptake would be expected to be most important for effect. It seems likely that peak serum levels during first passage may be more important than concentration–time factors with a drug that is so strongly protein–bound.

Dose–schedules for cisplatin, using a higher, intermittant dosage combined with radiation, may consequently have more potential for radiation enhancement. Recent studies incorporating this approach have achieved more durable survival results as shown in Table 1. Al–Sarraf, et al. [17] have used a schedule of 100 mg/m^2 every 3 weeks during radiation in 134 patients with inoperable head and neck cancer. They reported a complete response rate of 69% with highest response rates in nasopharyngeal and poorly differentiated carcinomas. Disease–free survival and overall survival results were 51% and 60% at one year and 39% and 55% at 2 years respectively. Frequent acute toxicities included leukopenia (83%), stomatitis (80%), vomiting (77%), and renal toxicity (52%). Compliance was a significant problem with only 60% of patients completing the planned treatment. Patient refusal (13%) and prohibitive toxicities (16%) were listed as the two principal reasons for failure to complete therapy. The authors thought these results were an improvement over prior Radiation Therapy Oncology Group (RTOG) experience.

An interesting application of this schedule of treatment has been presented by Ensley, et al. [18]. These authors have previously observed marked cross–resistance between cisplatin–containing induction chemotherapy and radiation [19]. They had noted a high response rate (97%)

Table 1. Cisplatin Phase II studies: effects of dose.

Cisplatin dose	% CR	Survival
Dose of ≤20 mg/m² daily × 5 or weekly [14]	18–75%	11–15 mo. median
100 mg/m² every 3 weeks [17]	69%	55% at 24 mo.
40 mg/m², d1–5, every 3 weeks [21]	100%	71% at 9 mo.

to radiation after partial response to induction therapy but marked resistance (only a 6% response rate) to subsequent radiation in chemotherapy non–responders. This cross–resistance has also been noted in animal models [20]. Nevertheless, using combined cisplatin and radiation in cisplatin/5–FU chemotherapy non–responders, Ensley et al. [18] observed 13 of 13 patients responding [18]. This marked difference from these authors' prior experience with radiation alone would strongly suggest synergism from the combination.

Wheeler, et al. [21] have used a more intense, high–dose schedule of cisplatin combined with radiation in a limited number of patients [21]. They gave cisplatin–40 mg/m² days 1–5 for 3 cycles to 17 patients, starting on day 1 of radiation (60–70 Gy in 7–9 weeks). Again, compliance and complications were problems with 65% completing the planned therapy. Nevertheless, all patients had complete responses. There were only 9 months of follow–up, but no local recurrences had occurred, while 5 patients developed distant metastases. Two (12%) died during treatment, and hematologic toxicity was the most frequent life–threatening toxicity. While the toxicity of this dose of cisplatin was considerable and would be expected to be intolerable to a significant number of unselected patients with head and neck cancer, the 100% complete response rate in those patients completing treatment is most impressive. These results certainly support a dose–effect relationship with cisplatin.

An alternative approach in administering cisplatin is to give it by prolonged infusion or daily injection during radiation. Forestiere, et al. [22] have examined the effects of prolonged (5–day) infusion on the serum concentration of cisplatin in comparison to those patients receiving 5 daily injections of the same dose of cisplatin [22]. Higher peak levels occurred with injection while a larger area under the concentration time curve was noted with infusion. Drug delivery and concentration within tumor was not measured, however, to know which approach might be optimal. No study of infusional cisplatin and radiation has been reported, but daily injection of 10 mg per day during radiation (60 Gy in 6 weeks) has been described [23]. In this study, 18 patients with stage II to IV head and neck cancer were treated. One half had complete responses and the rest partial responses. Renal toxicity with this regimen was particularly severe, however, with 2 treatment–related deaths from this cause. No follow–up data were supplied. The toxicity of this regimen without apparent improvement in anti–neoplastic activity make this schedule appear less promising.

Eisenberger, et al. [24] have studied carboplatin and radiation in unresectable head and neck cancer [24]. Carboplatin was given weekly at 60–100 mg/m^2 or at 400 mg/m^2 every 4 weeks during radiation. Ten of 22 evaluable patients in a cohort of 26 patients had complete responses. Follow–up was too limited to assess durability, but results were not different than those anticipated with radiation alone.

Despite the intense interest in cisplatin as single agent chemotherapy, 5-fluorouracil (5–FU) has become the most frequently used drug when combination chemotherapy and radiation has been used in recent years. Consequently, it is important to explore results of some older studies as background. First, 5–fluorouracil, given by bolus injection, has been shown to act as a radiation sensitizer in head and neck cancer, significantly improving survival [25]. More recently, Wiley et al. [26] analyzed 27 base of tongue lesions entered into that study [26]. They noted that the only long–term survivors were in the combined treatment arm. This benefit was seen despite more treatment interruptions and lower total dose of radiation in the group receiving 5–FU and radiation. They questioned whether modification of the conventional radiation fractionation to a planned split–course would be preferable, in order to allow preferential recovery of normal tissues.

In vitro studies performed by Bagshaw [27] and those by Byfield, et al. [28] have indicated a dose–response relationship for the radiation sensitizing properties of 5–FU. In addition, optimal sensitization requires exposure of cells after radiation for up to 48 hours. Development of high-dose infusional 5–FU allowed Byfield, et al. to take advantage of these principles. They described a planned split–course fractionation schedule for 5–FU and radiation in esophageal cancer and later reported a toxicity pilot study in head and neck cancer [29]. This incorporated an every–other–week treatment with combined radiation (2.5 Gy per day) for 4 days, and 5–Fu–20 to 30 mg/kg/day continued for 48 hours after the last radiation treatment. This was primarily a toxicity study with too few patients given the higher doses to define response, and with only as many as 6 cycles (60 Gy) given.

They described 10 of 14 evaluable stage III and IV patients having a complete response, but follow–up was too limited to assess durability of response. Two–year survival was approximately 55% based on the supplied Kaplan–Meier survival curve. The authors expressed concern that late fibrosis may have been increased over that expected from radiation alone.

Byfield et al. have since described a phase I study of twice daily fractionation of 2.5 Gy/fraction for 2 days plus 5–FU, 40 to 50 mg/kg/day for 3 days every other week to a maximum of 6 courses [30]. No response rates were reported with this regimen, but the schedule was found to be tolerable with mucositis as the dose–limiting toxicity.

Combination Chemotherapy and Radiation

While several combination chemotherapy regimens have been used for induction chemotherapy, very few drug combinations had been used concomitantly with radiation until Taylor, et al. [31] began using a modification of the Wayne State program of cisplatin and 5–FU with radiation in 1981.

The major contribution previously had been the introduction of alternating cycles of combination chemotherapy and radiation using split course fractionation of the radiation [7]. Alternating the chemotherapy and radiation was a way of integrating the two modalities of treatment without producing overwhelming normal tissue toxicity, despite using 2 mucous–membrane–toxic drugs (methotrexate and bleomycin). This treatment did produce more mucosal toxicity but also produced improved disease control as described above in two randomized studies. The disadvantage was that this schedule would not be expected to take optimal advantage of any radiation sensitizing properties of the chemotherapy.

The goal of the pilot study by Taylor, et al. was to give the two modalities concomitantly, to maximize any synergy that they might have. Giving cisplatin and 5–FU with radiation required compromise in treatment delivery, and the schedule proposed by Byfield for 5–FU and radiation seemed optimal [29]. With a week of treatment followed by a week of rest, any mucosal toxicity was due primarily to 5–FU dosage. This mucositis would generally clear quickly during the rest week and require relatively modest changes in 5–FU dosage to control, without modifying radiation.

The authors have recently updated their results in 53 unresectable patients followed for a median of 51 months with a range of 12 to 83 months [32]. All patients responded with the exception of one who had a massive stroke after his second cycle and was never reassessed. Median time to progression was 51 months. Median survival for all patients, including 7 deaths from other causes in patients without relapse, was 37 months. In this patient population with such advanced disease, only 25% of patients failed regionally, and another 15% failed at distant sites. Long–term analysis showed several patterns that the authors thought important. As in other studies, there was a marked decrease in disease control in those stage IV patients with N3 disease. It also appeared that delivery of 7 cycles (70 Gy) and receipt of at least 80% of the planned dose of 5–FU was important, as these patients had better disease control than those who had 6 cycles or less of 5–FU. Dose received of cisplatin did not appear to matter.

Surprisingly, partial responders did almost as well as complete responders with 47% remaining controlled versus 70% for complete responders. This finding is in contrast to most radiation therapy studies where partial responders do very badly, and this may have been due to the unreliability of clinical assessment of response. All but one patient with a partial response had at least 75% reduction in tumor mass, but bone destruction and large neck nodes would usually not normalize. Five of 9 patients with a clinical partial response who had a biopsy were histologically negative. In contrast, 2 of 6 patients with a clinical complete response who were biopsied were histologically positive.

Toxicity included a weight loss of more than 10% of body weight in 53% and severe mucositis in 52%. Myelotoxicity was generally easily managed with the every–other–week schedule. The toxicity of this regimen has been compared to induction cisplatin/5–FU chemotherapy followed by radiation in an ongoing randomized trial [33]. Severe mucositis and mean weight loss were not significantly different, although severe weight loss tended to be worse with simultaneous treatment (mean 11% vs. 7% respectively). On the other hand, renal dysfunction and untoward events tended to be more common with induction chemotherapy. Certainly there was no evidence for more unmanageable toxicity with the program of concomitant treatment.

Adelstein, et al. [34] have used cisplatin and 5–FU infusion in a different regimen with radiation in 54 patients [34]. They gave cisplatin–75 mg/m^2 on day 1 of a 3–week course of radiation (30 Gy) and 5–FU–1.0 gm/m^2 days 1–4. The chemotherapy was repeated 2 to 4 weeks after the end of radiation. Patients were then reassessed, with an option for surgery. This was followed with a second cycle given 12 weeks after the start of the first cycle. The entire treatment was completed in 18 to 24 weeks. In their series, 51% of the patients were operable and 51% had stage I–III disease.

Differences between this schedule and that by Taylor, et al. were that chemotherapy and radiation were not given entirely concomitantly, that dose intensity was less, and longer cycles of radiation were given, with a much longer (2.5 months) hiatus between cycles. Despite the reduced dose intensity, toxicity was comparable with a mean weight loss of 12% and slightly more frequent severe myelotoxicity, severe mucositis, and transient renal dysfunction. This may possibly have been due to continuing radiation for the week after combined treatment.

The results also were impressive with all patients responding. Fifty–six percent had a complete response after the first cycle of treatment. Ninety–four percent were considered disease–free at the end of treatment. With a median follow–up of 21 months, median survival had not been reached with a 71% disease–free survival by Kaplan–Meier estimate. In addition, 13 technically operable patients did not undergo surgery with only one recurrence during follow–up. While follow–up was not as long as the study by Taylor, et al., durability of response appeared to be also a characteristic of this approach, despite the long hiatus between cycles and relatively low total dose of radiation (60 Gy).

More recently, Adelstein, et al. [35] have presented preliminary information on a small randomized study of 48 patients receiving either their schedule of simultaneous chemotherapy and radiation and surgery or sequential cisplatin/5–FU infusion followed by surgery and radiation [35]. Patients who had a complete response to the first cycle of combined treatment or to induction chemotherapy had surgery deleted. Toxicities were stated to be similar, but there was a larger mean weight loss in the simultaneous arm (19.2% versus 10.1% respectively). There was a higher complete response rate (67% vs. 39%) in the simultaneous arm, leading to slightly more patients avoiding surgery (11 vs. 7) and improved disease–free survival (69% vs. 44%), ($p = 0.04$). No survival differences were apparent, however, with follow–up still very limited.

Wendt, et al. [36] have combined cisplatin/5–FU with leucovorin and radiation [36]. They gave cisplatin–60 mg/m^2 day 1, 5–FU–350 mg/m^2 bolus day 1 and then continuous infusion days 1–5, leucovorin–50 mg/m^2 bolus day 1 and 100 mg/m^2 continuous infusion days 1–5. The dose of 5–FU was determined to be optimally tolerable after doses from 100 to 500 mg/m^2 were tried. Radiation was 1.8 Gy twice daily, days 2–4 and 7–10. Each cycle was repeated every 3 weeks for 3 cycles to a total dose of 70.2 Gy in 8 weeks. They treated 34 patients with stage III or IV disease, but excluded patients over age 65. As in the other combinations with cisplatin/5–FU and radiation, all patients responded, 50% completely. The percentage of complete responses increased to 82% at 3 months of follow–up. A presentation of an updated series of 62 cases indicated a 48% estimated 4–year survival rate [37].

These studies all combine 5–FU infusion relatively intensively with radiation. All three are characterized by unusually durable responses and long–term survival. They support the concept of integrating chemotherapy with radiation even with a long hiatus between radiation cycles, and they indicate toxicity is not substantially different from sequential therapy. While single institution phase II trials are always open to patient selection biases and require confirmation by others, the consistency of these findings is encouraging.

Other trials with combined cisplatin, 5–FU and radiation have used schedules that have avoided concomitant exposure. A study by Bolla, et al., used cisplatin–20 mg/m^2 followed by 5–FU–400 mg/m^2 infused over 2 hours on days 1,2,5,6 of each cycle with 5–FU only given on days 3 and 4 [38]. Radiation (3 Gy) was given on days 3 and 4 before the 5–FU. Three cycles were given at 3–week intervals, followed by conventional radiation of 60 Gy over 6 weeks without chemotherapy. After the combined treatment, 47% responded with 11% complete responses. After all treatment, 30% had a complete response. With median follow–up 11 months, survival at one year was 38%, with a median of 10 months. The authors concluded the complete response rate and overall results were not different from those following radiation alone, but nevertheless are proceeding with a randomized trial.

A similar study used slightly different doses of cisplatin–15 mg/m^2, 5–FU–350 mg/m^2 and radiation–4 Gy/day, with treatment extended to 7 days and a 3–week interval between cycles for 3 cycles, followed by 56 Gy in 2 Gy fractions without chemotherapy [39]. Forty patients with stage III or IV disease (3 were M1) received treatment. A complete response occurred in

Table 2. Cisplatin, 5–fluorouracil and radiation. Effect of dose and schedule.

Study	% RT concomitant	5–FU by 24 hr. infusion	Median survival
Taylor, et al. [32]	100%	yes	37 mo.
Wendt, et al. [37]	38%	yes*	48% at 48 mo.
Adelstein, et al. [34]	33%	yes	64% at 21 mo**
Dionet, et al. [39]	30%	no	11 mo.
Bolla, et al. [38]	23%	no	10 mo.
Merlano, et al. [40]	0	no	11 mo.

* With leucovorin

** 51% of patients in this study were operable and stages I–III. Patients in all other studies were considered unresectable.

15% after concomitant treatment and 51% after all radiation. Six patients, 15%, remain alive and disease–free at 13 to 35 months follow–up.

A second group of 30 recurrent patients received only concomitant treatment for 3 to 6 cycles [39]. Only 10% achieved a complete response and 20% a partial response with a median survival of 6 months.

Merlano, et al. [40] have reported a phase II trial of five days of cisplatin and bolus 5–FU therapy alternating with 2 weeks of radiation [40]. Cisplatin–20 mg/m^2 and 5–FU–200 mg/m^2 were given daily for 5 days every 3 weeks for 4 cycles with 3 cycles of radiation (2 Gy/day) for 10 fractions sandwiched in between. The authors reported a 76% response rate in 34 patients with stage IV or recurrent disease after surgery. Forty–one percent had a complete response. With a limited follow–up of 21 months, only 8 patients remained alive and disease–free with a median survival of 47 weeks.

None of these last 3 trials have achieved results obviously different from those expected with radiation alone. Merlano, et al. had found the schedule of alternating treatment with chemotherapy and radiation to be better than sequential treatment when using vinblastine, bleomycin and methotrexate [9]. They treated a more advanced patient population than usually considered, with 50% of their patients being surgery failures. This makes comparison difficult. But the previous 2 studies, which both had avoided more intensive concomitant administration of 5–FU and radiation, show very limited survival results as well. The impact on survival is demonstrated in Table 2. These findings would again suggest that concomitant administration might be optimal for tumor control and survival.

Other drugs have been combined with 5–FU and radiation. Keane, et al. have combined mitomycin–C 10 mg/m^2 day 1, 5–FU–1.0 gm/m^2, days 1–4 with radiation–2.5 Gy for 5 days, weeks 1 and 2, followed by a 4 week rest and repeat of the entire cycle [41]. Fifty–seven stage I–IV patients were treated with disease–free status and survival at 1 year of 62% and 74% respectively and at 2 years of 51% and 66%. Others have also used mitomycin–C and 5–FU with radiation but insufficient follow–up data were reported to assess results.

Vokes, et al. [42] have combined hydroxyurea with 5–FU and radiation. This combination is of some interest with both drugs being established radiation sensitizers in human malignancies and both being metabolic inhibitors affecting DNA synthesis. In a dose–seeking study, they gave hydroxyurea–500 to 1,000 mg days 1–5, 2 hours before radiation (1.8 to 2 Gy/day) and 5–FU–800 mg/m^2 continuous infusion for 5 days, all given every other week for 4 cycles prior to surgery. They treated 16 very advanced patients with 11 recurrent and 5 stage IV. One had no measurable disease and 9 had complete responses. Follow–up was too short to address durability of response, but all 5 previously untreated patients were controlled.

Conclusions

Combining chemotherapy with radiation has achieved improved disease–free survival and, in a few series, survival over radiation alone. While the optimal regimen has yet to be established, 5–FU seems to be an important part of any such therapy. All such regimens have found a split course schedule for radiation mandatory for acceptable toxicity. The most effective regimens appear to be those that combine the 5–FU with radiation as completely as possible. An every–other–week schedule has been optimal in our hands as peak 5–FU mucosal toxicity can be anticipated in the 'off' week. Giving radiation during that time would appear to be escalating toxicity without taking advantage of synergistic interaction. Nevertheless, groups that have given radiation during that time also report prolonged survival results.

Despite the negative Intergroup study, substantial evidence suggests cisplatin can also improve therapeutic efficacy of radiation, especially if combined at higher dosage. Its synergistic interaction with 5–FU makes the combination of cisplatin, 5–FU and radiation a logical one. Concern over toxicity continues to dampen the enthusiasm of many oncologists, however. Addressing this concern are the early results of two randomized studies that have failed to identify increased toxicity from simultaneous treatment in comparison to sequential therapy giving the chemotherapy in the usual manner as induction treatment. Hopefully, these results, as they get disseminated, will encourage others to try this approach and confirm the excellent results already achieved.

The addition of other agents, especially leucovorin, hydroxyurea or some of the newer radiation enhancers that have also shown enhancement of chemotherapeutic effects are promising approaches to improve the therapeutic ratio of concomitant chemotherapy and radiation treatment. Advanced head and neck cancer carries a terrible prognosis with radiation alone, so much so that many radiation oncologists regard their therapy as palliative. Many less advanced cancers require extensive surgery that is dysfiguring and destroys speech and swallowing functions. The results of several reports on concomitant chemotherapy and radiation studies indicate that substantial inroads into both these tragedies are now available.

References

1. Taylor SG IV: Head and Neck Cancer. In: Cancer Chemotherapy and Biological Response Modifiers, Annual 11. Pinedo HM, Longo DL, Chabner BA (eds). Amsterdam: Elsevier Science Publishers BV, (in press).
2. Fu KK, Phillips TL, Silverberg IJ, Jacobs C, Goffinet DR, Chun C, Friedman MA, Kohler M, McWhirter K, Carter SK: Combined radiotherapy and chemotherapy with bleomycin and methotrexate for advanced inoperable head and neck cancer: Update of a Northern California Oncology Group randomized trial. J Clin Oncol 5:1410–1418, 1987.
3. Eschwege F, Sancho–Garnier H, Gerard JP, Madelain M, DeSaulty A, Jortay A, Cachin Y: Ten–year results of a randomized trial comparing radiotherapy and concomitant bleomycin to radiotherapy alone in epidermoid carcinomas of the oropharynx: Experience of the European Organization for Research and Treatment of Cancer. NCI Monogr 6:275–278, 1988.
4. Gupta NK, Pointon RCS, Wilkinson PM: A randomized clinical trial to contrast radiotherapy with radiotherapy ad methotrexate given synchronously in head and neck cancer. Clin Radiol 38:575–581, 1987.
5. Papac RJ, Weisberg JB, Son YH, et al.: Prospective randomized trial of radiation therapy ± mitomycin C in head and neck cancer. Proc Am Soc Clin Oncol 6:126, 1987.
6. Haselow RE: Presentation on Integrated Chemotherapy–Radiation Therapy to the Second Int Conf Head and Neck Cancer. DR Goffinet, moderator. Boston MA: 1988.
7. O'Connor AD, Clifford P, Dalley VM, Durden–Smith DJ, Edwards WG, Hollis BA: Advanced head and neck cancer treated by combined radiotherapy and VBM cytotoxic regimen—four year results. Clinical Otolaryngology 4:329–337, 1979.
8. Clifford P, Durden–Smith DJ, Peto J: A randomized trial of combined multidrug chemotherapy and radiotherapy in advanced squamous cell carcinoma of the head and neck. An interim report from the SECOG participants. Eur J Surg Oncol 12:289–295, 1986.
9. Merlano M, Rosso R, Sertoli MR, Bonelli L, Margarino G, Grimaldi A, Benasso M, Gardin G, Corvo R, Scarpati D, Barbieri A, Pallestrini E, Castiglia G, Santelli A, Scasso F, Bottero G, Ciurlo E, Fracchia P, Moratti M, Santi L: Sequential versus alternating chemotherapy and radiotherapy in stage III–IV squamous cell carcinoma of the head and neck: A phase III study. J Clin Oncol 6:627–632, 1988.
10. Corvò R, Merlano M, Scarpati D, Grimaldi A, Benasso M, Franzone P, Santelli A, Scasso F, Rosso R, Vitale V: Chemio—radioterapia sequenziale o alternata nella cura dei tumori avanzati della testa e del collo. La Radiologia Medica 75:653–659, 1988.
11. Zak M, Drobnik J: Effects of cisdichlorodiammineplatinum(II) on the post–irradiation lethality in mice after irradiation with x–rays. Strahlentherapie 142:112–115, 1971.
12. Dritsschilo A, Piro AJ, Kelman AD: The effect of cis-platinum on the repair of radiation damage in plateau phase chinese hamster (V–79) cells. Int J Radiat Oncol Biol Phys 5:1345–1349, 1979.
13. Douple EB, Richmond RC: Radiosensitization of hypoxic tumour cells by cis- and trans-dichlorodiammineplatinum(II). Int J Radiat Oncol Biol Phys 5:1369–1372, 1979.
14. Taylor IV SG, Griem K: Radiopotentiation by cisplatin in continuous infusion: Head and neck cancer. In: Concomitant Infusion Chemotherapy and Radiation. M Rothman and Rosenthal CJ (eds) New York: Springer–Verlag, (in press).
15. Mortimer JE, Taylor ME, Schulman S, Cummings C, Weymuller E Jr, Laramore G: Feasibility and efficacy of weekly intraarterial cisplatin in locally advanced (stage III and IV) head and neck cancer. J Clin Oncol 6:969–975, 1988.

16. Choi TK, Wei W, Lau WF, Lam KH: Regional chemotherapy through a saphenous vein graft for the treatment of head and neck cancer. Cancer 60:1432–1438, 1987.
17. Al-Sarraf M, Pajak TF, Marcial VA, Mowry P, Cooper JS, Stetz J, Ensley JF, Velez-Garcia E: Concurrent radiotherapy and chemotherapy with cisplatin in inoperable squamous cell carcinoma of the head and neck. Cancer 59:259–265, 1987.
18. Ensley J, Ahmad K, Kish J, Tapazoglou E, Jacobs J, Al–Sarraf M: Improved response to radiation and concurrent cisplatinum in patients with advanced head and neck cancers that fail induction chemotherapy. Proc Amer Soc Clin Oncol 8:168(652), 1989.
19. Ensley JR, Jacobs JE, Weaver A, Kinzie J, Crissman J, et al.: Correlation between response to cisplatinum-combination chemotherapy and subsequent radiotherapy in previously untreated patients with advanced squamous cell cancers of the head and neck. Cancer 545: 811–814, 1984.
20. Scwarz JL, Rotmensch J, Beckett MA, et al.: X–ray and cis–diamminedichloroplatinum(II) cross–resistance in human tumor cell clones. Cancer Res 48:5133–5135, 1988.
21. Wheeler R, Salter M, Stephens S, Hardy I, Peters G, Urist M, Maddox W: Simultaneous therapy with high-dose cisplatin and radiation for unresectable squamous cell cancer of the head and neck: A phase I–II study. NCI Monogr 6:339–341, 1988.
22. Forestiere AA, Belliveau JF, Goren MP, et al.: Pharmacokinetic and toxicity evaluation of five-day continuous infusion versus intermittent bolus cisdiamminedichloroplatinum(II) in head and neck cancer patients. Cancer Res 48:3869–3874, 1988.
23. Tobias JS, Smith BJ, Blackman G, Finn G: Concurrent daily cisplatin and radiotherapy in locally advanced squamous carcinoma of the head–and–neck and bronchus. Radiotherapy and Oncology 9:263–268, 1987.
24. Eisenberger M, Sinibaldi V, Jacobs M, Gray W: Simultaneous treatment with carboplatin (NSC–241–240) and radiotherapy in advanced unresectable squamous cell carcinomas of the head and neck. Cancer Treatment Reviews 15:3–7, 1988.
25. Lo TCM, Wiley AL Jr, Ansfield FJ, Brandenburg JH, Davis HL Jr, Gollin FF, Johnson RO, Ramirez G, Vermund H: Combined radiation therapy and 5–fluorouracil for advanced squamous cell carcinoma of the oral cavity and oropharynx: A randomized study. Am J Roentgenol 126:229–235, 1976.
26. Wiley AL Jr, Ramirez G, Johnson RO, Brandenburg JH, Lieberman LM, Lo TCM, Vermund H: Treatment of carcinoma of base of tongue with radiation therapy and 5–fluorouracil. Acta Radiologica Oncology 18:235–243, 1979.
27. Bagshaw MA, Doggett RLS: A clinical study of chemical radiosensitization. Front Radiation Ther Onc 4:164–173, 1969.
28. Byfield JE, Calabro–Jones PM, Klisak I, et al.: Pharmacologic requirements for obtaining sensitization of human tumor cells *in vitro* to combined 5–fluorouracil or ftorafur and x rays. Int J Radiat Oncol Biol Phys 8:1923–1933, 1988.
29. Byfield JE, Sharp TR, Frankel SS, Tang SG, Callipari FB: Phase I and II trial of five–day infused 5–fluorouracil and radiation in advanced cancer of the head and neck. J Clin Oncol 2:406–413, 1984.
30. Byfield JE, Frankel SS, Sharp TR, Hornbeck CL, Callipari FB: Phase I and pharmacologic study of 72 hour infused 5–fluorouracil and hyperfractionated cyclical radiation. Int J Radiation Oncology, Biol, Phys 22:791–800, 1985.
31. Taylor SG IV, Murthy AK, Showel JL, Caldarelli DD, Hutchinson JC Jr, Holinger LD, Kramer T, Kiel K: Improved control in advanced head and neck cancer with simultaneous radiation and cisplatin/5–FU chemotherapy. Cancer Treat Rep 69:933–939, 1985.
32. Taylor, SG IV, Murthy AK, Caldarelli DD, Showel JL, Kiel K, Griem KL, Mittal BB, Kies M, Hutchinson JC Jr, Holinger LD, Campanella R, Witt TR, Hoover S: Combined simultaneous cisplatin/fluorouracil chemotherapy and split course radiation in head and neck cancer. J Clin Oncol 7:846–856, 1989.
33. Taylor SG IV, Murthy AK, Showel JL, Griem K, Kies MS, Mittal B, Kiel K, Vannetzel JM, Rebischung JL: Comparison of toxicity in a randomized trial of sequential vs. simul-

taneous cisplatin/5–FU infusion and radiation therapy in head and neck cancer. Proc Amer Soc Clin Oncol 8:175(681), 1989.
34. Adelstein DJ, Sharan VM, Earle AS, Shah AC, Vlastou C, Haria CD, Carter SG, Damm C, Hines JD: Simultaneous radiotherapy and chemotherapy with 5–fluorouracil and cisplatin for locally confined squamous cell head and neck cancer. NCI Mongr 6:347–351, 1988.
35. Adelstein DJ, Sharan VM, Earle AS, Shah AC, Vlastou C, Haria CD, Damm C, Carter SG, Hines JD: A prospective randomized trial of simultaneous vs. sequential chemoradiotherapy for squamous cell head and neck cancer. Proc Amer Soc Clin Oncol 8:167(648), 1989.
36. Wendt TG, Wustrow TPU, Hartenstein RC, et al.: Accelerated split–course radiotherapy and simultaneous cis–dichlorodiammine–platinum and 5–fluorouracil chemotherapy with folinic acid enhancement for unresectable carcinoma of the head and neck. Radiother Oncol, 10:277–284, 1987.
37. Wendt TG, Hartenstein RC, Wustrow TP: 4–years–update of simultaneous chemoradiotherapy with 5–FU/folonic Acid/cisplatin and accelerated radiation in inoperable head and neck cancer. Proc Amer Soc Clin Oncol 8:169(658), 1989.
38. Bolla M, Borgel J, Guenoun A, Junien–Lavillauroy C, Dionet C, Vrousos C: Chemotherapy with low doses of radiation followed by definitive radiotherapy for advanced unresectable carcinoma of the head and neck. NCI Monogr 6:357–359, 1988.
39. Dionet C, Rozan R, Achard JL, Verrelle P, Dumesnil Y, Russier M, Lemesle Ph, Theron H, deLatour M, Mondie JM, Lafaye M, Bolla M, Chollet Ph: Sequential combination of 5–fluorouracil, cis–platinum and irradiation. 1. Advanced head and neck cancers. Radiotherapy and Oncology 11:123–131, 1988.
40. Merlano M, Grimaldi A, Benasso M, Bacigalupo A, Toma S, Scarpati D, Corvo R, Santelli A, Garaventa G, Rosso R: Alternating cisplatin–5–fluorouracil and radiotherapy in head and neck cancer. Am J Clin Oncol (CCT) 11:538–542, 1988.
41. Keane TJ, Harwood AR, Beale FA, Cummings BJ, Payne DG, et al.: A pilot study of mitomycin–C/5–fluorouracil infusion combined with split course radiation therapy for carcinomas of the larynx and hypopharynx. J Otolaryngol 15:286–288, 1986.
42. Vokes EE, Panje WR, Weichselbaum RR, Schilsky RL, Moran WJ, Awan AM, Guarnieri CM: Concomitant hydroxyurea, 5–fluorouracil, and radiation therapy for recurrent head and neck cancer: Early Results. Otolaryngol Head Neck Surg 98:295–298, 1988.

13. The Role of Induction Chemotherapy for Organ Preservation in Laryngeal Carcinoma

Isaiah W. Dimery, Charles D. Wendt, Alan M. Kramer, Robert M. Byers and Waun K. Hong

Laryngeal carcinoma is the most common head and neck tumor, representing 2% of all malignancies and 28% of head and neck malignancies. It was estimated that in 1989, that 12,300 new cases would be diagnosed and that 3,700 deaths from this disease would occur, according to the American Cancer Society [1]. The extent of disease of the glottic and supraglottic larynx, which is defined by the American Joint Committee on Cancer Staging System criteria [Tables 1 and 2] [2], determines the modality selected for definitive treatment. Early–stage tumors (T_1 and T_2) can be treated successfully with either definitive radiotherapy alone or partial laryngectomy, at least in the United States, whereas total laryngectomy, with or without postoperative radiotherapy, is considered to be the standard treatment for more advanced T_3 and T_4 tumors.

Voice preservation is a major concern in these patients. Conservative surgery (partial or subtotal laryngectomy) to preserve laryngeal function is possible but must meet stringent criteria to assure recovery of the patient to a functional capacity [3]. However, not only patients with early stage disease, but also selected patients with advanced stage laryngeal tumors may be good candidates for voice preserving surgery or definitive radiotherapy. Heretofore, the only curative option has been total laryngectomy with the re–establishment of vocal communication accomplished postoperatively by artificial means. Recently, through the use of induction chemotherapy with radiotherapy, laryngeal function can be preserved without any compromise in their cancer control and overall survival in certain selected patients with advanced supraglottic and glottic cancers. Herein, we review the therapy of laryngeal carcinoma from the standpoints of surgery and radiotherapy and then discuss the rationale for the incorporation of chemotherapy into the management of this disease for the preservation of anatomy and organ function.

Early Glottic Tumors

The standard therapy for laryngeal tumors is dependent upon the extent of the primary disease. Early stage T_1 and T_2 cancers of the glottis are equally

Jacobs, C. (ed): Carcinomas of the Head and Neck: Evaluation and Management.

Table 1. 1988 AJCC staging of carcinoma of the glottis.

T_1	Tumor limited to vocal cord(s) (may involve anterior or posterior commissures) with normal mobility
T_{1a}	Tumor limited to one vocal cord
T_{1b}	Tumor involves both vocal cords
T_2	Tumor extends to supraglottis and/or subglottis, and/or with impaired vocal cord mobility
T_3	Tumor limited to the larynx with vocal cord fixation
T_4	Tumor invades through thyroid cartilage and/or extends to other tissues beyond the larynx (e.g., oropharynx, soft tissues of neck)

Table 2. 1988 AJCC staging of carcinoma of the supraglottis.

T_1	Tumor limited to one subsite of supraglottis with normal vocal cord mobility
T_2	Tumor invades more than one subsite of supraglottis or glottis, with normal vocal cord mobility
T_3	Tumor limited to larynx with vocal cord fixation and/or invades postcricoid area, medial wall of pyriform sinus, or pre-epiglottic tissues
T_4	Tumor invades through thyroid cartilage and/or extends to other tissues beyond the larynx, e.g., oropharynx, soft tissues of neck

well–controlled with definitive radiotherapy or a conservative surgical approach, with control rates as high as 95% for T_1 cancers and 70% to 85% for stage T_2 lesions [4]. At M.D. Anderson Cancer Center, radiotherapy is the preferred initial therapy as the functional result of larynges treated with radiotherapy is superior to those treated with conservative surgery. In addition, radiotherapy failures may be successfully treated with salvage surgery, with a determinate (cause specific) survival of >90% for T_1 lesions and 70% to 80% for T_2 lesions [5–9].

Some irradiation failures may successfully be salvaged even with conservative surgery. For example, between January 1975 and December 1984, 46 patients at M.D. Anderson underwent surgery to conserve laryngeal function after either irradiation failure or for new cancer in a previously irradiated field. The various surgical procedures utilized included supraglottic laryngectomy, vertical hemilaryngectomy or laryngofissure, transoral glottic procedures, and subtotal laryngectomy. Local control was obtained in 9 of 10 patients undergoing supraglottic laryngectomy, and the 5–year determinate survival was 64%. Patients who underwent hemilaryngectomy or laryngofissure had an 81% 5–year survival. The overall 5–year survival, with a median follow–up of 2 years was 72%. A recent report described vertical hemilaryngectomy as the sole treatment modality in T_1 carcinoma of the glottic larynx resulting in an ultimate disease control rate of 95% [10]. The transoral glottic procedures were often inadequate as the first salvage procedure, but failures were successfully treated by additional surgery then yielding a 5–year survival of >90% [11].

Advanced Glottic Tumors

In the United States, standard therapy for advanced–stage glottic and supraglottic tumors is total laryngectomy with or without postoperative radiotherapy. In most other countries the preferred therapy is definitive radiotherapy with laryngectomy reserved for radiation failures. The advantage of the latter method of treatment is that a proportion of patients retain functioning larynges. Disadvantages of this method include the possibility that patients failing radiotherapy might not be treatable with surgery, and a potential increased risk exists of postoperative complications following laryngectomy in a previously irradiated bed.

With fixation or impaired mobility of the cord (classified as a T_3 lesion), cure rates may drop by as much as 20% below those obtained for T_2 lesions with radiotherapy alone [4]. The 5–year survival rate for patients with T_3 lesions treated with radiotherapy alone is as low as 25–30% in some early series [16]. This figure improves to 50% if salvage surgery is able to be performed at the time of recurrence [12,16,17]. More recently, using superior radiotherapeutic techniques, with definitive radiotherapy, local control is 50% to 67%; local control after surgical salvage is 69% to 89%, and determinate survival ranges from 57% to 74% [18–22].

Determinate survival after total laryngectomy for glottic cancers is 62%–90% for T_3 lesions and 36%–63% for T_4 tumors; for supraglottic tumors the 5–year determinate survival is 59%–66% for T_3 cancers and 31%–47% for T_4 tumors [23–27]. Thus, although irradiation gives the patient a chance of preserving laryngeal function, there is 5% to 25% increase in the probability of dying from disease. Vocal communication may be re–established in several ways including esophageal speech, duckbill (Blom–Singer) prosthesis [28] or electrolarynx.

Nonetheless, most T_2 and selected T_3 lesions can be successfully treated with radiotherapy alone with good tumor control. Some cases with advanced vocal cord lesions are more suitable than others for primary radiation. Favorable tumors are those confined to one vocal cord and predominately exophytic. Unfavorable tumors are large infiltrative tumors causing airway obstruction. Further, because frequent examinations are necessary after radiotherapy to detect recurrences before they become too extensive for surgical salvage, patients selected for radiotherapy must be anatomically easy to examine and must be reliable regarding frequent follow–up. Some groups have obtained a better cure rate with women than men [29–31]. The non-randomized, retrospectively analyzed treatment of 140 patients with $T_3N_0M_0$ glottic cancers at the Princess Margaret Hospital, Toronto from 1963–1977 was reported by Harwood et al. [29]. Patients were given either preoperative radiotherapy (50 to 55 Gy in 3 to 5 weeks) followed by a total laryngectomy (28 patients) or radical radiotherapy (50 to 55 Gy in 4 to 5 weeks) followed by salvage surgery (112 patients) [29]. The overall local control rate by radical radiotherapy was 51% at both 3 and 5 years. In the respective groups, 50% and 55% were alive at 5 years with 45% and 44% alive at 10 years. Forty–two percent versus 26% died of glottic cancer at 5 and 10 years in both groups [29]. Of particular note was the observation that half of the patients who received high–dose preoperative radiotherapy had no tumor at laryngectomy, and surgery was therefore unnecessary.

A twice–daily radiotherapy trial reported by Parsons et al., delivering 7,400–7,600 cGy in 120 cGy fractions to 21 previously untreated patients with T_3 true vocal cord carcinoma achieved local control in 12 of 18 (67%) evaluable patients, resulting in a 5–year rate of larynx preservation of 65% [32]. Three of six patients who underwent total laryngectomy for local recurrence remain alive 2.5 to 4 years after surgery. Severe complications of radiotherapy were encountered in 2 patients, and complications of salvage surgery occurred in 4 patients.

Supraglottic Tumors

Some supraglottic lesions can be treated with preservation of laryngeal function by supraglottic laryngectomy. Tumors without extension to the true vocal cord, anterior commissure, or both arytenoids, without vocal cord fixation and without thyroid or cricoid cartilage invasion, can be treated with supraglottic laryngectomy [33]. Because of a tendency toward aspiration in the postoperative period, patients must have adequate pulmonary reserve. Three–year determinate survivals of 70% for T_3 lesions and 64% for T_4 lesions have been obtained [34]. Major complications include postoperative infection, fistula formation, and difficulty with swallowing leading to aspiration pneumonia. A few patients never regain swallowing function and have to undergo complete laryngectomy [35].

Between 1974 and 1983, 34 patients at M.D. Anderson with a stage T_2 or T_3 supraglottic primary (13 and 21 patients, respectively) underwent supraglottic laryngectomy [36]. Only 3 of the 34 patients suffered local–regional failures. Five–year determinate survival was 89%. The functional results of therapy were evaluated 3 months after surgery at which time 14 (41%) of patients had symptoms of aspiration, 4 (12%) developed aspiration pneumonia, and 1 (3%) patient died of aspiration pneumonia. Two patients continued to require a nasogastric tube, and decannulation could not be performed in two others. Overall, 31 (91%) of the 34 patients remained disease–free above the clavicle and retained some laryngeal function for the duration of their lives [36].

Definitive radiotherapy has a high probability of controlling disease in selected stage T_3 supraglottic lesions as well. Unfortunately, cancers that have invaded the base of tongue, with vocal cord fixation, extensive invasion of the pyriform sinus, or extensive preepiglottic space invasion are unlikely to be controlled with radiotherapy alone [37]. Local control rates of 42% to

76% have been obtained with primary radiotherapy. With surgical salvage, the ultimate local control is 70% to 85% [38–40].

Conservative Surgical Alternatives

Partial laryngectomy as salvage treatment is possible in patients with T_{1-2} lesions who fail radiation therapy provided the disease is still limited to the confines of conservation surgery [41]. Approximately 40% of radiotherapy failures can be salvaged with partial laryngectomy [42,43] but with a resultant 20% to 30% rate of second recurrences [43–46] and with considerable morbidity. This second recurrence rate reflects the difficulty preoperatively or intraoperatively of assessing the extent of residual disease. Thus, the recurrent tumors in radiated tissues tend to be more extensive than the presurgical evaluations would disclose [47,48].

Hemilaryngectomy can be an alternative to total laryngectomy in selected patients with previously untreated stage T_3 glottic cancer. Tumors that are suitable for treatment with hemilaryngectomy should involve no more than one vocal cord plus one–third of the opposite vocal cord. The maximum subglottic extension is 8 to 9 mm anteriorly and 5 mm posteriorly. The tumor must not extend to both arytenoids [33]. Local control rates of 59% to 78% and determinate survivals of 68% to 85% have been obtained [49–51]. Complications following hemilaryngectomy include: infection, fistula, necrosis, aspiration and hemorrhage [35]. Patients who undergo vertical hemilaryngectomy have poor voice quality, but it is preferred to that provided after a total laryngectomy.

The options of conservative surgical therapy or definitive radiotherapy may be a viable alternative for a minority of patients with no increase in the risk of death from disease. For most patients, however, the option of definitive radiotherapy, which, although allowing some patients to preserve good laryngeal function, carries an increased risk of dying from cancer. In advanced laryngeal cancer, conservative surgery is in fact an alternative for only a selected minority of patients, and those who undergo such surgical procedures will sometimes have an inferior functional result. These studies, for the most part support the success and shortcomings of standard treatment for carcinoma of the larynx. However, voice preservation would be advantageous to the patient whose livelihood depends upon the use of their voice and who desires an alternative approach in the management of the cancer if there is no compromise in survival.

Chemotherapeutic Strategies

For the patient in whom standard management of his/her larynx cancer would necessitate a total laryngectomy if treated initially with surgery or who has a very low chance of tumor control if treated with radiation alone, the concept of induction chemotherapy may appear attractive.

A survey of the attitudes of a healthy volunteer population toward the reduced (presumed) quality of life resulting from a laryngectomy for stage T_3 carcinoma of the larynx led approximately 20 percent to indicate that they would choose radiotherapy alone as their treatment despite a possible reduction in survival (52). Although long–term survival data resulting from combination chemotherapy + radiotherapy are as yet not available, current information to be discussed suggests that survival approaches that of surgery + radiotherapy. Thus no trade–off for quantity of life would exist with chemotherapy, providing yet another therapeutic option for consideration.

The selection of an appropriate patient population for this combination treatment must be carefully considered. If, for example, there is a large, bulky tumor that has already destroyed the laryngeal skeleton, standard treatment modalities (total laryngectomy) should be adhered to because preserving the organ is no longer possible, and an attempt to do so may be at the expense of patient survival.

On the other hand, for patients with cancers which are marginally resectable with standard conservation procedures, and yet a total laryngectomy may be considered excessive, the use of induction chemotherapy may provide sufficient tumor reduction to allow either less surgery or improve the success with the use of definitive radiotherapy.

Medically, the approach to determining who will benefit from combined chemotherapy and radiotherapy with a minimum of toxicity is straightforward. Patients must be in reasonably good physical condition (Zubrod performance 0–2) and thus expected to tolerate several months of chemotherapy; they must show sufficient pulmonary function (for bleomycin–containing regimens) without significant airway obstruction to indicate possible problems during the administration of chemotherapy. Additionally, these patients must be closely followed to determine if salvage surgery is required. Follow–up by the same head and neck surgeon or otolaryngologist and radiotherapist is also quite essential since the larynx is usually altered to some degree during treatment. Subsequent well–meaning attempts to determine the presence or absence of recurrent disease by biopsy may result in edema or obstruction, necessitating tracheostomy and possibly a laryngectomy for biopsy–induced infection and chondronecrosis in the absence of disease.

Laryngeal preservation was initially conceptualized by Popkin and Hong when they identified 20 candidates among 110 patients with advanced laryngeal and hypopharyngeal carcinoma who were selected or elected to receive induction chemotherapy followed by radiotherapy instead of a total laryngectomy [53,54]. Seven of the candidates had refused laryngectomy; surgery was contraindicated in three; a nonsurgical approach was the preference of the physician in six; and the reasons for chemotherapy were various in the remaining four [53,54]. Chemotherapy with cisplatin and bleomycin, bleomycin alone, or cisplatin and 5–fluorouracil resulted in an objective response rate in 16 (80%), with 4 (20%) achieving complete remission. Thus, when chemotherapy was used in conjunction with sequential radiotherapy, 17 (85%) experienced complete response; the median disease–free survival time was 37 months for laryngeal cancer and 25 months for hypopharyngeal cancer [53,54].

Despite some positive data, it is not known if a role for the routine use of chemotherapy as induction treatment will become a standard of care. Early induction chemotherapy trials have demonstrated that survival of patients who have laryngeal carcinoma is significantly better than those with carcinoma of the oral cavity or hypopharynx as a primary tumor [55]. A positive impact on the treatment of head and neck cancer is, therefore, most likely to be seen in this particular site. However, a specific analysis of primary tumors of the larynx was not reported in this series. Recent experience had indicated that surgery may be circumvented, while the resulting survival rate is comparable to those who undergo laryngectomy; those with pyriform sinus or hypopharyngeal or base of tongue cancers respond less well to this treatment [56].

The introduction of induction chemotherapy into the multimodality approach of advanced head and neck cancer originating in various sites has led to widespread investigations utilizing chemotherapy followed by conventional surgery and/or radiation therapy to improve the survival rate. To date, these studies have uniformly failed to demonstrate significant improvement in the survival rates. Numerous studies, however, have confirmed the feasibility of this approach, identified highly active drug regimens and documented dramatic tumor response rates to induction chemotherapy in the majority of previously untreated patients with complete response rates in 30 to 40% of the patients. Prior induction chemotherapy trials have also demonstrated that survival rates are significantly increased in the subset of patients in whom complete tumor response is achieved. In a variety of solid tumors, the emphasis has increasingly been placed on decreasing the use of radical surgery, preserving the normal function and improving the quality of life. The successful outcome of induction chemotherapy in head and neck cancer could allow the preservation of voice, normal swallowing mechanism, and normal function of the neck muscles, in addition to providing better cosmetic outcome in most patients. If, as a result of the use of induction chemotherapy, a reduction in, or elimination of, the radical surgery in head and neck cancer were possible, the quality of life would be improved.

Several other studies demonstrated that response to induction chemotherapy predicts a further response with radiation treatment. Haines et al. [57,58] have reported using induction chemotherapy to facilitate laryngeal preservation in other tumors (for example, hypopharyngeal tumors) whose traditional treatment required laryngectomy. This approach preserved the larynx in 28 of 35 (80%) patients, and 14 (50%) had no evidence of disease at 18 months. Furthermore, a subset analysis of 73 laryngeal carcinomas treated at the Royal Marsden Hospital in London [59] demonstrated a 61% response to chemotherapy, after which 52 of these patients were given radiotherapy alone. The final complete remission rate was 79%. Patients in that series who achieved a complete response had a median survival of 7 years, which was not significantly different from that of patients treated with total laryngectomy followed by radiotherapy at the Royal Marsden [59].

This provocative and innovative approach for organ preservation was also investigated by Jacobs et al. from Stanford University [60]. Thirty head and neck cancer patients were treated with 3 cycles of cisplatinum and 5–FU followed by re–endoscopy and biopsy. Twelve patients (40%) achieved a pathologic complete response at the primary site and thereafter received only irradiation. At 2 years, relapse–free survival and overall survival for those 12 patients were 60 and 70% respectively. For all 30 patients at 2 years, relapse–free survival was 52% and overall survival was 53%. This study clearly demonstrated for the first time that eliminating surgery to treat with primary radiotherapy not only is feasible but also does not compromise the survival in patients who achieve a pathologic complete response.

Our current approach with neoadjuvant chemotherapy and radiotherapy in larynx preservation at M.D. Anderson Cancer Center consists of the combination of cisplatin–100 mg/m^2 on the first day plus 5–fluorouracil–1,000 mg/m^2 continuous infusion for 4 days with the addition of bleomycin–15 mg/m^2/day continuous infusion for 3 days [61]. Currently, 34 patients with locally advanced cancer of the larynx, hypopharynx and base of tongue have been entered into this nonrandomized pilot study. The overall response rate to chemotherapy was 26/34 or 76% (CR – 29%, PR – 47%). Twenty–three patients successfully completed radiotherapy with 15/23 (65%) rendered disease–free and 11/15 (73%) of these patients ultimately spared laryngectomy.

An example of representative treatment responses and survival outcome are described in the following two cases illustrated by figures 1 and 2. In the first case, the patient presented with $T_2N_0M_0$ tumor of the glottic larynx (with subglottic extension) (figure 1a). A 90% tumor reduction was achieved after the completion of 3 cycles of therapy (figure 1b). Following radiotherapy the patient achieved a complete response and continue in remission more than 3 years after initial diagnosis. In the second case, the patient initially had $T_3N_0M_0$ involvement of the supraglottic larynx including the left vocal cord (figure 2a) and received 3 cycles of chemotherapy after which a complete clinical response was documented (figure 2b). Despite no evidence of residual disease after radiotherapy, recurrence necessitated laryngectomy 26 months after initial diagnosis. The patient remains free of disease 6 months after salvage surgery. This approach to organ preservation is an emotional one for the medical oncologist, the surgeon, and the radiotherapist who realize that induction chemotherapy alone has not yet been shown to enhance long–term survival. Of greatest concern is the patient who does not want to sacrifice his voice. The initial antitumor response rates obtained

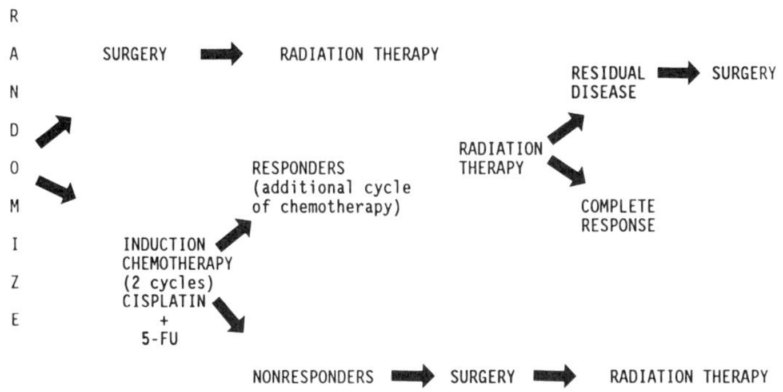

Figure 3. Protocol schema of the Veterans Administration Cooperative Laryngeal Study, begun in 1985.

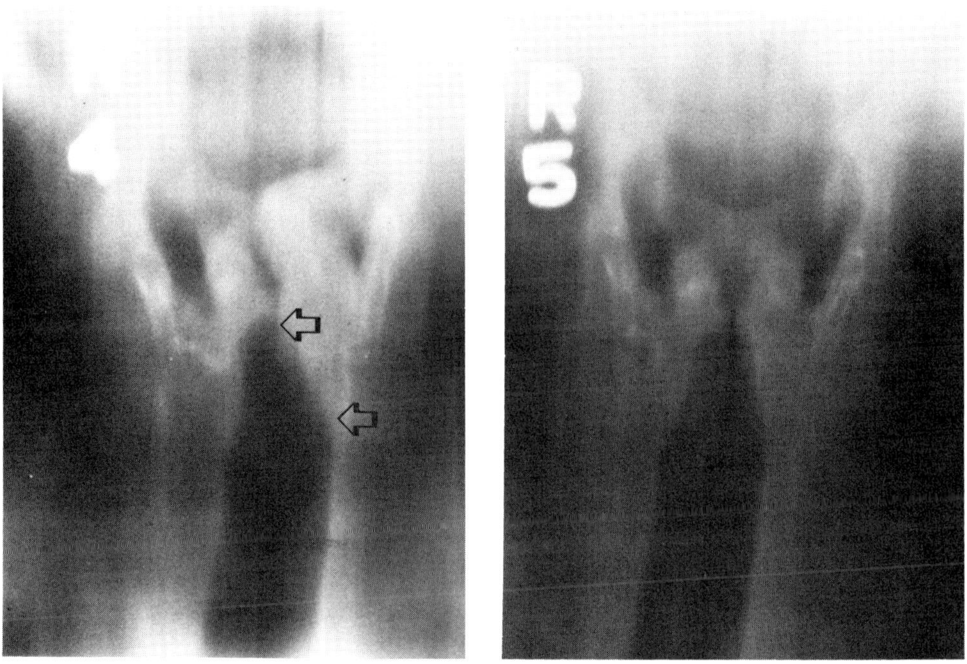

Figure 1. Laryngeal polytomography demonstrating the extent of the tumor (a) before T2NOMO and, (b) after chemotherapy. Note the degree of subglottic extension (arrows) before therapy. Reproduced with permission from Dimery et al. [60].

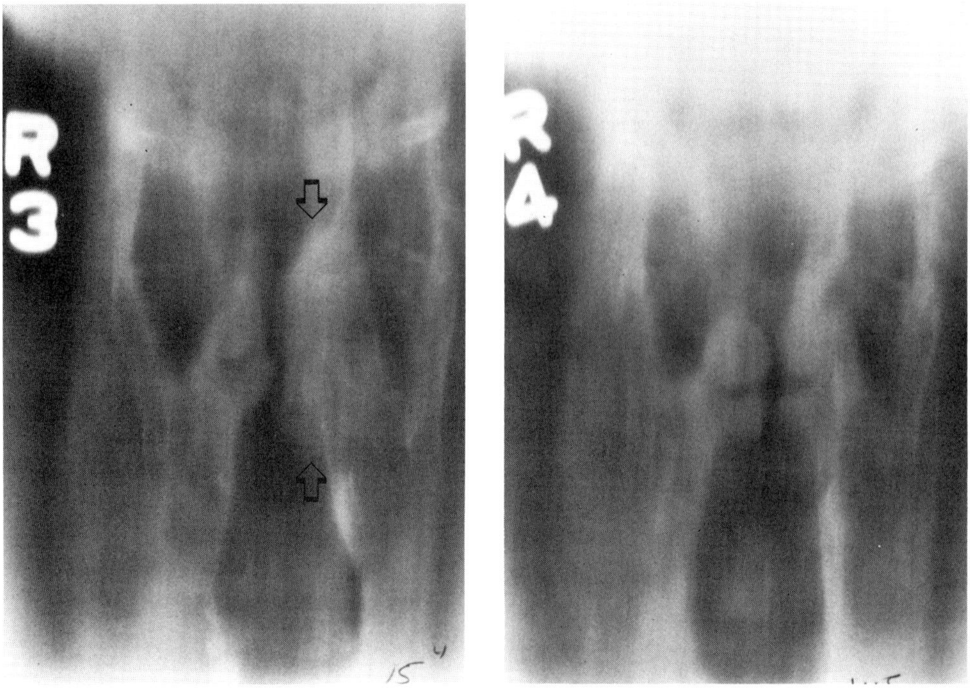

Figure 2. Laryngeal polytomography demonstrating (a) the extent (arrows) of the T3NOMO tumor involving the left glottic and supraglottic region, at presentation, and (b) complete disappearance of the tumor after chemotherapy. Reproduced with permission from Dimery et al. [60].

in these patients illustrate the potential oncologic, as well as, functional value of induction chemotherapy followed by radiation since it could spare selected individuals from total laryngectomy. The chemotherapy is well tolerated followed by a high–rate of complete response and was predictive of the patients' response to radiotherapy.

These issues for the potential role of induction chemotherapy in eliminating the need for functional, potentially debilitating surgical resection have been initially addressed on a broad national scale through the V.A. Cooperative Study Program in a prospective, randomized fashion the design of which is illustrated in figure 3 [62]. The V.A. Cooperative Study #268 entitled 'A new strategy to preserve the voice–box in advanced laryngeal cancers' was activated in January 1985 and was closed to patient accrual in March 1989. This trial compared traditional laryngectomy and postoperative radiation therapy to induction chemotherapy followed by definitive radiation therapy. The larynx was selected as the optimal tumor site to test this hypothesis because of the importance of larynx preservation for the quality of life and the effectiveness of radiation therapy (with salvage surgery) if necessary in treating minimum or microscopic disease post–chemotherapy.

Preliminary analysis of the results of this trial was presented at the 1989 American Society of Clinical Oncology meeting at San Francisco, CA [63]. At the end of March 1989, 332 patients had been randomized; 166 patients were assigned to surgery and radiation treatment, and 166 patients were assigned to chemotherapy and radiation therapy. Using combination induction chemotherapy and radiation therapy, the larynx can initially be preserved in two–thirds of the patients with advanced laryngeal cancer without compromising survival rate. Analysis of the interim data from the V.A. Study found that approximately 80% of the 166 patients who received induction chemotherapy had dramatic response to chemotherapy. The vast majority of patients achieved complete local control of their disease after radiation treatment. Patients whose laryngeal tumors did not regress during two courses of induction chemotherapy were sent to surgery for conventional treatment. The estimated actuarial two–year survival of each treatment group is exactly identical at 66%. In the chemotherapy arm of this V.A. Study, the majority of initial tumor failures were local and regional; however, a lower percentage of distant metastasis (16% vs. 49%) occurred in the chemotherapy arm compared to the surgical arm. Until the final report of this study is complete and until the results supporting this approach are confirmed, the use of chemotherapy and radiotherapy is considered experimental and should not be attempted outside of a formal protocol.

Conclusion

The approach to the treatment of head and neck cancer has changed dramatically in the past 10 years both in terms of surgical, radiotherapeutic and chemotherapeutic treatment modalities. Despite these advances, the overall survival of these patients has not been significantly improved, especially regarding advanced stage disease.

It remains to be shown conclusively whether induction chemotherapy, followed by radiotherapy for responding tumors, should be the standard of care in the treatment of head and neck cancers necessitating laryngectomy whether those are tumors of the larynx or of other anatomic sites (for example, base of tongue, hypopharynx). It appears that overall response and survival after this approach are inferior in the latter groups. The larynx, therefore, appears to be the ideal site upon which to concentrate our efforts in analyzing the ultimate usefulness and therapeutic outcome of this concept.

This chapter has provided an overview of the varied approaches used in the management of laryngeal carcinoma including their advantages and pitfalls. Now that multi–institutional randomized trials can be performed utilizing patient numbers never before achieved in the history of head and neck cancer trials, with accurate longitudinal follow–up assured, a new standard of care is evolving which will impact and benefit quality of life of all patients.

References

1. Silverberg E, Lubera JA: Cancer statistics, 1988. CA 39:3–20, 1989.
2. American Joint Committee on Cancer: Manuel for Staging of Cancer, ed 3. Beahrs OH, Hensun DE, Hutter RVP, Myers MH. (eds) Philadelphia: JB Lippincott, p 40, 1988.
3. Biller HF: The Joseph H. Ogura Memorial Lecture: Conservative surgery—past, present, and future. Laryngoscope 97:38–41, 1987.
4. Hendrickson FR: Radiation therapy treatment of larynx cancers. Cancer 55:2058–2061, 1985.
5. Smith RR, Caulk R, Jackson LC, Russell W: End results of 600 laryngeal cancers using the American Joint Committee's method of classification and end–result reporting. Surg Gynecol Obstet 113:435–444, 1961.
6. Howell–Burke D, Peters LJ, Oswald MJ: T_2 glottic carcinoma: 16 years experience at the University of Texas Cancer Center. Int J Radiat Oncol Biol Phys (in press).
7. Fletcher GH, Goepfert H: The role of irradiation in the treatment of cancer of the larynx. In: Cancer of the Larynx, vol 3. Ferlito A (ed) Boca Raton, FL: CRC Press, pp 70–114, 1984.
8. Wang CC: Radiation Therapy for Head and Neck Neoplasms. Boston: John Wright–PSG, 1983.
9. Fisher AJ, Caldarelli DD, Chacko DC, Holinger LD: Glottic cancer: Surgical salvage for radiation failure. Arch Otolaryngol Head Neck Surg 112:519–521, 1986.
10. Rothfield RE, Johnson JT, Myers EN, Wagner RL: The role of hemilaryngectomy in the management of T_1 vocal cord cancer. Arch Otolaryngeal Head Neck Surg 115:677–680, 1989.
11. Campbell BH, Goepfert H: Partial laryngectomy as a salvage procedure for radiation failure. In: Head and Neck Oncology: Clinical Management. Kagan AR, Miles JW (eds) Elmsford, NY: Pergamon Press, 1988 (in press).
12. Ennuyer A, Bataini P: Laryngeal carcinomas. Panel discussion on glottic tumors, VI. Laryngoscope 85:1467–1476, 1975.
13. Kirchner JA, Owen JR: Five hundred cancers of the larynx and pyriform sinus. Results of treatment by radiation and surgery. Laryngoscope 87:1288–1303, 1977.
14. Miller D: Management of glottic carcinomas. Panel discussion on glottic tumors. III. Laryngoscope 85:1435–1439, 1975.
15. Vermund H: Role of radiotherapy in cancer of the larynx as related to the TNM system of staging: a review. Cancer 25:485–504, 1970.
16. Wang CC: Treatment of squamous cell carcinoma of the larynx by radiation. Radiol Clin North Am 16:209–218, 1978.
17. Hawkins NV: The treatment of glottic carcinomas: An analysis of 800 cases. Panel discussion on glottic tumors, VIII. Laryngoscope 85:1485–1493, 1975.
18. Parsons JT, Mendenhall WM, Cassisi NJ, Issac JH, Million RR: Accelerated hyperfractionation for head and neck cancer. Int J Radiat Oncol Biol Phys (in press).
19. Wang CC: Treatment of glottic carcinoma by megavoltage radiation therapy and results AJR 120:157–163, 1974.
20. Stewart JG, Brown JR, Palmer MK, et al.: The management of glottic carcinoma by primary irradiation with surgery in reserve. Laryngoscope 85:1477–1484, 1975.
21. Mendenhall WM, Million RR, Sharkey DE: Stage T_3 squamous cell carcinoma of the glottic larynx treated with surgery and/or radiation therapy. Int J Radiat Oncol Biol Phys 10:357–363, 1984.

22. Terhaard HS, Wiggeraad RG, Hordijk GJ, et al.: Regression after 50 Gy as a selection for therapy in advanced laryngeal carcinoma. Int J Radiat Oncol Biol Phys 15:591–597, 1986.
23. Putney FJ, Chapman CE: Carcinoma of the larynx: Analysis of 311 cases treated surgically. Ann Otol Rhinol Laryngol 81:455–464, 1972.
24. Smith RR, Caulk R, Frazell E, Holinger PH, MacComb WS, Russel WO, Schulz MD, Tucker GF: Revision of the clinical staging system for cancer of the larynx. Cancer 31:72–80, 1973.
25. Yuen A, Medina JE, Goepfert H, Fletcher G: Management of stage T_3 and T_4 glottic carcinomas. Am J Surg 148:467–472, 1984.
26. Lindberg RD: Sites of first failure in head and neck cancer. Cancer Treat Symp 2:21–31, 1983.
27. DeSanto LW, Devine KD, Lillie JC: Cancers of the larynx: Glottic scanner. Surg Clin North Am 57:611–621, 1977.
28. Singer M, Blom E: An endoscopic technique for restoration of voice after laryngectomy. Ann Otol Rhinol Laryngol 89:529–533, 1980.
29. Harwood AR, Bryce DP, Rider WD: Management of T_3 glottic cancer. Arch Otolaryngol 106:697–699, 1980.
30. Wang CC: personal communication.
31. Jorgenson K, Hjelm–Hansen M, Anderson AP, et al.: Laryngeal cancer. I. Treatment results. Acta Radiol Oncol Radiat Phys Biol 18:262, 1979.
32. Parsons JT, Mendenhall WM, Mancuso AA, et al.: Twice–a–day radiotherapy for T_3 squamous cell carcinoma of the glottic larynx. Head Neck Surg 11:123–128, 1989.
33. Million RR, Cassisi NJ: Larynx. In: Management of Head and Neck Cancer: A Multidisciplinary Approach. Million RR (ed) Philadelphia: JB Lippincott, pp 315–364, 1984.
34. Ogura JH, Sessions DG, Spector GJ: Conservation surgery for epidermoid carcinoma of the supraglottic larynx. Laryngoscope 85:1808–1815, 1975.
35. Gall AM, Sessions DG, Ogura JH: Complications following surgery for cancer of the larynx and hypopharynx. Cancer 39:624–631, 1977.
36. Robbins TK, Davidson W, Peers LS, et al.: Conservation surgery for $T_2 + T_3$ carcinomas of the supraglottic larynx. Arch Otolaryngol Head and Neck Surg 114:421–426, 1988.
37. Fletcher GH, Jesse RH, Lindberg RD, et al.: The place of radiotherapy in the management of squamous cell carcinoma of the supraglottic larynx. AJR 108:19–26, 1970.
38. Bataini JP, Ennuger A, Porcet P, et al.: Treatment of supraglottic cancer by radical high dose radiotherapy. Cancer 33:1253–1302, 1974.
39. Harwood AR, Beale FA, Cummings BJ, et al.: Supraglottic laryngeal carcinoma: An analysis of dose–time–volume factors in 410 patients. Int J Radiat Oncol Biol Phys 9:311–319, 1983.
40. Mendenhall WM, Million RR, Cassisi NJ: Squamous cell carcinoma of the supraglottic larynx treated with radical irradiation: Analysis of treatment parameters and results. Int J Radiat Oncol Biol Phys 10:2223–2230, 1984.
41. Strauss M: Hemilaryngectomy rescue: surgery for radiation failure in early glottic carcinoma. Laryngoscope 98:317–320, 1988.
42. Ballantyne AJ, Fletcher GH: Surgical management of irradiation failure of non–fixed cancers of the glottic region. AJR 120:164–168, 1974.
43. Biller HF, Barnhill FR, Ogura JH, Perez CA: Hemilaryngectomy following radiation failure for carcinoma of the vocal cords. Laryngoscope 80:249–253, 1970.
44. Nichols RD, Stine PH, Greenwald KJ: Partial laryngectomy after radiation failure. Laryngoscope 90:571–575, 1980.
45. Sorensen H, Hansen HS, Thomsen KA: Partial laryngectomy following irradiation. Laryngoscope 90:1344–1349, 1980.
46. Czinger J: Vertical and horizontal partial resections of the larynx after radiotherapy. In: Functional Partial Laryngectomy: conservative surgery for carcinoma of the larynx. Wigand ME, Steiner W, Stell PM (eds) New York: Springer–Verlag, pp 280–284, 1984.

47. Brandenberg JH, Condon KG, Frank TW: Coronal sections of larynges from radiation therapy failures: a clinico–pathologic study. Otolaryngol–Head Neck Surg 95:213–218, 1986.
48. Kirchner JA: Pathways and pitfalls in partial laryngectomy. Ann Otol Rhinol Laryngol 93:301–305, 1984.
49. Lerous–Rubert J: La chirurgie conservative dans le cancer du larynx. Annales d'Oto-Laryngologic 74:40–74, 1957.
50. Kirchner JA, Som MA: Clinical significance of the fixed vocal cord. Laryngoscope 81:1029–1044, 1971.
51. Lesinski SG, Bauer WC, Ogura JH: Hemilaryngectomy for T_3 (fixed cord) epidermoid carcinoma of the larynx. Laryngoscope 86:1563–1571, 1976.
52. McNeil BJ, Werchelbaum R, Panker SG: Speech and Survival: Tradeoffs between quality and quantity of life in laryngeal cancer. N Engl J Med 305:982–987, 1981.
53. Popkin J, Hong WK, Dorman B, Vaughn C, Fofonoff S, Willett B, Karp D, Welch J, Strong S: Voice preservation with sequential chemotherapy and radiation therapy without laryngectomy in patients with operable Stage III, IV squamous cell carcinoma of the larynx and hypopharynx (abstract). Proc Am Soc Clin Oncol 4:149, 1985.
54. Hong WK, O'Doneghue GM, Sheetz S, et al.: Sequential response patterns to chemotherapy and radiotherapy in head and neck cancer: Potential impact of treatment in advanced laryngeal cancer. In: Primary Chemotherapy in Cancer Medicine. Wegener DJT, et al. (eds) New York: Alan R. Liss, pp 191–197, 1985.
55. The Head and Neck Contract Program. Adjuvant chemotherapy for advanced head and neck squamous carcinoma. Final report of the Head and Neck Contract Program. Cancer 60:301–311, 1987.
56. Karp D, Carter R, Vaughan C, Willett B, Heeren T, Calarese P, Zeitels S, Hong W: Voice preservation using induction chemotherapy plus radiation therapy as an alternative to laryngectomy in advanced head and neck cancer: long–term follow up (abstract). Proc Am Soc Clin Oncol 7:152, 1988.
57. Haines, IE, Bosl GJ, Pfister D, Gerold F, Shah J, Sessions R, Spiro R, Strong E, Vikram B: Larynx preservation in patients with advanced squamous cell cancer of the head and neck: recommendations for patient selection (abstract). Proc Am Soc Clin Oncol 6:133, 1987.
58. Haines I, Bosl GJ, Pfister D, Spiro D, Gerald F, Sessions R, Shah J, Strong E, Vikram B, Harrison L: Very high–dose cisplatin with bleomycin infusion as initial treatment of advanced head and neck cancer. J Clin Oncol 5:1594–1600, 1987.
59. Hill BT, Price LA: Induction combination chemotherapy without cisplatin followed by radiotherapy without radical surgery as definitive treatment for advanced epidermoid carcinoma of the larynx (Abstract JB). Presented at the Second International Congress on Neo–Adjuvant Chemotherapy, Feb. 19–21, 1988, Paris, France.
60. Jacobs C, Goffinet DR, Goffinet L, Kohler M, Fee WE: Chemotherapy as a substitute for surgery in the treatment of advanced resectable head and neck cancer. A report from the Northern California Oncology Group. Cancer 60:1178–1183, 1987.
61. Dimery IW, Kramer AM, Choksi AJ, Hong WK: Neoadjuvant chemotherapy and radiotherapy in larynx preservation. Clinical Case Reports from MD Anderson Cancer Center. Am J Clin Oncol 12(2):173–177, 1989.
62. Wolf GT, Hong WK, Fisher S, Spaulding M, Endicott J, Hillman R, Laramore G: A new strategy to preserve the larynx in the treatment of advanced laryngeal cancer. Preliminary report. (Abstract 1.4) Presented at the Second International Head and Neck Oncology Research Conference. Sept. 10–12, 1987, Arlington, Va.
63. Hong WK, Wolf GT, Fisher S, Spaulding M, Endicott J, Laramore G, et al.: Laryngeal preservation with induction chemotherapy (CT) and radiotherapy (XRT) in the treatment for advanced laryngeal cancer: Interim survival data of VACSP #268. VA Laryngeal Cancer Study Group. Proc Am Soc Clin Oncol (1989).

IV

Basic Biology and Etiology

14. Methodology and Clinical Applications of Cellular DNA Content Parameters Determined by Flow Cytometry in Squamous Cell Cancers of the Head and Neck

John F. Ensley, Zosia Maciorowski, Haline Pietraszkiewicz, Filippo deBraud and Wael Sakr.

Most patients with squamous cell carcinomas of the head and neck (SCCHN) present with incurable or recurrent disease, and many who are cured acquire unacceptable functional and cosmetic deficits as a consequence of conventional therapy [1,2]. Effective cytotoxic treatment regimens may eventually cure patients in advanced stages as well as prevent recurrences and reduce the undesirable consequences of conventional therapy in patients with earlier stages [3–5]. Overall and complete response (CR) rates in the range of 80–90% and 35–54% respectively, have been reported in advanced tumors [1]. CR rates above 80% have been described recently in pilot trials using intensive chemotherapy or concurrent chemo–radiotherapy [6–7]. Patients achieving clinical CR demonstrate survival advantages [1–5] which are particularly evident when therapy results in the eradication of microscopic disease [8]. Nevertheless, following initial treatment, 50% of the patients achieve less than a CR, and 50% of the CRs are associated with residual microscopic disease.

Patients who have similar tumor burdens and are comparable in terms of other important clinical features may differ widely in terms of treatment outcome. Clinical and morphological parameters alone are inadequate as predictors of treatment outcome following conventional [8] as well as cytotoxic therapy [9–12]. This is particularly true for an individual patient and very evident in even the most advanced stage (N_3 lymph node status) where up to 30% of these patients may achieve a CR with cytotoxic therapy [1–4]. The ability to predict the clinical outcome following therapy would allow: (a) better stratification of clinical trials, (b) the proper selection of stage I, II and certain stage III patients for adjuvant cytotoxic trials, (c) the design of more effective cytotoxic regimens for advanced tumors that are expected to be or become resistant, (d) the reduction of cytotoxic regimen intensity for advanced tumors that are very responsive, and (e) the study of response and resistance at the clinical and experimental level [9,10].

Cellular DNA content parameters have become important as prognostic indicators for hematological malignancies and a few solid tumors [13]. The DNA content parameter most commonly determined from DNA histograms is the DNA Index (DI) which compares the cellular DNA content of a

Jacobs, C. (ed): Carcinomas of the Head and Neck: Evaluation and Management.

sample to a known diploid standard which is arbitrarily defined as having a DI = 1.0 [13]. A second derived parameter is the percentage of cells synthesizing DNA, or the % S Phase Fraction (SPF) which is an estimate of the cells within the S phase region of the DNA histogram. Aneuploid DNA content (DI 1.1) has been predictive of poor survival in surgically treated, early stage tumors of the breast [14–15], bladder [16], prostate [17], kidney [18], colon [19] and lung [20]. Similar studies of SCCHN report survival advantages for patients with resectable early stage diploid SCCHN [21–28]. Few of these studies attempt to prospectively relate cellular DNA content parameters to cytotoxic response in advanced tumors; most are retrospective examinations of early stage tumors treated with surgery and/or radiation in which survival was the only endpoint. Recent investigations in childhood lymphoblastic leukemia [29], advanced lymphoma [30–32], medulloblastomas [33], neuroblastomas [34–36], breast cancer [37], advanced colon cancer [38], prostate cancer [39], sarcomas [40–44], and head and neck cancer [45,46] have indicated that aneuploid tumors or aneuploid subpopulations are more sensitive than diploid populations to cytotoxic therapy.

Solid Tumor Preparation for Flow Cytometry

The in vitro examination of individual cells from human solid tumors is hindered by inadequate techniques of specimen preparation. High yield, representative, viable, unaltered cell suspensions are prerequisites for quantitative determinations of solid tumor subpopulations by flow cytometry. Information regarding these quality control aspects of tumor preparation is rarely included when solid tumor flow cytometry studies are reported. Most large series have employed the same techniques of tumor dissociation, fixation and staining for all tumor specimens regardless of type [47–51].

Inadequacies in solid tumor preparation have been discussed by many investigators in this field, who stress that such techniques must be individualized for each tissue of interest [52–56]. It is encouraging that recent publications include such data or are entirely devoted to these concerns [57–65]. Techniques currently employed for human solid tumor dissociation include mechanical, chemical, enucleation, single and combination enzyme methods as well as tissue retrieval from formalin fixed–paraffin embedded (FFPE) blocks.

Enucleation techniques have been proposed as a means of circumventing difficult problems in solid tissue dissociation [66,67]. Unfortunately, few reports provide information regarding the important questions of nuclear loss or how representative the resultant nuclear suspensions are. In the original paper by Vindelov [66], nuclear losses were not evident following freeze–thawing JB–1 mouse ascites tumor in cell suspensions, but studies were not performed for human solid tumors. In Thornthwaite's paper [67], nuclear yields from normal C57BL/6J murine liver varied from 4.5 to

8.3×10^7/g depending on the length of exposure to Nuclear Isolation Medium. These values were not compared to theoretical yields nor were quantitative yields from human solid tumors measured. The theoretical cellular yield of CDF murine liver was determined to be 1.47×10^8/g by Petersen [68]. Following detergent nuclear isolation, nuclear yields dropped to 8.6×10^7/g, a 41.5% cell loss. Used as a theoretical yield for Thornthwaite's data, this would represent a 43% cellular loss.

The use of FFPE specimens for flow cytometric analysis is desirable because of the availability of archival material and retrospective analysis of clinical data as well as the possibility for microscopic examination of thin sections adjacent to areas that are investigated [69,70]. FFPE specimens are also convenient for multi–institutional and cooperative group flow cytometric trials. Although nearly all published flow cytometry trials in SCCHN have employed FFPE specimens, data relevant to validation of this technique for this tumor has not been provided.

We use this technique only when fresh material is not available or when tissue specimens are inadvertently placed in formalin. In addition to the loss of important size, plasma membrane, and cytoplasmic features, variations inherent in the tissue, the technique and institutional methodology are further drawbacks of this method. In certain tumors, adequate comparisons have been reported for FFPE and fresh specimens, although increased background and larger coefficients of variation are characteristic of suspensions from FFPE blocks [71–74]. Concern is raised by the report of aneuploid frequencies ranging from 86% [21] to 38% [27] in FFPE specimens of SCCHN. In addition to reviews that comment on the generic pitfalls associated with this technique [75,76], reports of specific aspects that are problematic include: representivity [77], section thickness [78], age of paraffin blocks [79], variations in tissue fixation that alter DNA staining characteristics, particularly decreased fluorochrome intercalation due to DNA cross–link formation caused by formalin [80], proteolytic enzyme alteration of subsequent DNA–dye interactions [81], and cellular subpopulations of interest with differential susceptibility to enzymatic treatment in different tissues [65,74,82]. In addition, the common practice of designating all DNA histograms from FFPE specimens with single G0/G1 peaks as diploid may underestimate the presence of aneuploid tumors [65] as shown recently in breast specimens where this practice would have underestimated the aneuploid frequency by 15% [75]. If DNA histograms from FFPE specimens are demonstrated to be comparable to fresh specimens, and proper diploid standards are used, FFPE SCCHN may be used to produce DNA histograms and may also be mixed with and compared to those from fresh ethanol fixed specimens [74].

Bijman et al. [83] compared several enzyme/chemical combinations in 26 patients with head and neck cancer, the majority being SCC. Nine combinations of enzymes and/or chemicals were employed. The yield ranged from 1.2×10^6 to 5.0×10^8 with an average of 6.5×10^7 cells per gram. The median value for viability was 60% which probably included mechanically released cells. No data regarding the quality of the DNA histograms (coefficient of variation, C.V.) are reported.

No single technique was superior for a particular tumor site or morphology although aneuploidal subpopulations were lost in specimens treated with collagenase alone. The study was hampered by small specimens (<300 mg) which prevented comparative determinations on each patient and other sample sizes (<50 mg) from which quantitative cellular yields were determined.

Tumor preparative studies using reproducible tumor models, either murine or human, that structurally resemble the tissue of interest may aide significantly in developing optimum techniques of tumor preparation for in vitro studies of human tumors. Comparative preparative data derived from a standard well–differentiated murine SCC, LC12, has been employed successfully to predict significant problems in SCCHN tumor dissociation [63]. These include lower cell yields, lower viability and loss of aneuploidal subpopulations seen in mechanical and nuclear preparations. Mechanical techniques, both manual and automated, resulted in low viable cell yields (3.4% theoretical), dye exclusion viabilities (15%), and loss of aneuploid cell content in 80% of the specimens. Total yields approaching theoretical LC12 cell content were possible with a variety of combinations and reached a maximum of $1.3–1.4 \times 10^8$/g (82% theoretical) and a dye exclusion viability of >90%. A collagenase based system was chosen due to the anticipated need for connective tissue dissolution in native human SCCHN which has a larger desmoplastic and stromal component than transplanted tumors. The addition of trypsin permitted the use of lower concentrations of collagenase. DNase was required to reduce cell clumping due to DNA inadvertently released from lysed cells during dissociation.

When applied to specimens of human SCCHN, the inferiority of mechanical dissociation and enucleation techniques was confirmed [64]. The average combined cell yields/g of tissue for these specimens was 7.4×10^7 with a mean dye exclusion viability of 91.4% for enzymatically released cells which allowed 65% fo these specimens to be successfully cultured. The lower cell yields for patient specimens relative to LC12 was expected due to the higher tumor component of transplanted neoplasms and the presence of specimens from patients with recurrent tumors which contain extensive fibrosis and scarring.

LC12 was also used to modify and validate the use of FFPE specimens for flow cytometric investigation of human SCCHN, demonstrating that high yield, reproducible DNA histograms of excellent technical quality can be achieved [74]. The average nuclear yield per gram of embedded tissue was 108.8×10^6 (66.5% of theoretical) which compared favorably with average yields from fresh LC12, 134×10^6 cells/g (82% of theoretical). With average nuclear yields of 2.1×10^6 per 35 micron tissue slice, adequate analysis was possible with 1 or 2 properly selected sections. Technical modifications were made which controlled for the effects of formalin fixation and proteolytic enzyme treatment on DNA fluorochrome staining intensity, and appropriate diploid standards were established. DNA histograms simultaneously obtained from fresh, ethanol fixed and FFPE SCCHN specimens were comparable with respect to morphology, DNA indices, % S phase and coefficients of variation.

It remains necessary to individualize the techniques of tumor preparation for each tissue of interest. Divergent results are often produced when tissue dissociation techniques are compared in different solid tumors. Studies similar to those for SCC were performed in human colon cancer where it was demonstrated that mechanical dissociations always contained the aneuploidal cell subpopulations, and enzymatic dissociation selectively destroyed such subpopulations [82].

Clinical Correlations of Cellular DNA Parameters

Correlations with Clinical and Morphological Features

Comparisons of the presenting clinical parameters (stage, size of primary, lymph node status, grade) and cellular DNA parameters of patients with SCCHN have been primarily retrospectively studied using tissue sections and formalin fixed, paraffin embedded (FFPE) blocks (Table 1). Using such specimens Johnson et al., reported an aneuploid frequency of 86% in 73 patients with advanced SCCHN treated with radiotherapy [21]. Tumor grade, as represented by cumulative scores of individual features of histopathology, did not correlate with DI and SPF individually, although specimens with high DI (>1.5) and SPF (>20%) were associated with poor histological grade and invasion.

Holm described 45 patients with SCC of the oral cavity, pharynx and larynx treated primarily with low dose preoperative radiation (4,000 cGy or less) followed by surgery and/or chemotherapy [22]. Using Feulgen stained thin section scanning microspectrophotometry, 10 patients (22%) were diploid and 35 (78%) were aneuploid. Stage did not correlate with DNA ploidy, but the number of tumor cells with increased DNA content (>50% cells with DNA > G^0/G_1 peak + 2SD) as associated with the presence of N_3 disease. Low scores for individual parameters of histopathology were associated with diploid tumors.

Goldsmith reported DNA content parameters from 48 FFPE specimens of patients with laryngeal SCC treated primarily with surgery and postoperative radiotherapy [23]. Patients entered onto the study were required to have negative surgical margins and adequate radiotherapy dosage (>5,000 cGy). Seventy percent of the tumors were defined as aneuploid or tetraploid, and no correlation of ploidy and clinical characteristics was performed.

Gussack reported 29 patients with laryngeal carcinomas treated with

Table 1. SCCHN flow cytometry clinical studies.

Author	Number patients	Type specimen	Yield $\times 10^6$/g	CV	% Aneuploid	Treatment	Endpoint correlated
Bijman [83]	37	Fresh	65	NP	51^d	NP	Technical
Johnson [21]	73	FFPE	NP	NP	86^c	R	Grade
Holm [22]	45	Fresh*	NP	NA	76^e	SRC	Survival
Goldsmith [23]	48	FFPE	NP	8.1	$70^{b,c,e}$	RS(–MAR)	'Outcome'
Gussack [24]	21	FFPE	NP	NP	57^f	SR	Survival.
Kaplan [25]	46	FFPE	NP	§10	41^b	S	Clinical
Sickle–Santanello [26]	15	FFPE	NP	NP	67^b	S(–MAR)	Survival
Farrar [27]	197	FFPE	NP	NP	38^b	SR	Survival
Kokal [28]	79	FFPE	NP	NP	51^b	S(–MAR)	DFS–SUR
Tytor [94]	51	FFPE	NP	5.3	62^b	R	Response
Ensley [45]	237	Fresh	70	4.1	72^d	SRC	Clinical

NP = not provided; NA = not applicable; * Feulgen DNA cytophotometry; FFPE = formalin fixed, paraffin embedded; S = surgery; R = radiation; C = chemotherapy; DFS = disease free survival; a = no standard; b = internal standard (monoclonals assumed diploid) c = arbitrary standard; d = lymphocyte standard; e = keratinocyte standard; f = standard unknown

surgery and postoperative radiation therapy [24]. Aneuploidy rates were reported as 57% in data obtained from FFPE blocks. Differences in ploidy for stage, size of the primary, nodal status or differentiation were not noted.

Kaplan described the cellular DNA content characteristics of 46 patients with SCC of oral cavity, pharynx and larynx from FFPE specimens treated with surgery [25]. The aneuploid frequency was only 41% and was associated with high surgical stage, tumors outside the oral cavity and large tumors but did not relate to nodal metastasis or morphological features.

Sickle–Santanello reported cellular DNA characteristics from FFPE blocks in 15 patients with early SCC of the tongue [26] and in a larger study of 195 patients with oral cavity tumors [27]. All patients were N_0, had negative surgical margins and were treated primarily with surgery. Sixty–seven percent and 37% of the tumors were aneuploid in the two studies respectively. Comparisons with presenting clinical parameters were not made.

Kokal, et al., presented FFPE data from 76 patients with SCC of the oral cavity, pharynx and larynx following margin negative surgery. Sixty–six percent were aneuploid and were associated with advanced stage and presence of lymph node invasion as well as extracapsular spread but not size of tumor or differentiation [28].

In our series, the correlation of clinical and morphological characteristics with cellular DNA content parameters were reported for the first 237 patients and are summarized in Table 2 [45]. These results have recently been updated for 346 patients and 479 fresh, whole cell specimens with similar results. The degree of aneuploidy and mean DI did not differ significantly with respect to the overall stage (I–IV) of the tumor, although trends were

Table 2. Association of DI and % aneuploidy with clinical parameters.

Variable	Number specimens	Mean DNA index	%Aneuploidy
Stage[a]			
I	9	1.54 ± .23	55.6
II	11	1.59 ± .14	63.6
III	65	1.51 ± .05	63.1
IV	111	1.52 ± .04	69.4
		p = .915[c]	p = .736[d]
IV N_{0-2}	88	1.56 ± .03	76
IV N_3	23	1.36 ± .10	43
		p = .03	p = .003
T[a]			
1	17	1.47 ± .13	64.7
2	31	1.45 ± .08	51.6
3	84	1.49 ± .05	66.7
4	64	1.60 ± .06	73.4
		p = .319[c]	p = .214[d]
N[a]			
0	78	1.60 ± .06	69.2
1	49	1.50 ± .06	67.4
2	46	1.48 ± .05	71.7
3	23	1.36 ± .10	43.5
		p = .020[e]	p = .030[e]
Morphology[b]			
Well	22	1.41 ± .10	50.0
Moderate	151	1.52 ± .04	67.6
Poor	110	1.43 ± .04	60.0
		p = .119[c]	p = .186[d]
Tumor source[a]			
Primary	175	1.54 ± .03	67.4
Lymph node	20	1.34 ± .07	55.0
		p = .045	p = .226
Treatment status[b]			
Untreated	196	1.52 ± .03	66.3
Recurrent	95	1.38 ± .04	53.7
		p = .010	p = .037

DI entries are mean ± standard error. [a] For untreated specimens only. [b] For all specimens; [c] For significance of the differences in mean DNA index across the four (or three) comparison groups, by Wilcoxon rank sum test.[d] For significance of the differences in aneuploidy rates across the four (three) comparison groups, by Chi-square test; [e] for N status where N_{0-2} is compared with N_3 (*) as defined by AJC criteria

evident and stage I and II are under–represented. Size of the primary tumor (T_0–T_4) was not associated with degree of DNA ploidy. Conventional grade (well, moderate or poor differentiation) designations also were not significantly associated with degree of DNA ploidy, although data for well–differentiated tumors was small. Importantly a significantly higher proportion of tumors associated at clinical presentation with N_3 lymph nodes were diploid than those with N_{0-2} status [45].

Although the conventional grades of SCCHN did not correlate with

Table 3. Parameters of Morphology Correlated FCM parameters

Histological Parameter	Diploid		Aneuploid		p Value
	Low Score 1 2	High Score 3 4	Low Score 1 2	High Score 3 4	
1. Keratinization	20(42)	28(58)	60(56)	47(44)	0.13
2. Nuclear Grade	34(71)	14(29)	43(40)	64(60)	0.005
3. Inflammatory Response	18(38)	30(62)	51(49)	53(51)	0.06
4. Stromal Response	29(62)	18(38)	82(78)	23(22)	0.035
5. Pattern of Invasion	36(75)	12(25)	58(54)	49(46)	0.01
6. Vascular Invasion	32(68)	15(32)	59(56)	46(44)	0.16
7. Mitotic Figures/HPF (1=0–3/HPF;4=3/HPF)	35(73)	13(27)	54(50)	53(50)	0.009

ploidy or SPF groups, interesting and significant differences were noted between diploid and aneuploid tumors when individual features of histopathology were examined in the first 155 specimens [84]. Each of the parameters in Table 3 was graded by assigning a semi–quantitative score from 1 to 4 (1 = well–differentiated, 4 = poorly differentiated) as defined by Jakobsson [85] and modified by Crissman [86]. Diploid tumors are characterized by well defined tumor–stromal interfaces, a high–degree of desmoplasia, a low–degree of inflammatory response, low nuclear grade and mitotic index when compared to aneuploid specimens. The tendency for diploid tumors to form well–defined tumor–stromal interfaces may explain the good outcome of surgically treated patients with diploid SCCHN as discussed in the following section.

Correlation with Survival in Patients Treated with Surgery

Retrospective data from FFPE specimens indicate that patients with diploid SCCHN have lower recurrence rates and superior survival following surgery as initial therapy [21–28]. Sickle–Santanello reported a survival advantage at 5 years for 33% of the patients with diploid tumors following surgery in 15 patients with locally invasive, lymph node negative SCC of the tongue [26]. The same group later reported 195 patients with localized SCCHN of the oral cavity treated with surgery ± radiation [27]. With a median follow–up of 63 months, survival advantages for diploid tumors approached but did not reach statistical significance ($p = 0.07$). With a minimum 12–month follow–up, Gussack reported a significant survival advantage (77% vs. 25%) for the diploid tumors in 29 patients with laryngeal cancer treated with surgery and radiation [24]. Kokal, et al., reported that DNA content was the single most important factor in predicting prognosis in resectable patients with SCCHN. Decreased recurrence rates and improved disease–free and absolute survival were reported for patients with diploid tumors [28].

This question is also being addressed prospectively with whole cell DNA

Table 4. Outcome of patients with advanced resectable SCCHN

Parameter	Diploid	Aneuploid
107 patients	34%	66%
Stage III & IV	97%	90%
Stage IV	47%	67%
T_4	28%	46%
Treated with Post–operative:		
Radiotherapy	89%	68%
Chemotherapy	20%	19%
Follow–up (months)		
Minimum	24	24
Maximum	69	76
Median	41	38
Recurrence rate	25%	51%
% Disease free (Alive + Dead)	81%	49%
Survival:		
Median Disease-free	36 months	15 months
Absolute	64%	39%

flow cytometry from fresh surgical specimens in a series of advanced, resectable SCCHN [46]. One hundred and seven patients have had a minimum follow–up of 24 months. Thirty eight tumors (34%) were diploid and 69 (66%) were aneuploid. There were no differences of age, sex or degree of lymph node involvement (N) in diploid and aneuploid groups. Advanced disease (stage III + IV) predominated in both groups (97%–90%), but a higher incidence of stage IV (67% vs. 47%) and T_4 (46% vs. 28%) were present in the aneuploid group. Postoperative radiation (RT) and/or chemotherapy (CH) was performed in similar percentages of the patients with diploid (RT 89%, CH 20%) and (RT 68%, CH 19%) aneuploid tumors. The recurrence rate was lower (25% vs. 51%) and the median disease–free survival better (36 mo vs. 15 mo) in the diploid group. Eighty one percent of the patients with diploid tumors remained disease–free compared with only 49% of the patients with aneuploid tumors. With a median follow–up of 41 and 38 months for diploid and aneuploid patients respectively, a higher percentage of the diploid patients are currently alive (64% vs. 39%).
This preliminary prospective data, summarized in Table 4, supports the retrospective reports of a better clinical outcome for patients with early staged, diploid SCCHN following surgery.

The 5–year local recurrence rates for patients with T_1 and T_2 SCCHN are considerably different (65% vs. 23%) for patients with positive margins versus negative margins [87]. It has been proposed that positive margins are a result of the multicentric origin of certain of these tumors which grow independently and coalesce to form macroscopic tumors [88]. The data from flow studies previously reviewed would suggest an alternate explanation. SCCHN that recur following surgery are predominately aneuploid, and aneuploid tumors have growth characteristics and stromal response patterns that make tumor–stromal interfaces indistinct and access to vascular structures more likely. The establishment of negative margins would, therefore, be more difficult to achieve and demonstrate for aneuploid tumors.

Correlation with Response in Patients Treated with Cytotoxic Therapy

Few flow cytometry studies related cellular DNA parameters to cytotoxic response in patients with advanced SCCHN. Serial measurements of ploidy using microdensitometry determinations of Feulgen stained tissue and autoradiographic determinations of percent labeled mitoses indicated that radioresistant SCCHN tumors tend to become more mature with lower percent labeled mitoses and DNA aneuploidy rates [89,90]. Cell lines established from metastatic or recurrent SCCHN tumors have been reported to have lower DI and chromosome numbers when compared to lines from non–metastatic or recurrent tumors [91].

In Holm's series, similar CR rates were reported for diploid and aneuploid tumors following preoperative radiotherapy (73% vs. 65%, respectively), although a larger (50% vs. 38%) but not significant proportion of patients with diploid tumors survived compared to those with aneuploid tumors [22]. An analysis of this data reveals that 80% of the diploid tumors received 4,000 cGy preoperative radiation and surgery, whereas nearly 50% of the aneuploid tumors did not receive surgery, and many (7 patients) also received inadequate dosages of radiation (<4000 cGy) or single agent chemotherapy (2 patients).

Goldsmith's report of 48 patients with advanced laryngeal SCC treated with postoperative radiation and surgery indicated that patients with aneuploid tumors responded better than diploid tumors and were associated with statistically significant survival advantage at 18 months ($p = 0.008$) which continued to be significant when stage and nodal status were examined by multifactorial analysis [23].

More recently, Franzen et al. reported that 73% of oral SCCHN with pretreatment aneuploid specimens achieved histological CR following radiotherapy compared with only 11% in patients with pretreatment diploid specimens [92].

Table 2 demonstrates that the mean DI and % aneuploidy are lower in tumor specimens from patients with recurrent tumors and untreated patients with the most advanced lymph node metastases, N_3 [45]. These are clinical characteristics that have predicted poor cytotoxic response and survival in past clinical trials [1–4]. These data suggest that the aneuploid cells are vulnerable to cytotoxic therapy. Diploid tumors may be less susceptible to cytotoxic therapy due to cellular kinetics or undefined characteristics that confer resistance independent of kinetic considerations.

Ploidy has been determined on pre– and post–treatment tumor specimens and prospectively correlated with clinical response and resistance in 128

Table 5. Ploidy and chemotherapy response.

Pre-treatment status	Post-treatment status						
		Clinical response			Histological response		
	DNA ploidy	CR	PR	NR	Positive		Negative
All patients:							
66% A 34% D	20% A, 80% D	46%	27%	24%	67%		33%
Diploid patients:	100% D	0%	30%	70%	100%		
Aneuploid patients:	16% A, 84% D	70%	30%	0%	52%		48%
						1/3 A+	
						2/3 D+	

A = Aneuploid population present; D = only diploid population present
+ = Histologically positive

previously untreated patients undergoing intensive cytotoxic therapy as initial treatment [93]. Table 5 indicates that the percentage of DNA aneuploid specimens in pre– and post–treatment specimens decreased from 66% to 20%. No complete responses and more importantly, no histological eradication of disease occurred in patients with pre–treatment diploid tumors. On the other hand, 70% of the patients with aneuploid pre–treatment specimens achieved complete responses with 48% associated with the eradication of microscopic disease. Therefore, unresponsive tumors from previously untreated, advanced patients with SCCHN tend to be DNA diploid.

This is consistent with the indirect evidence from comparisons of untreated and recurrent tumors. Similar data is emerging for advanced human tumors treated initially with cytotoxic therapy including childhood lymphoblastic leukemia [29], non–Hodgkin's lymphomas [30–32], advanced breast cancer [37], colon cancer treated with radiotherapy [38], neuroblastomas [34–36], medulloblastomas [33], and sarcomas treated with adjuvant chemotherapy [40–44].

Conclusions

Cytotoxic therapy may eventually reduce the recurrence rates and unacceptable functional and cosmetic sequelae following conventional therapy as well as achieve cures in patients with SCCHN that are currently incurable. The determination of cellular properties by flow cytometry will aid in the pretherapeutic prediction of treatment outcome in patients with early and advanced tumors and help unravel the mechanisms underlying response or resistance. Solid tumor flow cytometry trials must be preceded by careful development and validation of tissue preparative methodology, particularly with respect to the cellular parameter of interest. For SCCHN, enzymatic methods of dissociation are superior in terms of yields, viabilities, clonigenicity and maintenance of aneuploid populations. Specimens may be retrieved from FFPE blocks following modification of these techniques and development of appropriate diploid standards.

The flow cytometric characteristics of specimens of SCCHN vary considerably depending on the patient population chosen for study in terms of tumor burden, treatment history, and the endpoints correlated with such cellular parameters. Ploidy differences are associated with and may underlie histopathological patterns of growth and associated stromal response in this tumor. These patterns may account for the fact that early and even moderately (resectable) advanced diploid SCCHN tend to do well following surgery (local control) and disseminate less frequently. It is therefore reasonable to consider patients with resectable tumors containing aneuploid components for adjuvant trials with cytotoxic therapy.

The clinical groups that have been most unresponsive to both radiation and chemotherapy, recurrent tumors and those associated with N_3 lymph nodes, are predominantly diploid. Prospective studies indicate that the portions of advanced tumors that remain unresponsive to intermittent cytotoxic therapy also tend to be diploid. Therefore, patients with unresectable diploid tumors or who develop diploid remnants following cytotoxic therapy should be candidates for new treatment approaches. If feasible, such patients may be candidates for aggressive surgery following maximum clinical response. Other strategies such as low–dose continuous chemotherapy, concurrent chemo–radiotherapy or the use of approaches that are not based on cellular kinetics, such as immunotherapy, would also be suitable for investigation in this group of patients. The biological characteristics, clinical presentations, natural histories and response patterns of these tumors may be dictated in part by genetic differences associated with these ploidy classes. The addition of flow cytometric parameters to the conventional clinical categories of patients with SCCHN may permit the identification of subsets in both resectable and advanced patients that will fail these therapies and permit the testing of alternate treatment strategies in clinical trials.

Acknowledgments

Supported by grants from: NIH Grant CA 40498–01A1; Comprehensive Cancer Center Support Grant, NIH 2P30CA22453; Southwest Oncology Group Grant, NIH CA 32102, ± Department of Internal Medicine Fund for Medical Research and Education; Harper Hospital Medical Staff Trust Fund for Medical Research and Education and the Ben Kasle Flow Cytometry Laboratory, Wayne State University, Detroit, Michigan

References

1. Al–Sarraf M: Head and neck cancer. Chemotherapy Concepts. Seminars in Oncology 15:70–85, 1988.

2. Kish J, Ensley J, Al–Sarraf M: Clinical results of chemotherapy in recurrent head and neck carcinoma, Scientific and Clinical Perspective of Head and Neck Cancer Management Strategies for Cure, Jacobs J, Al–Sarraf M, Crissman J, Valeriote F (eds), Elsevier, New York: pp 199–211, 1987.
3. Ensley J, Kish J, Tapazoglou E, Jacobs J, Weaver A, Atkinson D, Ahmed K, Heilbrun L, Al–Sarraf M: The justification and strategies for the continued intensification of induction regimens in patients with advanced, untreated head and neck cancer. In: Head and Neck Oncology Research. Proceedings of the Second International Research Conference on Head and Neck Caner, Wolf GT and Carey T (eds). Amsterdam: Kugler Publishers, pp 313–323, 1988.
4. Ensley JF, Kish J, Tapazoglou E, Al–Sarraf M: Strategies for improvements in complete response rates with adjuvant combination chemotherapy in advanced head and neck cancer (SCC of H&N). Adjuvant Therapy of Cancer Vol V. Salmon SE (ed) Philadelphia: BC Decker, pp 101–111, 1987.
5. Ensley JF, Kish JA, Al–Sarraf M: The development of optimum induction chemotherapy regimens for advanced head and neck cancer: The Wayne State University Experience, In: Neo-Adjuvant Chemotherapy—First International Congress, Jacquillat C, Weil M, Khayat D (eds), London: John Libbey, pp 353–361, 1986.
6. Ensley J, Kish J, Tapazoglou E, Jacobs J, Weaver A, Atkinson, Ahmed K, Mathog R, Al–Sarraf M: An intensive, five course alternating combination chemotherapy induction regimen employed in patients with advanced, unresectable head and neck cancer. J Clin Oncol 6:1147–1153, 1988.
7. Al–Sarraf M, Pajak TF, Marcial VA, Mowry P, Cooper JS, Stetz J, Ensley JF, Velez–Garcia E: Concurrent radiotherapy and chemotherapy with cisplatin in inoperable squamous cell carcinoma of the head and neck. An RTOG study. Cancer 59:259–265, 1987.
8. Al–Kourainy K, Kish JA, Ensley JF, Tapazoglou E, Jacobs J, Weaver A, Crissman J, Cummings G, Al–Sarraf M: Achievement of superior survival for histologically negative vs. histologically positive clinically complete responders to cis–platinum combinations in patients with locally advanced head and neck cancer. Cancer 59:233–238, 1987.
9. Ensley JF, Kish JA, Al–Sarraf M: The pretherapeutic identification of prognostically important parameters predictive of tumor response in squamous cell cancers of the head and neck, Head and Neck Cancer, Vogl S (Editor), New York: Churchill Livingstone, pp 109–124, 1988.
10. Ensley JF, Maciorowski Z, Kish JA, Al–Sarraf M: The significance of pretreatment identification of prognostically important subgroups of squamous cell cancer of the head and neck, Scientific and Clinical Perspective of Head and Neck Cancer Management Strategies for Cure, Jacobs J, Al–Sarraf M, Crissman J, Valeriote F (eds), New York: Elsevier, pp 35–36, 1987.
11. Ensley J, Crissman J, Kish J, Jacobs J, Weaver A, Kinzie J, Cummings G, Al–Sarraf M: The impact of morphological analysis on response rates and survival in patients with squamous cell cancer of the head and neck. Cancer 57:711–717, 1986.
12. Ensley J, Crissman J, Kish J, Weaver A, Jacobs J, Cummings G, Al–Sarraf M: The correlation of individual parameters of tumor differentiation with response rate and survival in patients with advanced head and neck cancer treated with induction therapy. Cancer 63:1487–1492, 1989.
13. Barlogie B, Raber MN, Schumann J, Johnson TS, Drewinko B, Swartzendruber DE, Gohde W, Andreeff M, Freireich E: Flow cytometry in clinical cancer research. Cancer Res 43:3977–3982, 1983.
14. McDivitt RW, Stone KR, Craig B, Palmer JO, Meyer JS, Bauer WC: A proposed classification of breast cancer based on kinetic information. Cancer 57:269–276, 1986.
15. McGuire WL, Meyer JS, Barlogie B, Kute TE: Impact of flow cytometry on predicting recurrence and survival in breast cancer patients. In: Breast Cancer Research and Treatment. Boston: Martinus Nijhoff, pp 117–128, 1985.

16. Frankfort OS, Huben RP: Clinical applications of DNA flow cytometry for bladder tumors. Urol Supp 23:29–34, 1984.
17. Zetterberg A, Esposti PL: Prognostic significance of nuclear DNA levels in prostatic carcinoma. Scand J Urol Nephrol 55:53–58, 1980.
18. Otto LL, Baisch H, Hulano H, Kloppel G: Tumor cell deoxyribonucleic acid content and prognosis in human renal carcinoma. J Urol 132:237–239, 1984.
19. Wolley RC, Schreiber K, Koss LG, Karas M, Sherman A: DNA distribution in human colon carcinoma and its relationship to clinical behavior. J Natl Cancer Inst 69:15–22, 1982.
20. Volm M, Hahn EW, Mattern J, Vogt–Moykopf I: Independent flow cytometric prognostic factors for the survival of patients with non–small cell lung cancer: A five year follow–up study. Proc AACR 29:26, 1988.
21. Johnson TS, Williamson KD, Cramer MM, Peters LJ: Flow cytometric analysis of head and neck carcinoma DNA index and S phase from paraffin embedded sections: comparison with malignancy grading. Cytometry 6:461–480, 1985.
22. Holm LE: Cellular DNA amounts of squamous cell carcinomas of the head and neck region in relation to prognosis. Laryngoscope 92:1064–1069, 1982.
23. Goldsmith MM, Cresson DH, Postma DS, Askin FB, Arnold LW, Pillsbury HC: The significance of ploidy in laryngeal cancer. Am J Surg 152:396–402, 1986.
24. Gussack GS, Donelly K, Hester R, Dowling E: Flow cytometric DNA analysis of laryngeal carcinomas. In: Head and Neck Oncology Research. Proceedings of the Second International Research Conference on Head and Neck Cancer, 1987. Wolf GT and Carey T (eds). Amsterdam: Kugler Publishers, pp 241–249, 1988.
25. Kaplan AS, Caldarelli DD, Chacho MS, Bruce DR, Hutchninson J, Conway S, Coon JS: Retrospective DNA analysis of head and neck squamous cell carcinoma. Arch Otolaryngol Head and Neck Surg 112:1159–1162, 1986.
26. Sickle–Santanello BJ, Farrar WB, Dobson JL, O'Toole RV, Keyhani–Rofaghua S: Flow cytometry as a prognostic indicator in squamous cell carcinoma of the tongue. Am J Surg 152:393–395, 1986.
27. Farrar WB, Artman S, Sickle–Santanello B, et al.: Flow cytometric analysis of DNA content in squamous cell carcinomas of the oral cavity. In: Head and Neck Oncology Research. Proceedings of the Second International Research Conference on Head and Neck Cancer, 1987. Wolf GT and Carey T (eds). Amsterdam: Kugler Publishers, pp 197–203, 1988.
29. Look AT, Roberson PK, Williams DL, Bowman WP, Pui C–H, Ochs J, Abromowitch M, Kalwinski D, Dahl GV, George S, Murphy SB: Prognostic importance of blast cell DNA content in childhood acute lymphoblastic leukemia. Blood 65:1079–1086, 1985.
30. Woodbridge TN, Grierson HL, Pierson JL, Pauza ME, Collins MM, Armitage JO, Weisenburger DD, Purtilo DT: DNA Aneuploidy and low proliferative activity predict a favorable clinical outcome in diffuse large cell lymphoma. Proc AACR 28:131, 1987.
31. Bauer KD, Merkel DE, Winter JN, Marder RJ, Hauck WW, Wallemark CR, Williams TJ, Variakojis D: Prognostic implications of ploidy and proliferative activity in diffuse large cell lymphomas. Cancer Res 46:3173–3178, 1986.
32. Macarteny JC, Camplejohn RS, Alder J, Stone MG, Powell G: Prognostic importance of DNA flow cytometry in non–Hodgkin's lymphomas. J Clin Pathol 39:542–546, 1986.
33. Tomita T, Yasue M, Englehard HH, McLone DG, Gonzalez–Crussi F, Bauer KD: Flow cytometric DNA analysis of medulloblastomas. Prognostic implications of ploidy. Cancer 61:744–749, 1988.
34. Look AT, Hayes FA, Nitschke R, McWilliams NB, Green A: Cellular DNA content as a predictor of response to chemotherapy in infants with unresectable neurosarcomas. N Eng J Med 311:231–235, 1984.
35. Oppedal BR, Strom–Mathisen I, Lie SO, Brandtzaeg P: Prognostic factors in neuroblastomas: Clinical, histopathologic, and immunohistochemical features and DNA ploidy in relation to prognosis. Cancer 62:772–780, 1988.

36. Taylor SR, Blatt GM, Costantino JP, Roederer M, Murphy RF: Flow cytometric DNA analysis of neuroblastoma and ganglioneuroma: A 10–year restrospective study. Cancer 62:749–754, 1988.
37. Brifford M, Spyratos F, Tubiana–Hulin M, Pallud C, Mayras C, Filleul A, Rouesse J: Sequential cytopunctures during preoperative chemotherapy for primary breast cancer. Cytomorphologic changes, initial tumor ploidy, and tumor regression. Cancer 63:631–637, 1989.
38. Meyer JS, Priolea PG: S–Phase fractions of colorectal carcinomas related to pathologic and clinical features. Cancer 48:1221–1228, 1981.
39. Frankfort OS, Chin JL, Ensglander LS, Greco WR, Pontes JE, Rustum YM: Relationship between DNA ploidy, glandular differentiation and tumor spread in human prostate cancer. Cancer Res 45:1418–1423, 1985.
40. Kreicbergs A, Tribukait B, Williams J, et al.: DNA flow analysis of soft tissue tumors. Cancer 59:128–133, 1987.
41. Matsuno T, Gebhardt MC, Mankin HJ, Bell RS: Ploidic analysis in benign and malignant soft tissue tumors. Proc. 10th Annual Meeting Cell Kinetics Society, Santa Fe, New Mexico, March 18–21, p 14, 1986.
42. Bell RS, Mankin HJ, Gebhardt MC, Lee R: Disease–free survival and tumor ploidy in high-grade osteosarcoma. Proc. 10th Annual Meeting Cell Kinetics Society, Santa Fe, New Mexico, March 18–21, p 30, 1986.
43. Bauer HC, Kreicbergs A, Tribukait B: DNA microspectro–photometry of bone sarcomas in tissue sections as compared to imprint and flow DNA analysis. Cytometry 7:544–550, 1986.
44. Look AT, Douglass EC, Meyer WH: Clinical importance of near–diploid tumor stem cell lines in patients with osteosarcoma of an extremity. N Eng J Med 318:1567–1572, 1988.
45. Ensley JF, Maciorowski Z, Hassan M, Pietraszkiewicz H, Reading B, Heilbrun L: Characterization and clinical correlation of cellular DNA parameters in untreated and recurrent squamous cell cancers of the head and neck. Cytometry 10:334–338, 1989.
46. de Braud F, Ensley JF, Hassan M, Maciorowski Z, Pietraskiewicz H, Sakr W, Kish J, Tapazoglou E, Reed M, Al–Sarraf M: Prospective correlation of clinical outcome in patients with advanced, resectable squamous cell carcinomas of the head and neck (SCCHN) with DNA ploidy from fresh specimens. Proc AACR 30:1045, 1989.
47. Barlogie B, Drewinko B, Schumann J, Gohoe J, Dosik G, Latreille J, Johnston DA, Freireich EJ: Cellular DNA content as a marker of neoplasia in man. Am J Med 69:195–203, 1980.
48. Laerum OD, Farsund T. Clinical Application of Flow Cytometry. A Review. Cytometry 2:1–13, 1981.
49. Barlogie B, Johnson DA, Smallwood L, Rabner MN, Maddow AM, Latreille J, Swartzendruber DI, Drewinko B: Prognostic implications of ploidy and proliferative activity in human solid tumors. Cancer Gent Cytogenet 6:17–28, 1982.
50. Frankfurt OS, Slocum HK, Rustum YM, Arbor SG, Pavelic ZP, Petrelli N, Huben RP, Pontes EJ, Greco WR: Flow cytometric analysis of DNA aneuploidy in primary and metastatic human solid tumors. Cytometry 5:71–80, 1984.
51. Frankfurt OS, Greco WR, Slocum HK, Arbuck SG, Gamarra M, Pavelic ZP, Rustum YM: Proliferative characteristics of primary and metastatic human solid tumors by DNA flow cytometry. Cytometry 5:629–635, 1984.
52. Pretlow TG II, Weir EE, Zettergren JG: Problems connected with the separation of different kinds of cells. Int Rev Exp Pathol 14:91–204, 1975.
53. Pretlow TG II, Pretlow TP: Evaluation of data, problems and general approach. In: Cell Separation: Methods and Selected Applications. vol 1. Thomas G Pretlow II and Theresa P Pretlow (ed). New York: Academic Press, pp 31–40, 1982.
54. Waymouth C: Methods for obtaining cells in suspension from animal tissues. In: Cell Separation: Methods and Applications. Vol 1. Thomas G Pretlow II and Theresa P Pretlow (ed). New York: Academic Press, pp 1–30, 1982.

55. Waymouth C: To Disaggregate or not to disaggregate. Injury and cell disaggregation, transcient or permanent. In Vitro 30:97–111, 1974.
56. Brattain M: Tissue disaggregation. In: Flow Cytometry and Sorting. Melamed R, Mullaney P, Mendelsohn ML (ed). NY: Wiley & Sons, pp 193–203, 1979.
57. Wooley RC, Herz F, Dembitzer HM, Schreiber K, Koss LG: The monodisperse cervical smear. Quantitative analysis of cell dispersion with enzymatic and chemical agents. Anal Quant Cytol 1:43–49, 1979.
58. Chassevent, Dauer A, Bertrand G, Coic H, Geslin J, Bidabe M, George P, Larra F: Comparative flow DNA analysis of different cell suspensions of breast carcinoma. Cytometry 5:263–267, 1984.
59. Engelholm SA, Spang–Thomsen M, Brunner N, Nohr I, Vindelov LL: Disaggregation of human solid tumors by combined mechanical and enzymatic methods. Br Cancer 51:93–98, 1985.
60. McDivitt RW, Store KE, Meyer JS: A method for dissociation for viable human breast cancer cells that produces flow cytometric kinetic information similar to that obtained by thymidine labelling. Cancer Res 44:2628–2633, 1984.
61. Slocum HK, Pavelic ZP, Rustum YM, Craven PJ, Karakousis C, Takita H, Greco WR: Characterization of cells obtained by mechanical and enzymatic means from human melanoma, sarcoma and lung tumors. Cancer Res 41:1428–1434, 1981.
62. Slocum HK, Pavelic ZP, Kanter PM, Nowak HJ, Rustum YM: The soft agar clonogenicity and characterization of cells obtained from human solid tumors by mechanical and enzymatic means. Cancer Chemother Parmacol 6:219–225, 1981.
63. Ensley JF, Maciorowski Z, Pietraszkiewicz H, Klemic G, Kukuruga M, Sapareto S, Corbett T, Crissman JD: Solid tumor preparation for flow cytometry using a standard murine tumor model. Cytometry 8:479–487, 1987.
64. Ensley JF, Maciorowski Z, Pietraszkiewicz H, Hassan M, Kish J, Al–Sarraf M, Jacobs J, Weaver A, Atkinson D, Crissman J: Tumor preparation for clinical application of flow cytometry. Cytometry 8:488–493, 1987.
65. Ensley JF, Maciorowski Z, Hassan M, Pietraszkiewicz H, Kish J, Tapazoglou E, Jacobs J, Mathog R, Weaver A, Atkinson D, Binns P, Ahmed K, Al–Sarraf M, Weil S, Zarbo R, Crissman J: The potential and pitfalls of solid tumor flow cytometry with respect to squamous cell cancers of the head and neck. In: Head and Neck Oncology Research. Proceeding of the Second International Research Conference on Head and Neck Cancer. Wolf GT and Carey T (eds). Amsterdam: Kugler Publishers, pp 213–224, 1988.
66. Vindelov LL, Christensen IJ and Nissen NI: A detergent-trypsin method for the preparation of nuclei for flow cytometric DNA analysis. Cytometry 3:323–327, 1983.
67. Thornthwaite JT, Sugerbaker EV, Temple W: Preparation of tissue for DNA flow cytometric analysis. Cytometry 1:229–237, 1980.
68. Peterson SE: Flow cytometry of human colorectal tumors: Nuclear isolation by detergent technique. Cytometry 6:452–460, 1985.
69. Hedley DW: Flow cytometry using paraffin–embedded tissue: Five years on. Cytometry 10:229–241, 1989.
70. Bauer KD, Clevenger CV, Endow RK, Murad T, Epstein AL, Scarpelli DG: Simultaneous nuclear antigen and DNA content quantitation using paraffin–embedded colonic tissue and multiparameter flow cytometry. Cancer Res 46:2428–2434, 1986.
71. Nakamura K, Simon AL, Kasabian NG, Addonizio JC, Choudhury M, Nagamatsu GR, Rossi JA, Chiao JW: Flow cytometric analysis of relative mean DNA content of urogenital cancer cells in fresh and paraffin–embedded materials. Urology 30:333–336, 1987.
72. Camplejohn RS, Macarteney JC: Comparison of DNA flow cytometry from fresh and paraffin embedded samples of non–Hodgkin's lymphoma. J Clin Pathol 38:1096–1099, 1985.
73. Donova M, Mazzini G, Wilson G, Ucci G, Dionigi P, Riccardi A, Fiocca R: Ploidy and proliferative activity of human gastric carcinoma: a cytofluorometric study on fresh and on paraffin embedded material. Basic Appl Histochem 31:73–82, 1987.

74. Ensley J, Maciorowski Z, Ratanatharathorn V, Hassan M, Pietraszkiewicz H: The development and standardization of flow cytometric analysis of cellular DNA content from formalin fixed, paraffin embedded specimens of head and neck cancer using a murine standard, LC12. Proc AACR 28:129, 1987.
75. Kute TE, Gregory B, Galleshaw J, Hopkins M, Buss D, Case D: How reproducible are flow cytometry data from paraffin-embedded blocks? Cytometry 9:494–498, 1988.
76. Feichter GE, Goerttler: Pitfalls in the preparation of nuclear suspensions from paraffin-embedded tissue for flow cytometry (letter). Cytometry 7:616, 1986.
77. Qud PH, Hanselaar TG, Reubsaet–Veldhuizzen JA, Meijer JW, Gemmink AH, Pahlplatz MM, Beck HL, Vooijs GP: Extraction of nuclei from selected regions in paraffin-embedded tissue. Cytometry 7:595–600, 1986.
78. Stephenson RA, Gay H, Fair WR, Melamed MR: Effect of section thickness on quality of flow cytometric DNA content determinations in paraffin–embedded tissues. Cytometry 7:41–44, 1986.
79. Fossa SD, Thorud E, Shoaib MC, Pettersen EO: DNA flow cytometry of cells obtained from old paraffin–embedded specimens. A comparison with results of scanning absorption cytometry (a methodological study). Pathol Res Pract 181:200–205, 1986.
80. Schutte B, Reynders MMJ, Bouman FT, Blijham GH: Flow cytometric determination of DNA ploidy level in nuclei isolated from paraffin embedded tissue. Cytometry 6:26–30, 1985.
81. Eisenhut M, Chone B: Studies of the binding of ehidium bromide to cells before and after enzyme treatment. Histochemistry 62:207–220, 1979.
82. Ensley J, Maciorowski Z, Pietraszkiewicz H, Hassan M, Crissman J, Valdivieso M: Selective and consistent aneuploidal cellular subpopulation losses in enzymatically versus mechanically dissociated human colon specimens analysed by flow cytometry. Proc AACR 28:130, 1987.
83. Bijman J Th, Wagener DJ Th, van Rennes H, Wessels JMC, vandenBroek P: Flow cytometric evaluation of cell dispersion from human head and neck tumors. Cytometry 6:334–341, 1985.
84. Sakr W, Hassan M, Zarbo R, Ensley J, Crissman JD: DNA quantitation and histologic characteristics of squamous cell carcinomas of the upper aerodigestive tract. Arch Pathol and Lab Medicine 113:1009–1014, 1989.
85. Jakobsson PA: Histological grading of malignancy and prognosis in glottic carcinoma of the larynx, Workshop N. 14. In: Centennial Conference on Laryngeal Cancer. Alberti PW and Bryce DP (eds). New York: Appelton Century Crofts, pp 847–854, 1976.
86. Crissman JD, Liu Y, Gluckman JL, Cummings G: Prognostic value of histopathologic parameters in squamous cell carcinoma of the oropharynx. Cancer 54:2995–3001, 1984.
87. Looser KG, Shah JP, Strong EW: The significance of 'positive' margins in surgically resected epidermoid carcinomas. Head and Neck Surgery 1:107–111, 1978.
88. Slaughter DP, Southwick HW, Smejkal W: Field cancerization in oral stratified squamous epithelium; clinical implication of multicentric origins. Cancer 6:963–968, 1953.
89. Nervi C, Arcangeli G, Badaracco G, Cortese M, Morelli M, Starace G: The relevance of tumor size and cell kinetics as predictors of radiation response in head and neck cancer. Cancer 41:900–906, 1978.
90. Nervi C, Badaracco G, Morelli M, Starace G: Cytokinetic evaluation in human head and neck cancer by autoradiography and DNA cytofluorometry. Cancer 45:452–459, 1980.
91. Roa RA, Carey TE, Passamani PP, Greenwood JH, Hsu S, Riding EO, Schwartz DR, Wolf GT, Hudson JL: DNA content of human squamous cell carcinoma lines. Analysis by flow cytometry and chromosome enumeration. Arch Otolaryngol 111:565–575, 1985.
92. Franzen G, Olofsson J, Tytor M, Lintenberg C, Risberg B: Preoperative irradiation in oral cavity carcinoma. A study with special reference to DNA pattern, histological response and prognosis. ACTA ONCOL 26:349–355, 1987.
93. Ensley J, Maciorowski Z, Hassan M, Pietraszkiewicz H, Kish J, Tapazoglou E, Jacobs J, Weaver A, Mathog R, Sakr W, Al–Sarraf M: Prospective correlations of flow cytometry

(FCM) DNA parameters (DNA Index and % SPF) and cytotoxic response in previously untreated patients with advanced squamous cell cancers of the head and neck. Proc AACR 29:27, 1988.
94. Tytor M, Franzen G, Olofsson J, Brunk U, Nordenskjold B: DNA content, malignancy grading and prognosis in T1 and T2 oral cavity carcinomas. Br J Cancer 56:647–652, 1987.

15. Head and Neck Tumor Immunology
II. Humoral Immunity

Stimson P. Schantz, Howard E. Savage and Norris K. Lee

The field of head and neck tumor immunology is a rapidly progressing and growing discipline, a fact that restricts the ability to fit a meaningful review of the subject into a single article. This growth is illustrated by figure 1, which indicates the number of articles published between 1970 and 1987 that address the subject. Two sources, each with different perspectives, were utilized in compiling this information. Source one included all articles that address head and neck tumor immunology, from both a basic science and clinical perspective, identified from *Index Medicus*. Source two was derived by systematically reviewing five journals (as listed in the figure 1 legend) during the same period. Articles from the latter source were identified if the publication utilized an immune parameter to predict a particular clinical outcome, most commonly death with disease. Thus, the broad perspective of immunology is represented, as well as the perspective of clinically relevant immune monitoring. What is evident from figure 1 is the burgeoning number of articles published within the last 3 years. Indeed, two–thirds as many articles found within *Index Medicus* dealt with head and neck tumor immunology in the last 3 years (83) articles as in the entire preceding era.

Our approach, therefore, is to review head and neck immunology in a series of articles. We will focus on particular aspects of the field and hope to provide insight into current understanding of and directions for those aspects. Thus, our previous report on the subject must be considered [1]. The principal focus of that review was cellular immune functions, that is, determinants of cell–mediated immune destruction such as tumor immunogenicity, the significance of tumor antigens, the capacity of lymphocytes to stimulate rather than impede tumor growth, and the burgeoning information on both MHC–restricted and non–MHC–restricted cellular defense mechanisms. We have provided initial background information on the existence of two defense mechanisms in the head and neck cancer patient: a phylogenetically primitive system, the natural killer cell system, which appears to recognize principally not altered self–antigens but rather

Jacobs, C. (ed): Carcinomas of the Head and Neck: Evaluation and Management.

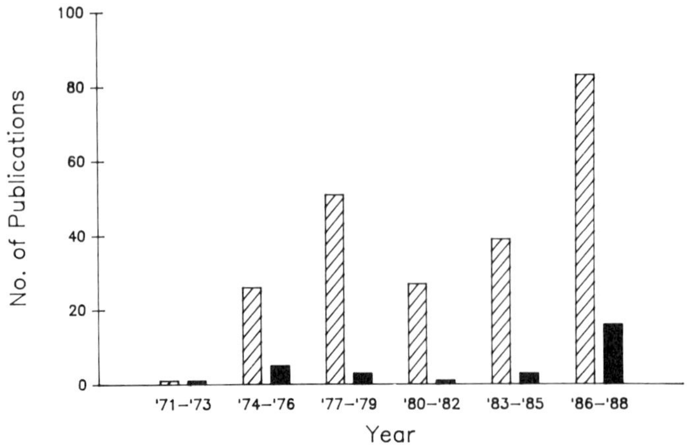

Figure 1. Number of publications related to head and neck tumor immunology from January 1, 1971 to January 1, 1989. Publications were identified from two sources: 1. articles that address head and neck tumor immunology from both a basic science and clinical perspective as listed in *Index Medicus*; 2. articles that address immune monitoring and clinical outcome as compiled from reviewing five journals in their entirety as published between 1971 and 1989 (Am J Surg, Arch Otolaryngol Head Neck Surg, Cancer, Head Neck Surg, and Otolaryngol Head Neck Surg).

nonself–antigens [2] and the more adaptive MHC–restricted T cell system. The latter makes its first appearance in more evolved animal species [3] and represents the classic cell–mediated effector mechanisms against tumor cells expressing altered (potentially tumor–specific) antigens on individual cancer cells. The existence of two defense mechanisms may serve the host in dealing with a heterogeneous cell population within a tumor mass, cell populations expressing different degrees of differentiation and tumor–associated antigens.

This chapter begins a discussion of a growing body of information on humoral immune components. We will address three aspects of humoral immunity as it relates to head and neck cancer. The first is the role of antibody in mediating tumor destruction. Principally, we will demonstrate the association of antibody to clinical outcome. We will then focus on the significance of circulating immune complexes (CIC), providing information as to the role of CIC in modulation of host defense mechanisms, as well as the potential clinical significance of CIC both on prognostication and in the design of therapeutic intervention. Finally, we will address burgeoning information on perspectives in humoral immunity that have not yet been addressed specifically in head and neck oncology but could be of clinical significance, namely, the use of monoclonal antibodies for drug delivery and immunoconjugate targeting and diagnosis.

Humoral Immune Status and Tumor Progression

The Significance of Circulating Antibodies

Distinct from measures of cellular immune status, circulating immunoglobulins are not characteristically deficient in the head and neck cancer patient. Indeed, one can more commonly identify a hypergammaglobulinemic state. This hypergammaglobulinemia characteristically revolves around elevated IgA levels, especially in patients with advanced disease [4–9]. Hughes first noted that head and neck cancer patients had elevated IgA a characteristic, likewise, expressed by patients with cancer of the skin, intestinal tract, lung, and uterus [4]. Results from these studies, however, reveal that the hypergammaglobulinemia is not confined to IgA. Elevations, though not as marked for IgA, have also been noted for IgG, IgE, as well as IgM classes [7–9]. The latter immunoglobulin is elevated primarily in young adults with head and neck cancer [9].

Not yet apparent is why the globulins, especially IgA, should be elevated at all. The elevated IgA levels identified in patients with advanced disease would suggest that tumor burden may be a critical factor [5–8]. Yet levels of immunoglobulin persist in those patients subsequently rendered disease free [10], a finding distinct from measures of other humoral substances such as CIC [10]. The significance of elevated IgA levels will most likely arise from investigations such as by Kutteh et al. [11]. The latter authors were assessing nonspecific stimulation of B cells and the resulting enhancement of IgA production. They noted that increased IgA production resulted from brief exposures to pokeweed mitogens, lipopolysacchsride, as well as Epstein–Barr virus. Thus, IgA production may simply represent nonspecific stimulation, perhaps by virally infected or transformed cells. It is relevant that numerous reports have demonstrated the potential role of virus in the generation of head and neck cancer [12–15]. It is, furthermore, relevant that Smith et al. noted that immunoglobulins from head and neck cancer patients crossreacted with viral particles from herpes simplex virus–type 1, a finding later confirmed by Shillitoe [12,14]. Elevations in antibody levels in head and neck cancer patients occur in response to viral antigens, expressed independently or in conjunction with tumor products.

Additional explanations for elevated circulating antibodies in head and neck cancer patients that imply a pathologic process (although not necessarily specific for head and neck cancer) include tissue destruction with superimposed infection, the maintenance of tolerance to oral antigens, and diminished transport function of the hepatobiliary system [16–20]. Regarding the latter explanation, head and cancer patients as a group have heavy alcohol consumption patterns that can result in hepatocellular destruction. One method of clearance of IgA that is either complexed to antigen or free–standing is through excretion within bile. Obstruction of biliary drainage, as occurs in cirrhosis or alcohol–induced hepatitis, can prevent IgA excretion. In such a setting, increased immunoglobulin may have no cancer–specific pathophysiologic implication but simply reflect parameters of a patient's general health status and the detrimental effect of chronic alcohol exposure.

Our principal purpose in presenting such information is to emphasize that although elevated circulating immunoglobulins provide a context for description of the head and neck cancer population (and provide prognostic implication), the biologic association between these cancers and immunoglobulins has yet to be explained. However, today's current predominant biologic conception is that elevated immunoglobulins, principally IgA, have a detrimental effect on host/tumor interaction and, therefore, promote tumor progression. IgA, as distinct from IgG or IgM, is incapable of binding tissue–damaging complement or mediating tumor lysis in conjunction with cellular effector mechanisms (principally, antibody–dependent killer cells). Thus, the major impact of IgA can be considered its function as a blocking agent [21–25], perhaps a physiologic response to control the detrimental effect of prolonged antigen stimulation [16]. Again, however, our understanding of this process is limited. Most recently Katz et al. have made use of the IgA–blocking theory in the design of a clinical trial [26]. In their study, patients with advanced recurrent disease underwent plasma exchange as part of their therapeutic regimen. The authors reported that disease regression induced by plasma exchange alone occurred in three of ten patients. Furthermore, results were most apparent in those individuals with elevated IgA. One effect of plasma exchange was in part reflected in a diminution of circulating IgA levels. Confirmation of these studies is needed. However, results support the contention that removal of IgA allows unblocking of an effective host response against tumors.

Although the pathophysiologic basis for elevated immunoglobulins in head and neck cancer patients remains to be seen, its clinical implication is more evident. Elevated immunoglobulins, principally elevated IgA, in previously untreated patients portend a worse prognosis [6–8]. Katz found that patients with previously untreated head and neck cancer and elevated IgA were more likely to die of their disease—an observation we confirmed (figure 2) [7,8]. Two additional prognostic features have been identified for patients with elevated IgA. Namely, concomitant measurement of IgE will provide a confounding influence when defining the risk of progressive disease. Those patients with elevated IgE were likely to fare well [7]. Thus, the ratio of IgE to IgA appears to be more descriptive than simply measuring IgA.

Second, levels of IgA when viewed in relationship to parameters of cellular immunity provide more information than either parameter alone, as shown when measurement of IgA was combined with an in vitro quantitative assessment of natural killer (NK) cell activity [8]. NK cell activity was previously noted to define the probability of disease–free survival in patients

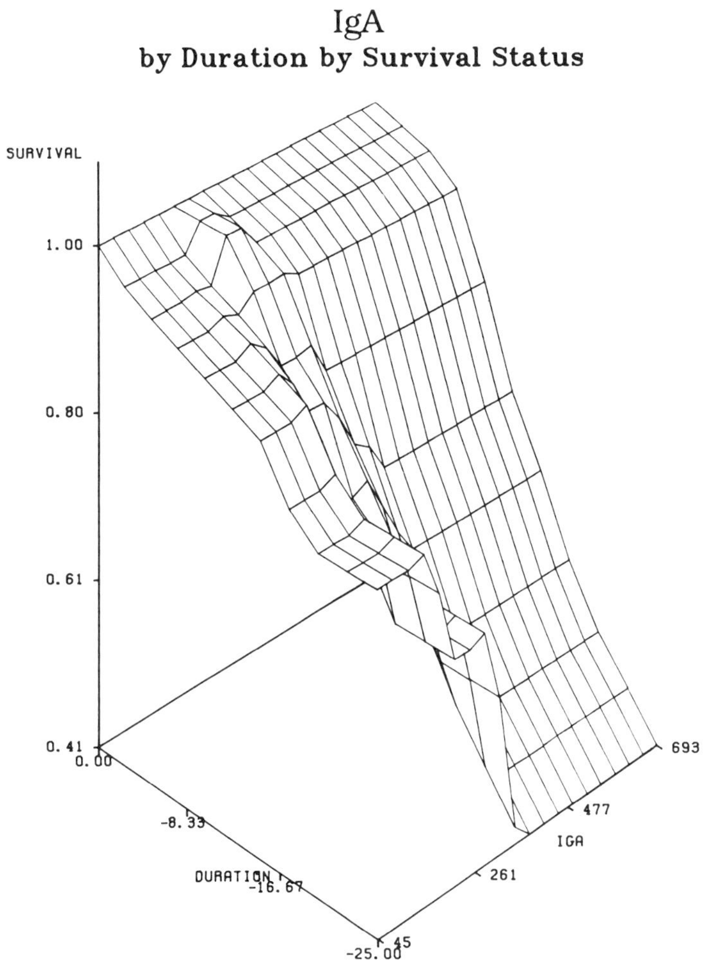

Figure 2. Relationship between disease-free survival in head and neck cancer patients and titers of circulating IgA. Duration from start of treatment is measured in months; IgA titers are measured in mg/dl. Increasing titers of IgA are associated with shorter survival (8) (by permission of the Laryngoscope).

with previously untreated head and neck cancer [1]. Those individuals with deficient function were more likely to die with disease. Perhaps most important about the measurement of natural killer cell activity is that it predicted patterns of recurrence, that is, low activity predicted a high–risk of disease relapse within regional lymph nodes and distant metastatic sites [1]. No relationship between NK cell function and local recurrence could be identified. Results suggested that NK cell function was important principally within peripheral blood. IgA, on the contrary, appeared to more readily predict death from disease than did NK cell function [8]. Yet quantitated

Table 1. Patients with elevated IgA: patterns of recurrence defined by natural killer (NK) cell cytotoxicity*,†

NK cell cytotoxicity	Total no. of patients	Total patients with recurrence	Recurrence patterns		
			L	R	D
≤60 LU	12	7	2	2	6
>60 LU	7	4	4	2	1

L = local; R = regional; D = distant; LU = lytic unit.
* As previously published [8].
† These 19 patients represent that group selected from a total population of 55 previously untreated head and neck cancer patients in whom IgA and NK cell activity had been assessed prior to treatment and longitudinal assessment. These 19 patients represent individuals with IgA levels >255 mg/dl as previously defined [8] and represent the population with the highest probability of dying with disease [8].

IgA levels failed to define patterns of recurrence. Table 1 shows results of combining NK cell function with IgA levels. Combining the two parameters was more effective in predicting disease course than either one alone. Results also show that patterns of recurrence were identified. Thus, a patient with elevated IgA is likely to die with disease. If he has concurrently low NK cell function, death will be principally a function of uncontrolled metastatic disease.

Circulating Immune Complexes (CIC)

CIC and Immune Response

Another area of increasing knowledge related to humoral immunity in the head and neck patient relates to the significance of CIC. The nature and function of CIC in cancer patients is dependent on many variables and has recently been reviewed by Phillips et al. [27]. These variables include type of immunoglobulin present, size of complex, complex formation in antigen or antibody excess or equivalence, and different antigens present in the complex. The complexes can be made of antigen–antibody, antibody–antibody, or a mixture of both. Formed complexes have the capacity to interact with complement, the clotting, kinin, and fibrinolytic systems, red blood cells, and platelets. The final makeup of the complex determines its function and fate within the host.

CIC have been reported to regulate a number of immune functions. Both direct and indirect evidence lends support for a downregulation of host immune response [27–35], as summarized in Table 2. The regulation of function appears to reside in the ability of CIC to react with Fc receptors or antigen receptors on T cells, B cells, and macrophages, thereby causing

Table 2. Reported suppressive functions of immune complexes

Cell function	Reference
T cell	
Suppression of T cell blastogenesis	30, 32, 33, 43–45
Induction of soluble FcR release from suppressor T cells followed by inhibition of antibody production	46–48
Blockage of T cell cytolytic activity	28, 35, 36
NK Cell	
Inhibition of natural killer cell activity	29, 49–51
Saturation of Fc receptors resulting in a decreased number of functional killer cells	52
B Cell	
Direct binding to FcR on B cells causing modulation of IgM/IgG antibody forming cells	37, 41
Induction of an immunoregulatory lymphokine in FcR+ cells that suppresses B cell proliferation	38, 39
Inhibition of B cell differentiation into IgG secreting cells	40
Inhibition of antibody response	42, 53
T and B Cells	
Depressed immune response to polyclonal mitogens	10
Blockage of normal leukocyte migration-inhibition	10
Suppression of proliferative response of lymphocytes to specific antigens or B and T cell mitogens	57
Macrophage	
Impairment of macrophage ability to phagocytose IgG-bound targets	54–56
Reduction of macrophage interleukin-1 production followed by a reduction of T helper cell interleukin-2	54–56
Inhibition of macrophage arming by cytophilic antitumor antibodies	34

modulation of both the primary and secondary host immune responses [27]. Hellstrom et al. noted the specific blocking effect of sera from tumor–bearing animals on immune lymphocytes [28]. The inhibition was tumor type specific, and the effect disappeared after tumor removal or absorption with the specific tumor cells. Later, Sjogren suggested that the inhibitory components were antigen–antibody complexes and inhibition was due to blocking of effector cell function and not to tumor masking [35]. Similar depression of natural killer cell function has been observed using syphilitic serum and immune complexes [29]. Thein et al. noted that CIC had the capacity to modulate the Fc–receptor phenotype and the proliferative capacity of Fc–IgG–receptor–positive lymphocytes in patients with systemic lupus erythematosus and rheumatoid arthritis [30]. They showed that Fc receptors were lost and Fc–IgM receptors expressed after lymphoid cells were cultured in the presence of immune complexes. Similar suppression of lymphocyte responsiveness by rheumatoid sera was found by Highton et al. [33]. The inhibitory activity in the sera could be removed by staphylococcal protein A absorption, suggesting that the inhibitory component was serum CIC [33]. CIC have been shown to inhibit macrophage function, as well. Rao et al. demonstrated that CIC injected into mice impaired the arming of macrophages by cytophilic antibody and that the Fc portion of the antibody was required for the suppressive effects of the immune complexes [34]. To counter the effects of CIC and suppressor factors, Israel et al. treated patients who had disseminated cancer with plasmapheresis, and 8 of 23 treated patients had partial objective responses after the removal of non-specific blocking factors [31].

CIC and Prognosis

In light of the adverse effect of CIC on cell–mediated immunity and the general consensus that the status of cell–mediated immunity is a critical determinant in head and neck tumor progression, it is important to note that CIC are elevated in head and neck cancer patients [10,59–67]. Using various methods of detection, CIC have been found elevated in patients with oral cancer, nasopharyngeal cancer, and laryngeal cancer when compared to normal populations [10,59–65]. Although evidence has been conflicting, most reports suggest that CIC reflect tumor burden in these patients and, therefore, could function potentially as both a tumor marker and/or a prognostic assay [10,61,63–67]. Mukhopadhyaya et al. [61] quantitated the CIC in untreated patients and in patients who had undergone radiation or surgery. Serial determinations showed that CIC remained high in patients with recurrent disease, while levels were reduced in patients with no evident disease. Saranath et al. noted similar results and showed that in patients with squamous cell carcinoma of the oral cavity, CIC correlated with tumor load [63]. Denaro et al. [65] noted that in laryngeal carcinoma, patients' preoperative values were much higher than those of normal controls. Yet there was not variation in CIC serum levels according to histologic types, presence or absence or lymphomonocytic infiltration, tumor stage or the course of monitoring [65]. They stated that the lack of correlation could be due to the relatively small quantity of tumor tissue involved in laryngeal carcinoma. Veltri et al. investigated multiple humoral and cellular functions in patients with squamous cell carcinoma of the head and neck [10]. In their study, the CIC levels never returned to normal values even after successful treatment. They suggest that the prolonged immunosuppressed state of head and neck cancer patients may be related to the continued presence of CIC. Maxim et al. also noted the persistence of CIC following radiation or surgery in head and neck cancer patients [64] and indicated that CIC might be related to the anergic state of these patients.

Our laboratory has recently examined the relationship between levels of CIC and response to induction chemotherapy [60]. We utilized as our assay system the complement (C1q) binding assay. In interpreting results of this assay, however, it should be realized that the test, as is true of most CIC assays, provides a quantitation of relatively nonspecific macromolecules that are capable of binding to complement. Whether these macromolecules are truly CIC (as is generally considered) cannot be stated with certainty. Nevertheless, the prognostic implication of these complement–binding sub-

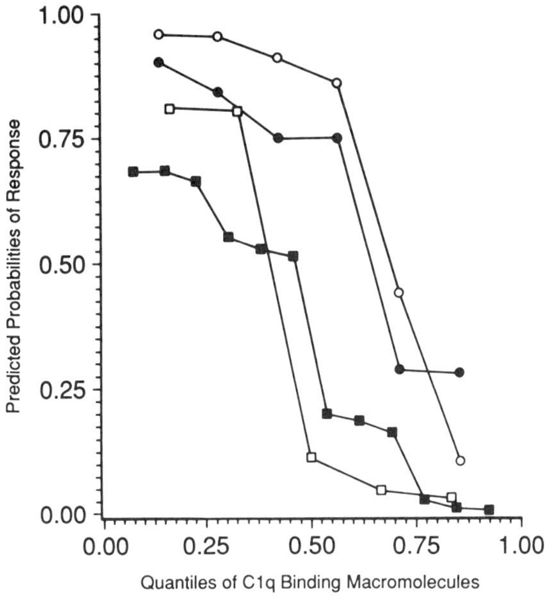

Figure 3. Quantiles of C1q BM and probability of response as estimated by logistic regression. Quantiles are estimated separately within each site and stage combination. The probability of response of those in the lowest quantile of C1q BM was estimated to be at least 70%, while the probability of response of those in the upper quantile is at most 30%. Open circle, Stage III, site–oral cavity/larynx; Closed circle, Stage III, site–pharynx; open square, Stage IV, site–oral cavity/larynx; closed square, stage IV, site–pharynx. A symbol is drawn for each patient in the stage–site group (60) (by permission of Cancer Res.).

stances was readily apparent. Those individuals with elevated levels of the C1q–binding macromolecules (C1qBM) were less likely to respond to induction chemotherapy (consisting primarily of *cis*–platinum, bleomycin, and 5–fluorouracil) than individuals with low levels. Furthermore, the prognostic results provided by measuring C1qBM were independent of the stage and site of patients' respective tumors. In a multivariate logistic regression analysis, the combined use of clinical staging and CIC measurement provided more information than either measure alone [60]. Figure 3 graphically depicts results from the regression analysis. The estimated size of the prognostic effect is striking. For all disease site and stage combinations for the 29 previously untreated patients in the study, the estimated antitumor response for those with the 25% lowest C1q values is at least 50% higher than for those with the 25% highest values.

This initial study has been extended to begin to answer questions raised: What is the true nature of C1qBM? Does the capacity to predict response to induction chemotherapy extend to other parameters of cellular immunity? What plausible and subsequently confirmable biologic explanations may account for the association? Recently, we have noted that by using an enzyme–linked immunosorbent assay system that C1qBM do contain (at least in part) aggregated immunoglobulins of the IgA, IgG, and IgM classes [66]. Furthermore, as the levels of C1qBM increase, so does the quantity of these aggregated immunoglobulins. Whether these immune complexes are composed of tumor antigens or represent antibody–antibody complexes such as those identified in testing for rheumatoid factor cannot yet be stated.

A recent multiparameter immune assessment of head and neck cancer patients examined whether response to induction chemotherapy was reflected in other parameters of host response [67]. Results showed no relationship to cell–mediated parameters, including in vitro lymphocyte–blastogenesis response to mitogens, NK cell activity, or lymphocyte subset quantitation. A significant relationship between response to chemotherapy and levels of total circulating immunoglobulin was, however, noted. Those patients with the highest levels of circulating IgG, IgA, and IgM were less likely to respond, with the principal determinant being IgG levels. However, in a multivariate analysis assessing all immune factors concurrently, only the quantitative measurement of CIC provided prognostic information.

Biologic explanations for the association of CIC and response to induction chemotherapy remain to be defined. One could hypothesize that the relationship is simply an associated phenomenon and that CIC may themselves play no direct role in influencing chemotherapeutic effect. The presence of those substances may reflect enhanced tumor kinetics, that is, enhanced cellular division, a shortened cell cycle, and an associated increase in tumor cell death. As tumor cells die, just as occurs with myocardial necrosis [68,69], cancer–related macromolecules capable of binding complement may be shed into the peripheral blood. The antitumor effect of chemotherapy utilized in this setting may simply fail to keep pace with tumor growth. Overall tumor mass may remain unaffected or even increase during therapy. Historically, the rapidly progressive disease in patients who fail chemotherapy has supported this hypothesis [70,71]. Recent longitudinal assessment shows patients with elevated C1qBM are more likely to die of their disease than those with low levels. Furthermore, and most important, the bad prognosis appears independent of treatment in these initially evaluated patients. Adverse prognosis was identified, as well, in those patients with elevated C1qBM who were treated with surgery and radiation without chemotherapy [66].

It should be reemphasized in interpreting these studies that, in most instances, the nature of the antigen and antibody in the immune complexes has not been determined. Thus, these tests lack specificity and are thereby limited in their clinical application. However, from the studies of Koneval et al. and Popovic et al. [72,73], it is clear that an autologous antitumor antibody response is being mounted. The immunoglobulins IgG, IgA, and IgM have been associated with the tumor cells and marginal tissues of patients with squamous cell carcinoma of the head and neck [72], and IgA and IgG immunoglobulins have been found in CIC of head and neck cancer patient [74,75]. Savage et al. [76] used immunoblotting technology to demonstrate autologous IgG, IgA, and IgM antibodies in the serum of head and neck cancer patients that reacted with antigens of defined molecular weight both in normal and tumor tissue. These reactive antigens may represent the antigen components of CIC. Vlock et al. also demonstrated autologous serum antibody activity to squamous cell carcinoma of the head and neck using the protein A hemadsorption assay [77]. Antibody reactivity to the tumor cells could be enhanced by dissociation of immune complexes using acidification and ultrafiltration of the patient sera [77]. Thus, continued research efforts on the nature and significance of CIC may help define the factors responsible for head and neck cancer progression. Appropriate new therapeutic approaches may become evident from such research, as well as an improved understanding of how to more effectively utilize current treatment modalities.

The Use of Monoclonal Antibodies in Cancer Diagnosis and Treatment

Manipulation of the humoral immune system has taken a quantum leap since the invention of monoclonal antibodies (mAb) and the introduction of hybridoma technology in 1975 [78]. The use of mAb has expanded into several areas of diagnostic and therapeutic research. Most of the advances have been made in fields other than head and neck tumor immunology. However, extrapolation and a wide perspective in the interpretation of mAb research in other tumor systems should shed light on the most promising avenues for mAb research in the field of head and neck cancers.

There are a variety of types of antigens to which a mAb can react. These include the classic tumor–associated antigens (TAA), but also include antigens associated with stages of differentiation (this category may overlap with TAA), oncogene products, or proteins associated with the metastatic process (for example, laminin receptor or type IV collagenase). They may be expressed either on the cell membrane or intracellularly; for diagnostic purposes, the location of the antigen does not matter, but most therapeutic uses depend on antigens being expressed on the cell membrane, that is, on the outside of the cell, accessible to mAb introduced intravenously. Whether for diagnosis or therapy, the sensitivity and specificity of these magic bullets are limited by certain factors inherent in the biology of solid tumors. The most important of these limitations is the fact that essentially all solid tumors are collections of a heterogeneous population of cancer cells. There is, therefore, variable expressivity of any given immunogenic antigen, both within each tumor and among all patients. Furthermore, in vitro testing of mAb and against cultured cell lines can be further complicated by antigenic modulation [79]. Such antigenic modulation is also seen in vivo, as a tumor cell can express different antigens depending on its cell cycle phase, environmental milieu, or even spatial relationship to neighboring cells [80].

Diagnosis

The possible diagnostic uses of mAb include immunohistopathologic analysis of tumor specimens, the detection of occult lesions, and the clinical monitoring of tumor burden. The pathologist's armamentarium of immunohistochemical probes is rapidly growing and has already made a significant impact on the accuracy of diagnosis of poorly differentiated tumors. A variety of commercially available mAb are in widespread use, directed against various antigens, such as keratins, vimentin, neuron–specific enolase. In tissue samples of limited volume (for example, effusions, and fine–needle aspirates), mAb can also be helpful in determining malignancy of cells that otherwise show few histologically significant signs. The development of highly specific mAb for head and neck cancers is actively being pursued. Ranken et al. [81], using a laryngeal carcinoma as an immunogenic source, have developed a mAb that reacts specifically against carcinomas of the head and neck region and related tissue such as cervical carcinoma, basal cells of normal squamous epithelium, and myoepithelial cells. Conversely, oncofetal antigen, a nonspecific antigen found in many different cancers, has also been identified recently in cells cultured from head and neck cancers [82]. Such information may be helpful in the study of tumor differentiation and oncogenesis.

Usage of mAb to monitor tumor burden may be dependent on presence of serum antigens, as is already widely utilized with carcinoembryonic antigen (CEA) and alpha–fetoprotein, or may require additional technology. Radioimmunodetection (RAID) falls into the latter category [83] and is based on the coupling of mAb to radionuclides for the detection of tumors previously difficult to image, whether because of size, location, or other factors. Radionuclides used include familiar imaging isotopes (I^{123}, In^{111}, Tc^{99m}), as well as newer isotopes [83]. Limitations of RAID are related to inherent factors of antibody physiology, such as binding and retention affinity and avidity, accessibility and density of antigen, and antigen expressivity. Other limiting factors depend on the radionuclide in use and largely depend on the ratio of tumor uptake to normal surrounding tissue uptake, for example, size of tumor, organ locale, depth, and photon yield. Some of these drawbacks have been overcome with newer innovations such as dual–isotope subtraction studies or use of Fab fragments instead of intact antibodies. The reader is referred to the review by Goldenberg for further discussion [83]. Specific uses in head and neck cancer diagnosis have yet to be reported.

Therapy

Since the introduction of hybridoma technology, the magic bullet theory of Ehrlich has seemed almost within reach [84]. Naturally occurring antibodies that recognize membrane receptors have been shown to directly affect physiologic function (for example, Graves' disease). Similarly, mAb can be manufactured to recognize normal membrane receptors and block physiologic function [85,86]. In addition to the relatively simplistic competitive blocking provided by these mAb, the conjugation of mAb to various compounds has expanded this field rapidly in the last several years. Coupling of mAb to toxins [87–90], effector cells [91], drugs [92], and radioisotopes [83, 92] have all been described; some of these techniques have been covered in the head and neck literature [93]. In addition, development of antiidiotypic immunoglobulins and manipulation of the idiotype/antiidiotype network is a theoretically viable arena [94–100].

Again, certain basic physiologic host factors are important in considering the efficacy of using mAb for delivery of therapy. Circulating antigen can theoretically bind mAb and thereby decrease the total mAb available for tumor binding. This possibility has been shown to be clinically insignificant in the case of CEA targeting [101]. Another factor shown to be important is the amount of tumor vascularity and the permeability of the tumor vasculature [102]. Delivery of the mAb to the tumor bed is dependent on adequate blood flow and may require as much as 24 hours of perfusion to reach therapeutically significant levels [83]. Cross-reactivity between the mAb and normal tissue has also been reported; Goldenberg et al. [103] have demonstrated granulocyte cross-reactivity that led to neutropenia. Most of the above mechanisms of tumor lysis require binding of mAb to every cell of the tumor for successful therapy. This requirement is viewed by some investigators as a serious drawback because the natural heterogeneity of solid tumors ensures that not all tumor cells will be targeted. Coupling to radioisotopes, however, does not depend on binding to every tumor cell. On the other hand, there is the increased danger of radiation damage to neighboring normal tissue.

Toxins used for binding to mAb include ricin A, diphtheria toxin fragment, abrin, *Pseudomonas* exotoxin A, and gelonin [87–90]. These compounds have been used against carcinomas originating in the colon, ovary, breast, prostate, and larynx [93]. Ozawa [87] has used gelonin coupled to a mAb that recognizes the epidermal growth factor [EGF] receptor, thereby increasing its specificity in recognizing cancers from tongue, gingiva, esophagus, and vulva.

Recruitment of the cellular immune system has also been attempted. Liu et al. [91] have combined a mAb recognizing a T cell receptor to a hormone that naturally targets the tumor cell. In this manner, they have brought the two cells into closer apposition and started the cell lysis mechanism.

Conjugation of mAb to cytotoxic drugs has also been tried in other tumor models. Doxorubicin, daunorubicin, methotrexate, vinblastine, and melphalan have all been used [92]. There is reduced toxicity to normal cells with this approach, but with each of the above-mentioned approaches there are the disadvantages of single cell killing for each mAb molecule. In addition, toxic drugs require that the mAb–conjugate be internalized to take effect, a prerequisite more often in hematopoeitic malignancies rather than solid tumors, in which the mAb–antigen complex is usually a stable membrane component.

The latter two drawbacks can be overcome by the use of radioisotopes as mAb conjugates. Such conjugates do not need an intracellular position for cell death; some isotopes can kill within a 50–cell radius. Cell killing is no longer tissue–specific, but the range of toxicity can be modulated by the use of different radioisotopes. Classically, I^{131} has been an isotope favored for clinical use because of the experience gained from its use for metastatic thyroid carcinoma. Its main disadvantage is bone marrow toxicity from its high–energy emissions. Currently, there is much research into other radioisotopes, mainly alpha–emitters that would have less toxicity for neighboring tissues. For more complete discussion of radioisotopes and their properties, the articles by Schlom [92], Foon [90], and Goldenberg [83] should be consulted.

Adjunctive Measures

Certain characteristics of antigen–to–antibody interactions will always pose problems, but newer technology and innovations hold promise in surmounting these stumbling blocks. The heterogeneity of antigen expression, both in solid tumor populations and over the life span of any particular cancer cell, is a major nemesis to mAb therapy. Inroads against this problem have been discovered by Greiner et al. [104,105], who have demonstrated upregulation of surface expression of TAA after incubation with recombinant alpha–interferon. Through fluorescence–activated cell sorter analysis, they have confirmed that the increase in surface antigen is due to both an increased density of antigen/cell and an increased percentage of cells expressing that antigen. This information is one example of immunomodulation that will be a helpful future adjunct to mAb therapy.

The patient's immune system poses another obstacle. Because most mAb are obtained by mounting an immune response in a mouse, mAb may elicit an anti–murine–immunoglobulin response in the patient [106,107]. Several methods attempt to abrogate that response. Antibody fragments (Fab' fragment usually) have been used in lieu of the intact antibody. This approach has been shown to alter binding properties but does not apparently change the specificity of targeting [108]. Using recombinant techniques, chimeric mAb have been generated, consisting of constant regions from human immunoglobulins and hypervariable regions from murine–based hybridoma mAb [109–111]. With the majority of the antibody molecule consisting of human amino acid sequences, the anti–murine response should, theoretically, be reduced.

Conclusion

We have focused on the status of and directions for humoral immune system research into circulating immunoglobulins and their biologic and clinical relevance, CIC, and the use of monoclonal antibodies in diagnosis and treatment. In many instances, we have compiled information from investigations in disease processes other than head and neck cancer that have implications for all neoplasias. What is most evident in the review process is the multiplicity of factors which define each clinical or biologic question that deals with humoral components. Thus, although CIC or circulating IgA, for example, may define a particular clinical outcome reflective of host/tumor interaction, that definition is limited. The use of these assays will not and should not be expected to provide information applicable to all patients with head and neck cancer. To have this expectation is to misunderstand the heterogeneity of host/tumor interactions that govern head and neck cancer growth. Ultimately, the use of the humoral system in clinical oncology will require individualization based on the understanding of a disease process for a particular head and neck cancer patient. It is the capacity to speak of this individualization with commonly understood definitions and rationale that will allow for treatment advances.

References

1. Schantz SP, Guillamondegui OM: Developing perspectives in head and neck tumor immunology. Prob Gen Surg 5:99–112, 1988.
2. Karre K, Ljunggren HG, Piontek G, Kiessling R: Selective rejection of H–2–deficient lymphoma variants suggests alternative immune defence strategy. Nature 319:675–678, 1986.
3. Savary CA, Lotzova E: Phylogeny and ontogeny of NK cells. In: Lotzova E, Herberman RB (eds). Immunobiology of natural killer cells. Vol I. Boca Raton, FL: CRC Press, pp 89–107, 1986.
4. Hughes NR: Serum concentrations of G, A, and M immunoglobulins in patients with carcinoma, melanoma, and sarcoma. JNCI 46:1015–1028, 1971.
5. Watanabe T, Iglehart JD, Bolognesi DP, Cox EB, Vaughn A, Hudson WR: Elevated serum secretory immunoglobulin A levels in patients with head and neck carcinoma. Otolaryngol Head Neck Surg 91:136–142, 1983.
6. Brown AM, Lally ET, Frankel A, Harwick P, Davis LW, Rominger CJ: The association of the IgA levels of serum and whole saliva with the progression of oral cancer. Cancer 35:1154–1162, 1975.
7. Katz AE: Immunobiologic staging of patients with carcinoma of the head and neck. Laryngoscope 93:445–463, 1983.
8. Schantz SP, Liu FJ, Taylor DL, Beddingfield N, Weber RS: The relationship of circulating IgA to cellular immunity in head and neck cancer patients. Laryngoscope 98:671–678, 1988.
9. Schantz SP, Liu FJ: An immunologic profile of young adults with head and neck cancer. Cancer (in press).

10. Veltri RW, Rodman SM, Maxim PE, Baseler MW, Sprinkle PM: Immune complexes, serum proteins, cell-mediated immunity, and immune regulation in patients with squamous cell carcinoma of the head and neck. Cancer 57:2295–2308, 1986.
11. Kutteh WH, Koopman WJ, et al.: Production of predominantly polymeric IgA by human peripheral blood lymphocytes stimulated in-vitro with mitogens. J Exp Med 152:1424–1429, 1980.
12. Shillitoe EJ, Silverman S: Oral cancer and herpes simplex virus: A review. Oral Surg 48:216–24, 1979.
13. deVilliers EM, Weidauer H, Otto H, zurHausen H: Papilloma-virus DNA in human tongue carcinomas. Int J Cancer 36:575–578, 1985.
14. Smith HG, Horowitz N, Silverman NA, et al.: Humoral immunity to herpes simplex viral-induced antigens in smokers. Cancer 38:1152–1162, 1976.
15. Shillitoe EJ, Hwang CBC, Silverman S Jr, Greenspan JS: Examination of oral cancer tissue for the presence of the proteins ICP4, ICP5, ICP6, ICP8, and gB of herpes simplex virus type 1. JNCI 76:371–374, 1986.
16. Bienenstock J, Befus AD: Some thoughts on the biologic role of immunoglobulin A. Gastroenterology 84:178–185, 1983.
17. Griffiss JM: Biologic function of the serum IgA system: Modulation of complement mediated effector mechanisms and conservation of antigenic mass. Ann NY Acad Sci 409:697–707, 1983.
18. Russell MW, Brown TA, Mestecky J: Role of serum IgA: Hepatobiliary transport of circulating antigen. J Exp Med 153:968–976, 1981.
19. Stokes C, Swarbrick ET: Induction of tolerance after oral feeding of soluble protein antigen. Biochem Soc Trans 5:1573, 1977.
20. Vaz NM, Maia LCS, Hanson DG, Lynch JM: Inhibition of homocytotrophic antibody response in adult inbred mice by previous feeding of the specific antigen. J Allergy Clin Immunol 60:110–115, 1977.
21. Wilton JMA: Suppression by IgA of IgG-mediated phagocytosis by human polymorphonuclear leucocytes. Clin Exp Immunol 34:423–428, 1978.
22. Griffiss JM: Bactericidal activity of meningococcal antisera: blocking by IgA of lytic antibody in human convalescent sera. J Immunol 114:1779–1784, 1975.
23. Russell-Jones GL, Ey PL, Reynolds BL: The ability of IgA to inhibit complement mediated lysis of target red blood cells sensitized with IgG antibody. Mol Immunol 17:1173–1180, 1980.
24. O'Neill PA, Romsdahl MM: IgA as a blocking factor in human malignant melanoma. Immunol. Commun. 3:427–438, 1974.
25. Sipos J, Gabor V, Toth Z: Inhibition of leukocyte migration by tumor-associated antigens and its modification by serum: IgA as a blocking factor. Neoplasma 25:181–188, 1978.
26. Katz DE, Seder RH, Keggins JJ, et al.: Plasmapheresis in patients with advanced carcinoma of the head and neck. In: Wolf GT, Carey TE (eds). Head and Neck Oncology Research. Amsterdam: Kugler and Ghedini, pp 151–157, 1988.
27. Phillips TM, Holohan TV, Korac S, More NS, Queen WD: The pathophysiology of circulating immune complexes: their role in host-tumor interactions and removal by immunoadsorption therapy. Contemp Top Immunobiol 15:111–137, 1985.
28. Hellstrom KE, Hellstrom I, Snyder HW, Balint JP, Jones FR: Blocking (suppressor) factors, immune complexes, and extracorporeal immunoadsorption in tumor immunity. Contemp Top Immunobiol 15:213–238, 1985.
29. Jensen JR, Jorgensen AS, Thestrup-Pedersen K: Depression of natural killer cell activity by syphilitic serum and immune complexes. British Journal of Venereal Disease 58:298–301, 1982.
30. Thein M, Renger D, Deicher H, Pichler WJ: Alteration of Fc-receptor phenotype and proliferative capacity of Fc-IgG-receptor positive lymphocytes through interaction with soluble immune complexes of patients with SLE or RA. Rheumatol Int 5:127–132, 1985.

31. Israel L, Edelstein R, Mannoni P, Radot E, Greenspan EM: Plasmapheresis in patients with disseminated cancer: clinical results and correlation with changes in serum protein. The concept of nonspecific blocking factors. Cancer 40:3146–3154, 1977.
32. Osaki Y, Koga S, Maeta M, Shimizu N, Kanayama H, Hamazoe R: Circulating immune complexes in gastric cancer patients and their effect on lymphocyte mitogensis (the first report). Jpn J Surg 14:524–526, 1984.
33. Highton J, Panayi GS, Shepherd P, Wooley P: Effect of sera from patients with rheumatoid arthritis on normal lymphocytes: a possible immunoregulatory role for immune complexes: Ann Rheum Dis 41:563–568, 1982.
34. Rao VS, Grodzicki RL, Mitchell MS: Specific in vivo inhibition of macrophage receptors for cytophylic antibody by soluble immune complexes. Cancer Res 39:174–182, 1979.
35. Sjogren HO, Helstrom I, Bansal SC, Hellstrom K: Suggestive evidence that the blocking antibodies of tumor-bearing individuals may be antigen–antibody complexes. Proc Nat Acad Sci USA 686:1372–1375, 1971.
36. Blair PB, Lane M–A, Yagi MJ: Blocking of spleen cell activity against target mammary cells by viral antigens. J Immunol 115:190–194, 1975.
37. Oberbarnscheidt J, Kolsh E: Direct blockade of antigen–reactive B lymphocytes by immune complexes. An off signal for precursors of IgM–producing cells provided by the linkage of antigen– and Fc–receptors. Immunology 35:151–157, 1978.
38. Suzuki T, Miyama–Inaba M, Masuda T, Uchino H, Ishii K: Monoclonal SBF produced by a hybridoma: in–vitro and in–vivo suppression of B tumour–cell proliferation. Immunology 50:595–603, 1983.
39. Miyama–Inaba M, Suzuki T, Paku Y–H, Masuda T: Feedback regulation of immune responses by immune complexes; possible involvement of a suppressive lymphokine by FcR–gamma bearing B cells. J Immunol 128:882–887, 1982.
40. Tsokos GC, Berger M, Balow JE: Modulation of human B cell immunoglobulin secretion by the C3b component of complement. J Immunol 132:622–626, 1984.
41. Park Y–H, Miyama–Inaba M, Suzuki T, Masuda T, Yoshida Y, Uchino H: Immunological characterization of FcR gamma bearing and nonbearing B cells: functional modulation of immune complexes. Cell Immunol 83:340–350, 1984.
42. Pisko EJ, Foster SL, White RE, Panetti M, Turner RA: Suppression of a pokeweed mitogen–stimulated plaque-forming cell response by a human B lymphocyte–derived aggregated IgG–stimulated suppressor factor: suppressive B cell factor (SBF). J Immunol 136:2141–2150, 1986.
43. Hotta R, Kuriki J, Kakumu S: Loss of suppressor T cell function and circulating immune complexes in chronic active liver diseases. Clin Exp Immunol 46:375–381, 1981.
44. Tanaka F, Yonemoto RH, Waldman SR: Blocking factors in sera of breast cancer patients. Cancer 43:838–847, 1979.
45. Samarut C, Cordier G, Revillard JP: Insoluble immune complexes suppress mitogen–induced proliferation of human T lymphocytes bearing Fc receptors. Cell Immunol 42:18–27, 1979.
46. Gisler RH, Fridman WH: Suppression of in vitro antibody synthesis by immunoglobulin–binding factor. J Exp Med 142:507–511, 1975.
47. Fridman WH, Rabourdin–Combe C, Neauport–Sautes C, Gisler RH: Characterization and function of the T cell Fc gamma receptor. Immunol Rev 56:52–88, 1981.
48. Bich–Thuy LT, Banchereau J, Revillard JP: Suppression of polyclonal human B cell activation by IgG binding factors: interference with the maturation of Ig–containing cells into Ig-secreting cells. Cell Immunol 87:231–239, 1984.
49. Karsh J, Dorval G, Osterland CK: Natural cytotoxicity in rheumatoid arthritis and systemic lupus erythematosus. Clin Immunol Immunopathol 19:437–446, 1981.
50. Sibbitt WL, Froelich CJ, Bankhurst AD: Abnormal interferon modulation of natural cytotoxicity in systemic lupus erythematosus: Relation to suppressive serum factors. Arthritis Rheum 26:1452–1459, 1983.

51. Pedersen BK, Thomsen BS, Nielsen H: Inhibition of natural killer cell activity by antigen–antibody complexes. Allergy 41:568–574, 1986.
52. Endo Y, Aratake Y, Yamamoto I, Nakagawa H, Kuribayashi T, Ohtaki S: Peripheral K cells in Graves' disease and Hashimoto's thyroiditis in relation to circulating immune complexes. Clin Endocrinol 18:187–194, 1983.
53. Caufield MJ, Shaffer D: Immunoregulation by antigen/antibody complexes. I. Specific immunosuppression induced in vivo with immune complexes formed in antibody excess. J Immunol 183:3680–3683, 1987.
54. Targowski SP, Klucinski W: Effect of immune complexes from mastitic milk on blocking of Fc receptors and phagocytosis. Infect Immun 47:484–488, 1985.
55. Michl J, Unkeless JC, Pieczonka MM, Silverstein SC: Modulation of Fc receptors on mononuclear phagocytes by immobilized antigen–antibody complexes: quantitative analysis of the relationship between ligand number and Fc receptor response. J Exp Med 157:1746–1757, 1983.
56. Pinching AJ: Inhibition of complement–dependent phagocytosis by monocytes following pre–incubation with immune complexes and interaction with plasma. Clin Exp Immunol 51:83–90, 1983.
57. Kilburn DC, Fairhurst M, Levy JG, Whitney RB: Synergism between immune complexes and serum from tumor–bearing mice in the suppression of mitogen responses. J Immunol 117:1612–1617, 1976.
58. Sjogren HO, Hellstrom I, Bansal SC, Warner GA, Hellstrom KE. Elution of blocking antibodies from human tumors, capable of abrogating tumor–cell destruction by specifically immune lymphocytes. Int J Cancer 9:274–283, 1972.
59. Scully C, Barkas T, Boyle P, McGregor IA, Ward–Booth P: Immune complexes in oral cancer. IRSC Med Sci 9:872, 1981.
60. Schantz SP, Savage HE, Brown BW, Reuben JM, Hong WK, Rossen RD: Association of levels of circulating C1q binding macromolecules with induction chemotherapy responses in head and neck cancer patients. Cancer Res 48:5868–5873, 1988.
61. Mukhopadhyaya R, Rao RS, Fakih AR, Gangal SG: Detection of circulating immune complexes in patients with squamous cell carcinoma of the oral cavity. J Clin Lab Immunol 21:189–193, 1986.
62. Chatterjee R, Guha S: Circulating immune complexes in sera of patients with oral cancer. J Clin Lab Immunol 15:145–147, 1984.
63. Saranath D, Mukhopadhyaya R, Rao RS, Fakih AR, Naik SL, Gangal SG: Cell–mediated immune status in patients with squamous cell carcinoma of the oral cavity. Cancer 56:1062–1070, 1985.
64. Maxim PE, Veltri RW, Sprinkle PM, Pusateri RJ: Soluble immune complexes in sera from head and neck cancer patients: A preliminary report. Ann Otol Rhinol Laryngol 86:428–423, 1978.
65. Denaro A, Caruso R, Rosi M, D'Arrigo C, Malaponte G, Mazzarino MC, Cutrona D: Circulating immunocomplexes and laryngeal carcinoma. Arch Otolaryngol 111:595–597, 1985.
66. Schantz SP, Savage H, Young G, Hong WK: C1q binding macromolecules and survival in head and neck cancer patients (Abstract). Proc Amer Soc Clin Oncol 8:170, 1989.
67. Schantz SP, Savage HE, Racz T, et al.: Immunologic determinants of head and neck cancer response to induction chemotherapy. J Clin Oncol (in-press).
68. Pinckard RN, Olson MS, Giclas PC, Terry R, Boyer JT, O'Rourke RA: Consumption of classical complement components by heart subcellular membranes in vitro and in patients after acute myocardial infarction. J Clin Invest 56:70–76, 1975.
69. Rossen RD, Michael LH, Kagiyama A, Savage HE, Hanson G, Reisberg MA, Moake JN, Kim SH, Self D, Weakley S, Giannini E, Entman ML. Mechanism of complement activation following coronary artery occlusion: evidence that myocardial ischemia in dogs causes release of constitutents of myocardial subcellular origin that complex with human C1q in vivo. Circ Res 1988; 62:572–584, 1988.

70. Elias EG, Chretien PB, Monnard E, Khan T, Bouchelle WH, Wiernik PH, Lipson SP, Hande KR, Zentai T: Chemotherapy prior to local therapy in advanced squamous cell carcinoma fo the head and neck. Preliminary assessment of an intensive drug regimen. Cancer 43:1025–1031, 1979.
71. Ervin TJ, Clark JR, Weichselbaum RR, Fallon BG, Miller D, Fabiran RL, Posner MR, Norris CM, Tuttle SA, Schoenfeld DA, Prue KN, Frei E III: An analysis of induction and adjuvant chemotherapy in the multidisciplinary treatment of squamous cell carcinoma of the head and neck. J Clin Oncol 5:10–20, 1987.
72. Konoval T, Applebaum E, Popovic D, et al.: Demonstration of immunoglobulin of tumor and marginal tissues of squamous cell carcinomas in the head and neck. JNCI 59:1089–1097, 1977.
73. Popovic D, Gill L, Sisson G, Applebaum E, Anderson B: Detection and localization of tumor–associated immune components of head and neck squamous cell carcinomas. Tr Am Acad Opthalmol Otolaryngol 82:119–130, 1976.
74. Heimer R, Klein G: Circulating immune complexes in sera of patients with Burkitt's lymphoma and nasopharyngeal carcinoma. Int J Cancer 18:310–316, 1976.
75. Baseler MW, Maxim PE, Veltri RW: Circulating IgA immune complexes in head and neck cancer, nasopharyngeal carcinoma, lung cancer and colon cancer. Cancer 59:1727–1731, 1987.
76. Savage HE, Schantz SP, Sacks PG, Birdsall HH, Rosen RD: Serum antibodies from head and neck cancer patients provide molecular probes to identify and characterize antigens in autologous and allogeneic tumor cells. In: Wolf GT, Carey TE (eds), Head and Neck Oncology Research. Amsterdam: Kugler and Ghedini, pp 109–119, 1988.
77. Vlock DR, Scalise D, Schwartz DR, et al.: Incidence of serum antibody reactivity to autologous head and neck cancer cell lines and augmentation of antibody reactivity following acid disassociation and ultrafiltration. Cancer Res 49:1361–1365, 1989.
78. Kohler M, Milstein C: 1975. Continuous cultures of fused cells secreting antibody of predefined specificity. Nature 256:494–497, 1975.
79. Hand P, Nuti M, Colcher D, Schlom J: Definition of antigenic heterogeneity and modulation among human mammary carcinoma cell populations using monoclonal antibodies to tumor associated antigens. Cancer Res 43:728–735, 1983.
80. Kufe DW, Nadler L, Sargent L, Shapiro H, Hand P, Austin F, Colcher D, Schlom J: Biological behavior of human breast carcinoma–associated antigens expressed during cellular proliferation. Cancer Res 43:851–857, 1983.
81. Ranken R, White CF, Gottfried TG, Yonkovich SJ, Blazek BE, Moss MS, Fee WE Jr, Liu YSV. Reactivity of monoclonal antibody 17.13. with human squamous cell carcinoma and its application to tumor diagnosis. Cancer Res 47:5684–5690, 1987.
82. Gussack GS, Rohrer SD, Hester RB, Liu PI, Coggin JH: Human squamous cell carcinoma lines express oncofetal 44–kD polypeptide defined by monoclonal antibody to mouse fetus. Cancer 62:283–290, 1988.
83. Goldenberg DM: Targeting of cancer with radiolabeled antibodies. Arch Pathol Lab Med 112:580–587, 1988.
84. Himmelweit F (ed): The Collected Papers of Paul Ehrlich. Vol. 2: Immunology and Cancer Research. New York: Pergamon Press, 1957.
85. Gorczynski RM, Kennedy M, Polidoulis I, Price GB: Altered tumor growth in vivo after immunization of mice with anti–tumor antibodies. Cancer Res 44:3291–3298, 1984.
86. Trowbridge IS: Therapeutic potential of monoclonal antibodies that block biological function. In: Boss BD, Langman R, Trowbridge I, Dulbecco R (eds), Monoclonal Antibodies and Cancer, Orlando:Academic Press, pp 53–61, 1983.
87. Ozawa S, Ueda M, Ando N, Abe O, Minoshima S, Shimizu N: Selective killing of squamous carcinoma cells by an immunotoxin that recognizes the EGF receptor. Int J Cancer 43:152–157, 1989.
88. Gilliland DG, Steplewski Z, Collier RJ, Mitchell KF, Chang TH, Koprowski H: Antibody–directed cytotoxic agents: use of monoclonal antibody to direct the action of

toxin A chains to colorectal carcinoma cells. Proc Natl Acad Sci USA 77:4539–4543, 1980.
89. Vitteta ES, Fulton RJ, May RD, Till M, Uhr JW: Redesigning nature's poisons to create anti–tumor reagents. Science 238:1098–1104, 1987.
90. Foon KA: Biological response modifiers: The new immunotherapy. Cancer Res 49:1621–1639, 1989.
91. Liu MA, Nussbaum SR, Eisen HN: Hormone conjugated with antibody to CD3 mediates cytotoxic T–cell lysis of human melanoma cells. Science 239:395–398, 1988.
92. Schlom J: Basic principles and applications of monoclonal antibodies in the management of carcinomas: the Richard and Hinda Rosenthal Foundation Award lecture. Cancer Res 46:3225–3238, 1986.
93. Zenner HP: Selective killing of laryngeal carcinoma cells by a monoclonal immunotoxin. Ann Otol Rhinol Laryngol 95:115–120, 1986.
94. Lindenmann J: Speculations on idiotypes and homobodies. Annales d'Immunologie 124:171–184, 1973.
95. Jerne NK: Idiotypic networks and other preconceived ideas. Immunol Rev 79:5–24, 1984.
96. Nepom GT, Nelson KA, Holbeck SL, Hellstrom I, Hellstrom KE: Induction of immunity to a human tumor marker by in vivo administration of anti–idiotypic antibodies in mice. Proc Natl Acad Sci USA 81:2864–2867, 1984.
97. Bottomly K: All idiotypes are equal, but some are more equal than others. Immunol Rev 79:45–61, 1984.
98. Coutinho A, Forni L, Homberg D, Ivars F, Vaz N: From an antigen–centered, clonal perspective of immune responses to an organism–centered, network perspective of autonomous activity in a self–referential immune system. Immunol Rev 79:151–168, 1984.
99. Kennedy RC, Zhou EM, Lanford RE, Chanh TC, Bona CA: Possible role of anti–idiotypic antibodies in the induction of tumor immunity. J Clin Invest 80:1217–1224, 1987.
100. Nepom GT, Hellstrom KE: Anti–idiotypic antibodies and the induction of specific tumor immunity. Cancer Metastasis Rev 6:489–502, 1987.
101. Goldenberg DM, Kim EE, DeLand FH: Radioimmunodetection of cancer with radioactive antibodies to carcinoembryonic antigen. Cancer Res 40:2984–2992, 1980.
102. Sands H, Shah HA, Jones PL, Neacy W, Gallagher BM: Non–immunological factors affecting the localization of monoclonal antibodies in xenografts of human breast and colon tumors. In: Ceriani RL (ed), Monoclonal Antibodies and Breast Cancer, Boston: Martinus Nijhoff, pp 303–315, 1985.
103. Goldenberg DM, Ford EH, Primus FJ, Goldenberg H, Alger EA, DeJager RL: Clinical evaluation of CEA monoclonal antibodies for cancer radioimmunodetection (Abstract). Proc Am Assoc Cancer Res 27:336, 1986.
104. Greiner JW, Guadagni F, Noguchi P, Pestka S, Colcher D, Fisher PB, Schlom J: Recombinant interferon enhances monoclonal antibody–targeting of carcinoma lesions in vivo. Science 235:895–898, 1987.
105. Greiner JW, Fisher PB, Pestka S, Schlom J: Differential effects of recombinant human leukocyte interferons on cell surface antigen expression. Cancer Res 46:4984–4990, 1986.
106. Schroff RW, Stevenson HC: Human immune responses to murine monoclonal antibodies. In: Foon KA, Morgan AC Jr (eds), Monoclonal Antibody Therapy of Human Cancer, Boston:Martinus Nijhoff, pp 121–138, 1985.
107. Schroff RW, Foon KA, Beatty SM, Oldham RK, Morgan AC Jr: Human anti–murine immunoglobulin responses in patients receiving monoclonal antibody therapy. Cancer Res 45:879–885, 1985.
108. Carrasquillo JA, Krohn KA, Beaumier P, McGuffin RW, Brown JP, Hellstrom KE, Hellstrom I, Larson SM: Diagnosis of and therapy for solid tumors with radiolabeled antibodies and immune fragments. Cancer Treat Rep 68:317–328, 1984.
109. Morrison SL, Johnson MJ, Herzenberg LA, Oi VT: Chimeric human antibody molecules: Mouse antigen–binding domains with human constant region domains. Proc Natl Acad Sci USA 81:6851–6855, 1984.

110. Morrison SL: Transfectomas provide novel chimeric antibodies. Science 229:1202–1207, 1985.
111. Steplewski Z, Sun LK, Shearman CW, Ghrayeb J, Daddona P, Koprowski H: Biological activity of human–mouse IgG1, IgG2, IgG3, and IgG4 chimeric monoclonal antibodies with antitumor specificity. Proc Natl Acad Sci USA 85:4852–4856, 1988.

16. Etiologic Considerations for Head and Neck Squamous Cancers

Charlotte D. Jacobs

Squamous cancers of the head and neck region represent approximately 5% of neoplasms in the United States. In 1989, there will be an estimated 43,000 new cases and 12,000 deaths from this disease (Table 1) [1]. There are regional differences in the U.S. with mortality being highest for men in northeastern cities and higher for women in the rural Southeast, predominantly from snuff use [2]. This disease has an even greater impact worldwide. Half of the cancers in Bombay are of oral cavity and pharyngeal origin. In France, the mortality from head and neck cancer is three times that in American males. A particularly high incidence of nasal cavity/sinus cancer has been reported in Uganda and Zimbabwe, related to the use of transnasal snuff with a high concentration of carcinogens. The incidence of nasopharyngeal cancer, while low in the United States (0.7/100,000), is 15.8/100,000 for Hong Kong citizens, representing a major health problem [2,3].

These cancers usually occur in the 50 to 60 age group, and the rate increases with age, with the exception of nasopharyngeal carcinoma where the incidence levels off after approximately age 50. Head and neck squamous cancers occur three times more frequently in men than in women. What was once a disease of white males, however, is now changing, and for women and nonwhite males, the death rate from oral cavity, oropharyngeal, and laryngeal cancers is increasing [4].

Even if a patient is cured of head and neck cancer, approximately twenty percent will develop a second primary, usually in the head and neck region, lung, or esophagus, and usually of squamous histology [5]. These may be synchronous or metachronous with a mean time to development of 2.6 years from the first cancer. This high rate is explained by continued exposure to carcinogens and the concept of field cancerization, causing widespread dysplasia with premalignant and malignant epithelial changes throughout the oral cavity and pharynx [6].

In studying factors that may be of etiologic significance in the disease process, several types of epidemiology trials are used. A case–control study investigates the excess of a particular factor, such as tobacco use, among cancer patients; whereas a cohort study investigates excess cancers among

Jacobs, C. (ed): Carcinomas of the Head and Neck: Evaluation and Management.

Table 1. Estimated new cases of head and neck cancer in the United States—1989.*

	Number of Cases (×1000)		
Site	Men	Women	Total
Larynx	10.0	2.3	12.3
Pharynx	6.0	2.7	8.7
Tongue	3.9	2.1	6.0
Lip	3.7	0.5	4.2
Oral Cavity (Other)	7.0	4.7	11.7

* from Cancer Statistics [1]

persons with a particular exposure history, such as smokers [4]. Relative risk (RR) refers to the ratio of the incidence of disease among persons with a particular exposure history divided by the incidence of disease among nonexposed populations [7].

Head and neck squamous cancer is one malignancy for which there is a strong relationship to multiple etiologic factors. The association of this disease with tobacco use, alcoholic beverages, industrial carcinogens, radiation exposure, diet, genetic predisposition, and viruses will be discussed in this chapter, along with efforts directed toward cancer prevention.

Tobacco

The association between tobacco and head and neck cancer is not new. Its relationship to lip and oral cavity cancer was reported by the mid 1880s [8]. Most head and neck cancer sites have been associated with cigarette smoking, the only exceptions being paranasal sinus, nasal cavity, and nasopharynx, where data is conflicting [7–12]. The relative risk of developing head and neck cancer is increased with the number of cigarettes smoked per day (Table 2). The risk of dying from laryngeal cancer is increased 32-fold and oral cavity 12-fold in persons smoking more than 40 cigarettes per day [11]. The type of tobacco influences risk as well. Among Uruguayan males, the use of dark tobacco produces a relative risk for laryngeal cancer 2.5 times that from use of light tobacco and 35 times that of not smoking [13]. Dark tobacco is more carcinogenic than light tobacco and is held in the oropharynx for longer time periods. Filtered cigarettes lower the risk, predominantly in heavy smokers [12]. In patient groups who have stopped smoking, it takes up to sixteen years for the risk to decrease to that of nonsmokers. For those who continue to smoke, the incidence of second primaries is as high as 40%, compared to 6% for those who quit smoking [14].

Cigarette smoke contains approximately 4,000 compounds. The carcinogenic activity is mainly contained in the tar fraction where aromatic

Table 2. Relative risk for head and neck cancer by tobacco product.*

Site	Cigarettes/Day 20–40	Cigarettes/Day > 40	Pipe	Smokeless Tobacco
Larynx	10.2–14.8	21.1–34.4	5.2	7.3
Pharynx	12.9–20	24	10	4.1
Lip	2.5	3.1	3.8	
Tongue	6.9	12	5.3	2.3
Oral Cavity	6.2–13.7	9.5–21.9	8.7–11	11.2
Sinus	2	4.9		33
Nasopharynx	1.8	4.2		5.3

* from Schottenfeld [2], Wynder et al. [12], Stockwell et al [20], Wynder et al. [77], Tuyns et al. [78]

hydrocarbons and nitrosamines have been measured [2]. Tobacco is a relatively weak carcinogen which requires prolonged exposure for its initiators (the hydrocarbons) and promoters (phenols) to render their effects [15]. Three–quarters of oral cavity cancers occur over ten percent of the oral mucosa. They commonly arise in a horseshoe–shaped area which begins at the anterior floor of mouth and extends along the gingival sulcus and lateral oral tongue to the retromolar trigone and anterior tonsillar pillar. It has been postulated that carcinogens concentrate in areas of pooled saliva [8]. Tobacco smoke also alters immunologic response which may contribute to its carcinogenicity [16].

Cigar and pipe smoke also appear to be carcinogenic [11,12]. Death from oral cavity cancers is increased 3 to 4–fold with cigar or pipe use, and laryngeal cancers are increased 10–fold from cigars. As little as one to five cigars or pipe bowls per day increases the risk of developing these cancers. Studies now show an increased incidence of oropharyngeal and hypopharyngeal cancers in pipe smokers as well.

A disproportionate number of young patients with head and neck cancers are routine users of marijuana [17]. It has been estimated that 17.5 million American adults and 2.5 million teenagers are regular marijuana smokers. Marijuana smoke produces greater amounts of primary irritants to the tracheobronchial tree than tobacco smoke. There is a 70% higher concentration of benzpyrene in marijuana smoke than in tobacco smoke, and a 50% higher concentration of aromatic hydrocarbons.

Smokeless tobacco, predominantly snuff and chewing tobacco, have become quite popular in recent years [8,9,18,19]. An estimated 11 to 22 million Americans use one of these products regularly. The average age of users is 18 to 30 years, but they are being used with increasing frequency by children. Smokeless tobacco has been associated with an increased risk of cancers of the oral cavity, oropharynx, and larynx [20]. Snuff consists of cured and ground tobacco and contains three major chemical carcinogens, including benzpyrene and several nitrosamines [8,9]. Levels of carcinogens exceed those found in cigarettes, probably from the process of curing and fermentation. The risk of oropharyngeal cancer is increased in relationship to the dose, length of exposure, and site of exposure. In the southern United States, the incidence of gum and buccal mucosa cancers is four times greater among snuff users [18]. In the last decade, the mortality from tongue cancer for young men, ages 10 to 29, has doubled in the United States, probably the result of increased use of chewing tobacco in children [21].

The prevalence and anatomic distribution of tobacco–related cancers vary widely with geographic location. In the United States, cancers of the oral cavity represent 3% of all malignancies; whereas in Bombay they represent 50%. In India, Hong Kong, the Philippines, and South Vietnam, betel nut is frequently mixed with slaked lime and tobacco to form a quid [8]. This quid is tucked in the gingivobuccal sulcus and held for long time periods. Cancers tend to appear in the area of the buccal mucosa in which the betel nut is placed.

There are particular districts in India where the incidence of hard palate cancer is 47 times that of the general population [8]. This increased risk is related to a practice called reverse smoking. Women make homemade cigars, or chuttas, and hold the burning end in the mouth to puff. Cancers occur in the area of the hard palate where the chutta is directed.

Alcoholic Beverages

Cancers of the oral cavity, oropharynx and larynx have been associated with use of alcoholic beverages [2,4,7,8,10]. Those areas that have the greatest exposure, such as oral cavity and oropharyngeal sites, have a greater risk than those sites which are not directly exposed to alcohol, such as the larynx [10]. In interpreting data from these case–control and cohort studies, one must adjust for tobacco use. In 1962, a large retrospective trial of 4,000 males did show a significant association between alcohol use and oropharyngeal cancer, controlling for tobacco use [22]. Another case–control study showed that the relative risk for oral cavity cancer rose from 3.3 in those persons consuming less than six whisky equivalents (WEs) daily to 15.2 for those who consumed greater than 6 WEs daily [23]. In fact, the risk for cancer was higher for those who drank six or more WEs daily than those who smoked 40 or more cigarettes per day. Several trials have now shown an increased relative risk for drinkers who do not use tobacco [7,24].

There is a positive association of head and neck cancer with different kinds of alcoholic beverages, including beer, wine, and hard liquor. Data concerning the type of alcoholic drink with highest risk are conflicting. In some trials, beer or wine consumption has been shown to have a higher risk [23]; whereas in other trials, whisky had the highest relative risk for cancer [7]. Perhaps different types of alcoholic beverages produce varying effects at different sites. In a case–control study of 2,000 Frenchmen, site–specific differences were demonstrated [24]. Wine consumption was higher among patients with oral cavity cancers; a higher proportion of aniseed spirit consumption was found among those with supraglottic cancers; and patients with glottic cancers consumed a higher amount of whisky. This suggests that the pathogenesis of alcohol–induced carcinomas may vary with site.

Several possible mechanisms for alcohol–induced cancers have been postulated [7,8,25]. There may be a local effect from direct contact with oral mucosa, alcohol causing a chemical burn. This could increase cell membrane permeability to tobacco carcinogens for which alcohol would also act as a solvent. Carcinogens have been found in low levels in some alcoholic beverages. These include nitrosamines, polycyclic hydrocarbons, fusel oil, and asbestos fibers. Nutritional deficiencies found in alcoholics could in themselves cause abnormal integrity of the oral mucosa, increasing permeability to carcinogens. In addition, alcohol and nutritional deficiencies could suppress immunity. Alcohol can cause induction of microsomal enzymes in the liver which could enhance the conversion of procarcinogens to carcinogens, and alcohol damage to the liver could decrease its ability to detoxify carcinogens.

Most trials show an increased incidence of cancer among smokers who drink, and at every level of tobacco use, the relative risk for cancer increases with alcohol consumption [7]. The risk of cancers of the oral cavity, hypopharynx, oropharynx, and larynx are elevated by combinations of alcohol and tobacco use above what is expected from either alone. This raises the question as to whether their effects are additive or syngeristic [4,7].

Persons exposed to a risk factor have a probability of developing the associated disease which is greater than the probability of persons not exposed by a certain amount (x). If a person has a relative risk (RR), for example, of developing tongue cancer of 6.5 because of tobacco use, and a nonsmoker has no risk ($RR = 1$), then the probability of developing tongue cancer for the smoker is increased by $x = 6.5 \quad 1 = 5.5$. If there is another risk factor which increases the probability of tongue cancer by 4.5(y), and the two factors are independent, then the excess risk is additive ($x + y = 10$). If the excess risk is greater than $x + y$, the two factors may be synergistic; if less than $x + y$, antagonistic.

In re–analyzing previously published data, Rothman found the RR for oral cancers in heavy smokers who were nondrinkers to be 2.43 ($x = 2.43 - 1$) (Table 3) [26]. The RR for heavy drinkers who were nonsmokers was 2.33 ($y = 2.33 - 1$). The sum of the increased probabilities was 2.76. The RR, however, of persons with heavy smoking and drinking history was 15.5, suggesting synergy. Rothman was cautious in his interpretation of the data and pointed out that the same analysis performed on data of others did not support a synergistic effect.

Applying maximum–likelihood techniques to facilitate the estimated index of interaction, Flanders and Rothman found that exposure to alcohol

Table 3. Synergism between tobacco/alcohol.*

Relative risk:	
tobacco without alcohol use	= 2.43
alcohol use without tobacco	= 2.33
tobacco + alcohol use	= 15.5
Independent variables:	
RR = base risk + excess for tobacco + excess for alcohol	
RR = 1.0 + (2.43 − 1.0) + (2.33 − 1.0) = 3.76	
Synergism: 15.5 > 3.76	

* Rothman and Keller [26], Blitzer [4]

and tobacco increased the risk of laryngeal cancer 50% more than that expected from additive effect [27]. A study from Uruguay also found the combined risk for laryngeal cancers to be more than 100 times higher than either risk factor alone [13]. But others in calculating risks associated with the two factors have found them to be independent, without evidence for synergism [28]. It has been estimated that if one could eliminate all tobacco and alcohol use, the incidence of cancers of the hypopharynx, larynx, oropharynx, and oral cavity would fall to one–quarter of their current level [4,26].

Mouthwash has been implicated as an etiologic factor in oral cavity cancer as well [7]. Alcohol content varies from 14 to 28 percent in commercial mouthwashes. Several case–control studies show conflicting data, however. One trial demonstrated an RR of 3.6 for oral cavity cancer in nonsmoking, nondrinking women who frequently used mouthwash [29]; whereas in another study of women with oral and pharyngeal cancers, the RR was only 1.9 in nonsmokers [30].

Industrial Carcinogens

A large number of trials have implicated a variety of occupational risk factors, particularly for nasal cavity, sinus, and laryngeal cancers (Table 4) [4,7,8]. One of the strongest associations is that of nickel exposure and nasal cavity cancer [31–33]. These squamous cancers tend to originate on the lateral nasal wall and spread locally to involve paranasal sinuses. In one report from Norway, the incidence of laryngeal cancer among nickel refinery workers was 3.9 times that expected, and cancer of the nasal cavity and sinuses was 28 times that expected [33]. The latency period ranged from 18 to 36 years, and the incidence varied with duration of exposure and type of work. For example, electrolytic workers who had been at their occupation for greater than 15 years had an incidence of nasal cavity cancer 250 times that expected. Sunderman has demonstrated the induction of cancer in

Table 4. Industrial carcinogens and head and neck cancer.*

Site	Industrial exposure	Range of relative risks
Nasal Cavity/Sinus	Nickel Refining	1.9–88.9
	Woodworking	1.5–8.1
	Mineral Oils	2.8
	Leather Working	3.0–9.8
	Chromium	2.7
Larynx	Asbestos	1.8–9.0
	Mustard Gas	4.0–9.3
	Textile Fiber	2.0–5.6
	Sulfuric Acid	5.2–13.4
	Metal Processing	5.3–8.5
Oral Cavity/Pharynx	Vulcanization	3.9
	Nickel dust	4.1
	Isopropyl oils	3.2–4.0

* from Cann et al. [7]

animals from nickel dust, pellets, and a variety of nickel compounds, including nickel carbonyl [32].

In a Norwegian study of histopathological changes, biopsies of nasal mucosa were performed on 318 active nickel workers, 15 retired workers, and 57 controls [34]. Epithelial dysplasia was found in 12% of active workers and 47% of retired workers. The incidence of dysplasia was related to age, length of exposure, and type of nickel–refining work. Data on contribution of smoking were inconclusive, but hand–rolled cigarettes were found to contain a substantial amount of nickel carbonyl. The concentration of nickel in biopsy specimens from workers exposed to insoluble nickel salts in dust was higher than the concentration in biopsies from those exposed to aerosols containing water–soluble salts [35]. The latency period for development of cancer was longer for those in the electrolytic departments who were exposed to aerosols than for workers in the roasting–smelting departments who were exposed to dust.

In several reports, asbestos exposure appeared to double the risk of laryngeal cancer [7]. In case–control studies, after controlling for alcohol use and smoking, the RR ranged from 1.8 to 9.0. In a recent review, however, of nine published case–control studies, Chan and Gee found that in those studies which properly adjusted for smoking and alcohol, the causal relationship between asbestos exposure and laryngeal cancer was tenuous [36]. They pointed out that in most longitudinal studies where dose, latency period, and incidence can be more accurately assessed, there were no excess deaths in asbestos workers from laryngeal cancer. They concluded that current data does not support a causal relationship between asbestos exposure and larynx cancer.

A variety of other industrial carcinogens have been associated with head and neck cancer. An increased incidence of cancers of the oropharynx has been reported in textile workers, and dust from carding wool and cotton has been implicated [7,8]. The high frequency of lip cancer in Canadian fishermen has been postulated to be related to exposure to tar compounds. Wood workers have been reported to have an increased incidence of adenocarcinomas of the sinuses, although squamous cancers have been reported as well, with a particularly high RR for smokers exposed to soft wood dust. The risk of sinonasal cancers is also increased in leather workers, particularly those who prepare and finish soles. Other occupational exposures with reported relationship to nasal cavity and sinus cancers include chromium, isopropyl alcohol, and mineral oils. Persons working in the manufacturing of mustard gas in the United States and Japan have been reported to have an increased risk of cancers of the pharynx, larynx, and sinuses. Mustard gas is a highly irritating chemical, and those parts of the respiratory tract that are exposed to high concentrations are particularly at risk. An increased incidence of laryngeal cancer has been found with exposure to isopropyl oils and sulfuric acid, and in those occupations which involve metal processing, textile fiber processing and vulcanization processes.

Radiation Exposure

Actinic radiation is associated with skin and lip cancers [8]. Most lip carcinomas occur on the lower lip in elderly, Caucasian males, following extensive exposure to sunlight. Thus, this cancer is more common in rural settings and in occupations involving outdoor work, such as fishing and farming.

Although malignancies of the thyroid, parathyroid, and salivary glands develop with increased frequency following ionizing radiation to the head and neck for benign conditions and in atomic bomb survivors, the data for head and neck cancer is more tenuous [8]. There is an increased mortality from pharyngeal cancer in patients who received spinal radiation for ankylosing spondylitis [37]. And among a group of 3,000 patients irradiated for thyrotoxicosis, cancer of the pharynx is ten times more common. In one series of 5,000 persons exposed to radium in their work, eleven developed malignant tumors of the paranasal sinuses, thought to be due to radon trapped in the sinuses and alpha particles emitted from radium deposited in bone [38]. Only three, however, were squamous cancers. There is no reported increased rate of head and neck cancers in children who received radiation therapy for tinea capis or for thymic enlargement, although they are at risk for cancers of the thyroid and salivary glands. The incidence of squamous cancers of the lip, nasal cavity, sinuses, larynx, oral cavity, and pharynx was determined in atomic bomb survivors and was not found to be increased over expected [39]. Thus, there does not appear to be a strong association between exposure to ionizing radiation and the development of head and neck squamous cancers.

Dietary Factors

One of the earliest associations of a dietary deficiency, Plummer–Vinson syndrome, and head and neck cancers were reported in the 1930s in Sweden [40]. This syndrome, which occurs most often in women residing in rural areas, is characterized by dysphagia from hypopharyngeal and esophageal webs and strictures, plus sideropenic anemia. These precancerous lesions lead to a high mortality rate from pharyngeal and hypopharyngeal cancers. Diets in the areas of highest incidence lack fruits and green vegetables. Dietary deficiency of vitamin C appears to interfere with iron absorption and also increases the risk of cancer. Riboflavin deficiencies have been noted as well. Since flour in Sweden has been fortified with iron and vitamins, the incidence of these cancers is decreasing.

Deficiencies of vitamins C and A have been implicated as etiologic factors for head and neck squamous cancers [2,7,10]. Vitamin C with its anitoxidant properties may inhibit the metabolism of carcinogens and decrease formation of nitrosamines. Multiple mechanisms of action have been postulated for retinoids (natural and synthetic compounds with vitamin A activity) to account for their regulation of cellular proliferation and differentiation [41].

Epidemiologic studies in humans which evaluate nutritional factors are predominantly of four types: 1) prospective dietary studies in which a group of patients have dietary intake tabulated and are followed to determine the incidence of cancer; 2) retrospective dietary studies where patients with cancer are asked to recall their dietary histories; 3) prospective studies of blood vitamin levels in which samples are stored and patients followed for development of disease; 4) retrospective blood vitamin levels where vitamin levels are measured on patients who have developed cancers.

In retrospective serologic studies, low serum vitamin A levels have been noted in patients with nasopharyngeal and oral cancers. Studies from India have reported lower serum levels of vitamin A and carotene in patients with oral cavity and oropharyngeal cancers than in controls [42]. The problems with retrospective studies of blood levels include the questionable relationship between a single level and nutritional status, and the influence of disease upon the serum level.

Early retrospective dietary–recall studies demonstrated little difference in diet between patients with oral cavity cancers and controls, although more recent studies suggest that diets low in vitamin A and vitamin C are associated with cancers of the oral cavity and larynx [43,44]. In one large case–control study of 871 patients, cancers of the oral cavity and pharynx were correlated with diet [45]. Adjusting for tobacco and alcohol use, the authors found an inverse relationship between fruit intake and risk of these cancers. Persons in the highest quartile of fruit intake had half the risk of those in the lowest quartile. Neither vitamin C, carotene, nor fiber could account for this relationship, since these nutrients are also found in vegetables, and diets high in vegetables did not afford protection. The authors postulated that cooking may have diminished nutritional value for vegetables or that other constituents were responsible. The investigators found no relationship with other vitamins or with diets high in nitrate-containing meats, pickled or smoked food.

The Southeast has the highest mortality in the United States from pharyngeal and oral cavity cancers. A case–control study of 227 women in North Carolina was conducted to explore the relationship between diet and these cancers [46]. Controlling for tobacco and alcohol use, there was a protective effect of diets high in fruits and vegetables. The investigators felt that their findings were consistent with numerous animal studies showing inhibition of carcinogenesis by retinoids and vitamin C.

It is premature to draw final conclusions from these studies since there is a limitation of the capacity to recall prior dietary history. Diets are complex and difficult to assess and validate, such that there are often inaccuracies in translation from foods to nutrients.

Genetic Predisposition

With the exception of nasopharyngeal carcinoma, squamous cancers of the head and neck do not appear to have a familial association. There are suggestions, however, that there may be populations with a genetic predisposition to this disease. The chief carcinogens in tobacco are polycyclic aromatic hydrocarbons: These must be activated in cells to exert a carcinogenic effect. This activation is carried out by an enzyme system called aryl hydrocarbon hydroxylase (AHH) which hydroxylates polycyclic aromatic hydrocarbons to epoxides, which, in turn, form covalent bonds with RNA and DNA [47]. Mitogen–stimulated human lymphocyte studies of AHH activity show individual variation which has a single autosomal locus of genetic control, and three phenotypes of AHH inducibility (low, medium, and high) have been described [48]. Thus, there may be genetic differences in susceptibility to smoke carcinogens.

One of the first associations of AHH activity and malignancy was that noted in lung cancer tissue in which a significant percent contained high AHH inducibility [49]. AHH inducibility has been determined in lymphocytes from 90 patients with laryngeal cancer, and a significantly higher proportion had high levels (21%) compared to normal controls (11%) [50]. The calculated relative risk for development of laryngeal cancer was 2.6 times higher in people with high AHH levels compared to those with low levels, and 1.5 times higher for those with intermediate levels of AHH. In another trial of 41 patients with laryngeal cancer, the frequency of high AHH inducibility was 36.6%, compared to 8.8% for controls [51]. AHH inducibility may be of value in understanding carcinogenesis and in identifying those persons at high risk for development of laryngeal cancer.

Nasopharyngeal Carcinoma

Nasopharyngeal cancer is a major health problem in China where the incidence rate is 18 cases per 100,000 [4,52,53]. This malignancy occurs with a frequency in Chinese 25 times that of Caucasians. It is particularly prevalent in the southern provinces where it is the most common cancer among persons between the ages of 15 and 34. In Shanghai, more than 700 new cases per year are seen at one cancer hospital. Race alone cannot explain geographical differences since the incidence of this cancer is relatively low in Korea. Americans with Chinese ancestry have an incidence halfway between native Chinese and Caucasians. There are several factors which have been implicated in the etiology of nasopharyngeal cancer: genetic predisposition, environmental exposure, diet, tobacco use, and the Epstein–Barr virus.

Given the high–incidence rate in this particular population, a genetic cause or susceptibility has been sought [4,52]. Familial aggregation may reflect an inborn susceptibility, but even in endemic areas, familial clustering is uncommon. The risk for nasopharyngeal cancer has been shown to be associated with an HLA specific haplotype (HLA–A2, BW46) [54], although data from other trials have not confirmed this. There may also be a predisposition in persons with particular blood groups. In two nasopharyngeal carcinoma cell lines, involvement of band q25 of a 3q+ marker chromosome has been described [55]. At present, however, there is no evidence that nasopharynx cancer is solely related to a particular genetic state. It may develop in persons with a certain physical characteristics as determined by genetic composition, or perhaps those with the same genetic susceptibility have similar environmental risk factors.

Even though nasopharyngeal cancer may be racially determined, environmental factors appear to be present as well. There is an increased risk for nasopharyngeal cancer among Caucasians born and raised in high–risk areas. Several studies have suggested the role of smoke in poorly ventilated homes [53,56]. The inefficient combustion of fossil fuels as occurs in indoor cooking on wood fires yields large particles which may be trapped in the upper airways. There are two observations which argue against inhaled domestic carcinogens as an etiologic agent. One is the high rate of nasopharyngeal carcinoma among populations in Hong Kong who live on open boats where ventilation is not a problem. Secondly, nasopharyngeal carcinoma occurs more frequently in men; whereas women do most of the cooking.

The role of cigarette smoking in nasopharyngeal carcinoma is still not clear. In one U.S. case–control study, patients with nasopharyngeal cancer smoked a greater number of cigarettes per day compared to healthy controls [57]. The odds ratio, however, was relatively small. Other trials have been inconclusive [53].

Ho has suggested that the high rate of nasopharyngeal carcinoma among Cantonese may be related to their consumption of salted fish [58]. At least three case–control studies have supported this hypothesis. Chinese immigrants in Los Angeles who consumed salted fish more than once a week had a relative risk of 3.1 compared to those who had no salted fish in their diet [59]. In Hong Kong, a history of using salted fish for weaning infants has been found more often in households with nasopharyngeal cancer than in those without this malignancy [60]. In a study of Malaysian Chinese, daily childhood consumption of salted fish carried a relative risk of 17.4 compared to those without salted fish in their diet [61]. There are supportive experimental findings as well. Mutagenic activity and nitrosamines have been demonstrated in salted fish, and extracts from salted fish can cause nasal cavity cancer in animals [60]. The diet in southern China contains other preserved foods which may be implicated as well. A strong association between nasopharyngeal cancer and exposure before age two to salted duck eggs, salted mustard greens, chung choi, and fermented black bean paste has been reported [62]. Nitrosamines have been detected in these foods as well.

One etiologic agent that is highly suspect is the Epstein-Barr virus (EBV) [2,52,63,64,65–67]. There are several observations which support this. First, the epithelial cells of patients with nasopharyngeal carcinoma contain the EBV genome, and after tumor tissue is grafted into nude mice, the EBV genome can be demonstrated in epithelial cells. Patients with nasopharynx cancer have increased secretion of IgA anti–EBV viral capsid antigen (VCA) in their saliva. Almost all patients with nasopharynx cancer have elevated IgG antibodies to VCA (Table 5). Titers are increased in relationship to tumor burden, and decrease following effective therapy [64]. These antibodies, however, can be demonstrated in patients with other head and neck cancers and in healthy controls. Approximately 65–85% of patients have elevated IgA anti–VCA, as do 20–30% of patients with other head and neck squamous cancers [63,64]. The IgA and IgG early antigens (EA) induced by EBV have two different patterns of immunofluoresence—a diffuse staining of both the nucleus and cytoplasm and a restricted staining of cytoplasm only. Anti–diffuse activity is the most useful in evaluating nasopharyngeal cancer. IgA anti–diffuse antibodies have the greatest specificity but least sensitivity of the various antibodies [64]. Elevated titers can be measured in 47% of patients with nasopharynx cancer and in 62% of those with cervical metastases [52]. Less than 2% of patients with other head and neck cancers will have IgA anti–diffuse reactivity. When one combines IgA anti–VCA, and IgG and IgA anti–diffuse early antigen, the probability of a diagnosis of nasopharyngeal cancer is twelve times that of other malignancies of the head and neck region. Patients with nasopharynx cancer have increased antibodies against nuclear antigen (EBNA) as well.

There is no *in vitro* evidence that EBV virus actually induces nasopharyngeal cancer. Although Koch's postulate has not been fulfilled, it is still likely that Epstein–Barr virus does play a role in the genesis of this cancer. It is not clear whether EBV is associated with nasopharynx cancer as a passenger

Table 5. Epstein–Barr virus serology.*

% Positive antibody+	Nasopharynx cancer	Other head & neck cancer	Controls
VCA (IgG)	100	93–100	90–98
VCA (IgA)	65–83	14–36	2–9
EA (IgG)	73–90	9–31	18–29
EA (IgA)	47–57	2	0

* from Neel et al. [62], Ringborg et al. [64], Pearson et al. [79], Desgranges et al. [80]
† VCA = viral capsid antigen, EA = early antigen

in neoplastic tissue since EBV is a permanent residence of the pharynx in most individuals after they have had an infection, or whether it is an etiologic cofactor. Nasopharyngeal cancer may result from an interaction of genetic, chemical, and viral factors. Lymphoblastoid Raji cells, bearing latent EBV genomes, have been activated by extracts of dried fish [66].

Cancer Prevention

In the United States, approximately 75% of all cancers of the oral cavity, oropharynx and larynx are related to tobacco and alcohol use [68]. There are other important etiologic factors, and they too should be pursued in prevention programs. Several strategies for cancer control have been used for head and neck cancers, including education, screening of high–risk groups, vaccines, and chemoprevention.

One example of a successful education program took place in the 1970s in a major Norwegian nickel refinery [31]. As has been noted in the section on industrial carcinogens, an epidemiologic study demonstrated an association between nickel refining and nasal cavity/paranasal sinus cancers. Based on these observations, modifications were made in several policies at the plant. Nickel plasma levels were followed, and if they increased, workers were transferred to low–risk areas. Airborn contamination was reduced by changing to a closed system. Workers were educated on the use of masks, nasal irrigation, and hand washing before rolling cigarettes. In more recent years, cancer of the sinuses has declined by 50% in this area.

In India, an intervention study was performed among 36,000 tobacco users [69]. In a house–to–house survey, tobacco chewers and smokers were identified from three rural areas of India. Patients were interviewed and examined for evidence of leukoplakia or other precancerous lesions. An intervention group and control group were followed for five years. The intervention group received information by film, posters, radio, and newspaper articles in selected districts. In two such regions, there were significantly more people who discontinued tobacco use compared to the control districts. The five–year adjusted incidence rate of leukoplakia was significantly lower in the study regions.

Education is desperately needed in the United States. Tobacco use, especially smokeless tobacco, is increasing in frequency among children and high school students. Formal classroom instruction by health professionals has demonstrated a successful increase in students' knowledge of health hazards [70]. It is yet to be shown if education will lead to a decrease in number of smokers in the future.

Screening is not a very cost–effective approach in the United States, since squamous carcinomas of the head and neck represent a small percentage of all malignancies. But screening is of more importance in countries where these represent a major health hazard. In one Chinese trial testing serum for IgA anti–VCA among 148,000 persons, 3,500 were positive, and 87 of those were subsequently shown to have nasopharyngeal cancer, many in early stages [71]. In another trial, a serological survey was conducted using antibody to EBV–specific DNase activity [67]. Ninety–eight hundred samples were collected from high–risk areas, and 12% were positive. Among the group, 12 patients with nasopharyngeal cancer were identified yielding a detection rate of 1.3%. IgA anti–VCA and antibodies to EBV DNase may be complimentary in screening attempts for nasopharyngeal carcinoma.

Because of the association of EBV and nasopharyngeal carcinoma, an attractive approach is the development of a vaccine to prevent this disease. A vaccine has been derived from the high molecular weight glycoprotein component of the EBV membrane antigen [72,73]. It can give complete protection against EBV infections in animals. The membrance–antigen gene has been cloned, making the development of a vaccine possible.

A new approach to the prevention of head and neck cancer is the inhibition of carcinogenesis with chemopreventive agents. Retinoids, synthetic analogues of vitamin A, have several proposed mechanisms of action for cancer reduction [41,74]: interaction with an inhibition of cancer initiators, antipromotion effects, direct effects on cellular protein synthesis, competition with promoting agents for control of cellular differentiation, inhibition of transforming growth factors, stimulation of humoral and cellular immunity, restoration of contact inhibition and cellular adhesiveness to premalignant cells, and effects on protein synthesis and cellular differentiation through intracellular retinol and retinoic acid binding proteins.

Retinoids have been investigated for the management of leukoplakia. These white plaques on oral mucus membranes represent hyperkeratosis with a rate of malignant transformation ranging from 4–18%. Trials of retinoids in oral leukoplakia demonstrate a response rate of approximately 80% (Table 6) [74]. Relapses, however, occur within one to two months after cessation of treatment. In a placebo controlled trial, 13–cis retinoic acid was given daily for three months [75]. Seventy–one percent of patients in the treatment arm experienced reduction of leukoplakia compared to 9% in the placebo group. Toxicities of vitamin A include mucocutaneous

Table 6. Activity of retinoids for oral leucoplakia.*

	Isotretinoin	Tretinoin	Etretinate
No. Patients	48	27	48
Response (%)	67–87	59	72–100
Relapse (%)	55	57	48–51
Toxicity Limitation (%)	4–8	11	0–1

* From Lippman [41], et al.

changes, musculoskeletal disturbances, hyperlipidemia and other toxicities which are related to the type of retinoid, dose, and length of treatment.

N–acetyl–cystein (NAC), a precursor of intracellular glutathione, has antioxidant properties and can inhibit carcinogens found in cigarette smoke. Trials are underway investigating its use to prevent second primaries in head and neck cancer [76].

Conclusion

Squamous cancers of the head and neck are a devastating group of diseases for which there are known etiologic factors. Since the causative factors are known, significant efforts should be made toward cancer prevention. In the meantime, further epidemiologic investigations need to be performed to identify other etiologic factors and to more fully understand those with an associated risk.

References

1. Cancer Statistics. CA 39:3–20, 1989.
2. Schottenfeld D: Epidemiology, etiology, and pathogenesis of head and neck cancer. In: Head and Neck Cancer. Chretien PB, John ME, Shedd DP, Strong EW, Ward PH (eds), Philadelphia: BC Decker, pp 6–18, 1985.
3. Gastpar H, Wilmes E, Wolf H: Epidemiologic, etiologic and immunologic aspects of nasopharyngeal carcinoma (NPC). J Med 12:257–284, 1981.
4. Blitzer PH: Epidemiology of head and neck cancer. Semin Oncol 15:2–9, 1988.
5. Karp DD, Guralnik E, Guidice LA: Multiple primary cancers: a prevelant and increasing problem. Proc Amer Soc Clin Onc 4:13, 1985.
6. Strong MS, Incze J, Vaughan CW: Field cancerization in the aerodigestive tract—its etiology, manifestation, and significance. J Otolaryngol 13:1–6, 1984.
7. Cann CI, Fried MP, Rothman KJ: Epidemiology of squamous cell cancer of the head and neck. Otolaryngol Clin North Am 18:367–388, 1985.
8. Baden E: Prevention of cancer of the oral cavity and pharynx. CA 37:49–62, 1987.
9. Spitz MR, Newell GR: Descriptive epidemiology of squamous cell carcinoma of the upper aerodigestive tract. Cancer Bull 39:79–81, 1987.
10. Keane WM, Atkins JP, Wetmore R, Vidas M: Epidemiology of head and neck cancer. Laryngoscope 91:2037–2045, 1981.

11. Kahn HA: The Dorn study of smoking and mortality among US veterans: report on 8½ years of observation. J Natl Cancer Inst 19:1–125, 1966.
12. Wynder EL, Stellman SD: Comparative epidemiology of tobacco-related cancers. Cancer Res 37:4608–4622, 1977.
13. De Stefani E, Correa P, Oreggia F, et al.: Risk factors for laryngeal cancer. Cancer 60:3087–3091, 1987.
14. Moore C: Cigarette smoking and cancer of the mouth, pharynx, and larynx: a continuing study. JAMA 218:553–558, 1971.
15. Vaughan CW, Homburger F, Shapshey SM, Soto E, Bernfeld P: Carcinogenesis in the upper aerodigestive tract. Otolaryngol Clin North Am 13:403–412, 1980.
16. Weiss JF, Chretien PB: Interrelationship of immune response, circulating proteins, and etiologic factors for head and neck cancer. In: Head and Neck Cancer. Chretien PB, Johns ME, Shedd DR, Strong EW, Ward PH (eds), Philadelphia: BC Decker, pp 559–563, 1985.
17. Donald PJ: Marijuana smoking—possible cause of head and neck carcinoma in young patients. Otolaryngol Head Neck Surg 94:517–521, 1986.
18. Winn DM, Blot WJ, Shy CM, et al.: Snuff dipping and oral cancer among women in the Southern United States. N Engl J Med 304:745–749, 1981.
19. National Institutes of Health consensus development conference statement: health implications of smokeless tobacco use. Jan 13–15, 1986. CA 36:310–316.
20. Stockwell HG, Lyman GH: Impact of smoking and smokeless tobacco on the risk of cancer of the head and neck. Head Neck Surg. 9:104–110, 1986.
21. Depue RH: Rising mortality from cancer of the tongue in young white males. N Engl J Med 315:647, 1986.
22. Schwartz D, Lellouch J, Flamant R, et al.: Alcool et cancer. Resultats d'une enquete retrospective. Rev Franc Etude Clin Biol 7:590–604, 1962.
23. Mashberg A, Garfinkel L, Harris S: Alcohol as a primary risk factor in oral squamous carcinoma. CA 31: 146–155, 1981.
24. Ledere A, Brugere J, Luce D, Point D, Guenel P: Type of alcoholic beverage and cancer of the upper respiratory and digestive tract. Eur J Cancer Clin Oncol 23:529–534, 1987.
25. McCoy GD, Hecht SS, Wynder EL: The roles of tobacco, alcohol, and diet in the etiology of upper alimentary and respiratory tract cancers. Prev Med 9:622–629, 1980.
26. Rothman K, Keller A: Effect of the joint exposure to alcohol and tobacco on the risk of cancer of the mouth and pharynx. J Chron Dis 25:711–716, 1972.
27. Flanders WD, Rothman KJ: Interaction of alcohol and tobacco in laryngeal cancer. Am J Epidemiol 115:371–379, 1982.
28. Hinds MW, Kolonel LN, Lee J, Hirohata T: Associations between cancer incidence and alcohol/cigarette consumption among five ethnic groups in Hawaii. Br J Cancer 41:929–940, 1980.
29. Wynder EL, Hultberg S, Jacobsson F, et al.: Oral cancer and mouthwash. JNCI 70:255–260, 1983.
30. Blot WJ, Winn DM, Fraumeni JF: Oral cancer and mouthwash. JNCI 70:251–253, 1983.
31. Barton R Th, Hogetveit A Ch: Nickel-related cancers of the respiratory tract. Cancer 45:3061–3064, 1980.
32. Sunderman FW Jr: Nickel carcinogenesis. Dis Chest 54:41–48, 1968.
33. Pedersen EA, Hogetveit AC, Andersen A: Cancer of the respiratory organs among workers at a nickel refinery in Norway. Int J Cancer 12:32–41, 1973.
34. Torjussen W, Solberg LA, Hogetveit AC: Histopathological changes of the nasal mucosa in active and retired nickel workers. Br J Cancer 40:568–580, 1979.
35. Torjussen W, Haug FMS, Olsen A, Andersen I: Concentration and distribution of heavy metals in nasal mucosa of nickel-exposed workers. Acta Otolaryngol 86:449–463, 1977.
36. Chan CK, Gee JBL: Asbestos exposure and laryngeal cancer: An analysis of the epidemiologic evidence. J Occup Med 30:23–27, 1988.
37. Court Brown WM, Poll R: Mortality from cancer and other causes after radiation for ankylosing spondylitis. Br Med J 2:1327–1332, 1965.

38. Goolden AWG: Radiation Cancer. A Review with special reference to radiation tumours in the pharynx, larynx, and thyroid. Br J Radiol 30:626–640, 1957.
39. Pinkston JA, Wakabuyashi T, Yamamoto T, et al.: Cancer of the head and neck in atomic bomb survivors: Hiroshima and Nagasaki, 1957–1976. Cancer 48:2172–2178, 1981.
40. Larsson LG, Sandstrom A, Westling P: Relationship of Plummer–Vinson disease to cancer of the upper alimentary tract in Sweden. Cancer Res 35:3308–3316, 1975.
41. Lippman SM, Kessler JF, Meyskens FL Jr: Retinoids as preventive and therapeutic anticancer agents (parts I, II). Cancer Treat Rep 71:391–405, 493–515, 1987.
42. Chaudhy NA, Jafarey NA, Ibrahim K: Plasma vitamin A and carotene levels in relation to the clinical stages of carcinoma of the oral cavity and oropharynx. JPMA 30:221–223, 1980.
43. Marshall J, Graham S, Mettlin C, Shedd D, Swanson M: Diet in the epidemiology of oral cancer. Nutr Cancer 3:145–149, 1982.
44. Graham S, Mettlio C, Marshall J, Privre R, Rzepka T, Shedd D: Dietary factors in the epidemiology of cancer of the larynx. Am J of Epidemiol 113:675–680, 1981.
45. McLaughlin JK, Gridley G, Block G, et al.: Dietary factors in oral and pharyngeal cancer. JNCI 80:1237–1243, 1988.
46. Winn DM, Ziegler RG, Pickle LW, Gridley G, Blot WJ, Hoover RN: Diet in the etiology of oral and pharyngeal cancer among women from the Southern United States. Cancer Res 44:1216–1222, 1984.
47. Grover PL, Slims P: K–region epoxides of polycyclic hydrocarbons. Reactions with nucleic acids and polyribonucleotides. Biochem Pharmacol 22:661–666, 1973.
48. Kellerman G, Layten–Kellerman M, Shaw CR: Genetic variation of aryl hydrocarbon hydroxylese in human lymphocytes. Am J Human Genet 25:327–331, 1973.
49. Kellerman G, Shaw CR, Layten–Kellerman M: Aryl hydrocarbon hydroxylase inducibility and bronchogenic carcinoma. N Eng J Med 289:934–937, 1973.
50. Brandenburg JH, Kellerman G: Aryl hydrocarbon hydroxylase inducibility in laryngeal carcinoma. Arch Otolaryngol 104:151–152, 1978.
51. Korsgaard R, Trell E, Kitzing P, et al.: Arylhydrocarbonhydroxylase inducibility and smoking habits in patients with laryngeal carcinomas. Acta Otolaryngol (Stockh) 98:368–373, 1984.
52. Fedder M, Gonzalez MF: Nasopharyngeal carcinoma. Am J Med 79:365–369, 1985.
53. Henderson BE, Louie E, Jing JSH, Buell P, Gardner M: Risk factors associated with nasopharyngeal carcinoma. N Engl J Med 295:1101–1106, 1976.
54. Simon MJ, Wee GB, Chan SH, Shanmugaratnam K: Provable identification of an HL–A second–lucus antigen associated with high risk of nasopharyngeal carcinoma. Lancet 1:142–143, 1975.
55. Mitleman F, Mark–Vendel E, Mineur A, Giovanella B, Klein G: A 3q+ marker chromosome in EBV–carrying nasopharyngeal carcinomas. Int J Cancer 32:651–655, 1983.
56. Miller D: The etiology of nasopharyngeal cancer and its management. Otolaryngol Clin North Am 13:167–175, 1980.
57. Mabuchi K, Bross DS, Kessler II: Cigarette smoking and nasopharyngeal carcinoma. Cancer 55:2874–2876, 1985.
58. Ho JHC. Nasopharyngeal carcinoma (NPC). Adv Cancer Res 15:57–92, 1972.
59. Henderson BE, Louis E: Discussion of risk factors for nasopharyngeal carcinoma. IARC Sci Publ 20:251–260, 1978.
60. Yu MC, Ho JHC, Lai SH, Henderson BE: Cantonese–style salted fish as a cause of nasopharyngeal carcinoma: report of a case–control study in Hong Kong. Cancer Res 46:956–961, 1986.
61. Armstrong RW, Armstrong MJ, Yu MC, Henderson BE: Salted fish and inhalants as risk factors for nasopharyngeal carcinoma in Malaysian Chinese. Cancer Res 43:2967–2970, 1983.
62. Yu MC, Mo CC, Chong WX, Yeh FS, Henderson BE: Preserved foods and nasopharyngeal carcinoma: A case–control study in Guangxi, China. Cancer Res 48:1954–1959, 1988.
63. Neel HB, Pearson GR, Taylor WF: Antibodies to Epstein–Barr virus in patients with

nasopharyngeal carcinoma and incomparison groups. Ann Otol Rhinol Laryngol 93:477–482, 1984.
64. Ringborg U, Henle W, Henle G, et al.: Epstein-Barr virus—specific serodiagnostic tests in carcinomas of the head and neck. Cancer 52:1237–1243, 1983.
65. Fey SJ, Larsen PM: DNA viruses and human cancer. Cancer Letters 41:1–18, 1988.
66. Shao YM, Poirior S, Ohshime H: Epstein–Barr virus activation in raji cells by extracts of preserved food from high–risk areas for nasopharyngeal carcinoma. Carcinogenesis 9:1455–1457, 1988.
67. Chen JY, Chen CJ, Liu MY, et al.: Antibody to Epstein-Barr verus specific DNase as a marker for field survey of patients with nasopharyngeal carcinoma in Taiwan. J Med Virol 27:269–273, 1989.
68. Thomas DB: Sinonasal, nasopharyngeal, oral, pharyngeal, laryngeal, and esophageal cancers: epidemiology and opportunities for primary prevention. In Head and Neck Cancer. Chretien PB, John ME, Shedd DP, Strong EW, Ward PH (eds), Philadelphia: BC Decker, pp 585–91, 1985.
69. Gupta PC, Pindborg JJ, Bhonsle RB, et al.: Intervention study for primary prevention of oral cancer among 36,000 Indian tobacco users. Lancet May 31:1235–1239, 1986.
70. Williams NJ, Arreola M, Covington JS, Arheart K, Mills K: Adolescent smokeless tobacco use: relationship between epidemiologic and cognitive factors. Prog Clin Biol Res 293:211–220, 1989.
71. Zeng Y, Zhang LG, Li HY, et al.: Serological mass survey for early detection of nasopharyngeal carcinoma in Wuzhou City, China. Cancer 29:139–141, 1982.
72. Epstein MA: Recent studies on a vaccine to prevent EB virus-associated cancers. Br J Cancer 54:1–5, 1986.
73. Epstein MA: Vaccination against Epstein–Barr virus: current progress and future strategies. The Lancet 1:1425–1427, 1986.
74. Goodman DS: Vitamin A and retinoids in health and disease. N Engl J Med 310:1023–12031, 1984.
75. Hong WK, Endicott J, Itri L, et al.: 13–cis retinoic acid in the treatment of oral leucoplakia. N Engl J Med 315:1501–1505, 1986.
76. DeVres N, Snow GB: Prevention of second primary cancers in head and neck cancer patients: new perspectives. AM J Otolaryngol 9:151–154, 1988.
77. Wynder EL, Covey LS, Mabuchi K, Mushinski M: Environmental factors in cancer of the larynx. Cancer 38:1591–1601, 1976.
78. Tuyns AJ, Esteve J, Raymond L, et al.: Cancer of the larynx/hypopharynx, tobacco and alcohol: IARC international case–control study in Turin and Varese (Italy), Zaragoza and Navarra (Spain), Geneva (Switzerland) and Calvados (France). Int J Cancer 41:483–491, 1988.
79. Pearson GR, Weiland LH, Neel HB, et al.: Application of Epstein–Barr virus (EBV) serology to the diagnosis of North American nasopharyngeal carcinoma. Cancer 51:260–268, 1983.
80. Desgranges C, De–The G: Epstein-Barr virus specific IgA serum antibodies in nasopharyngeal and other respiratory carcinomas. Int J Cancer 24:555–559, 1979.

Index